Long-term Conditions

A Guide for Nurses and Healthcare Professionals

Long-term Conditions

A Guide for Nurses and Healthcare Professionals

Edited by

Sue Randall

RGN, RHV, BSc (Hons), MSc, PGCE (HE)

Senior Lecturer
Pathway Leader Long-term Conditions
Department of Nursing, Midwifery and Healthcare
Faculty of Health and Life Sciences
Coventry University, UK

and

Helen Ford

RGN, BSc (Hons), MSc, PGCE (HE)

Senior Lecturer
Department of Nursing, Midwifery and Healthcare
Faculty of Health and Life Sciences
Coventry University, UK

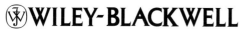

WILEY-BLACKWELL

A John Wiley & Sons, Ltd., Publication

Library of Congress Cataloging-in-Publication Data

Long-term conditions : a guide for nurses and healthcare professionals / edited by Sue Randall and Helen Ford.
    p. ; cm.
  Includes bibliographical references and index.
  ISBN 978-1-4443-3249-0 (pbk. : alk. paper)
1. Long-term care of the sick. 2. Chronic diseases-Nursing. I. Randall, Sue, editor. II. Ford, Helen, 1967- editor.
  [DNLM: 1. Long-Term Care-methods. 2. Chronic Disease-nursing. 3. Palliative Care-methods. WX 162]
  RT120.L64L66 2011
  362.16-dc22

                                                                                    2010048240

A catalogue record for this book is available from the British Library.

Set in 9/12.5 pt Interstate Light by Aptara® Inc., New Delhi, India

Printed and bound in Malaysia by Vivar Printing Sdn Bhd

1 2011

This book is dedicated to my family in recognition of their unwavering support for me, even when my work appears to take priority over my family.

So for my Mum and Dad, Joy and David Gill, my brother and his wife, Steve and Isobel Gill, and my beautiful nieces Sarah and Lauren, thank you.

For Tanya Hughes, whose friendship from the other side of the world keeps me sane, especially when others are asleep.

Last, but certainly not least, a very particular mention is needed for my husband Duncan Randall and my two very special boys, Matthew and Harry, who put up with lot!

Thank you all, so much. It means everything to know you are all there.

Sue Randall

I would like to dedicate this book to my lovely family: Andy, Imogen and Thomas. Thank you for your patience, support and ability to de-stress me by reminding me that there is a whole other world out there!

Thanks are also due to all the people involved in the reading of chapters, for their feedback and comments. Tony Privitera, in particular, was invaluable with his comments for the first draft of Chapter 1.

Both Sue and I are also grateful to the staff of Wiley for their support during the writing and editing of this book. The chapter contributors also deserve a mention, for their diligence in responding to the often-tight deadlines.

Helen Ford

Contents

Contributors

Darren Awang

Darren Awang is Course Director for the MSc in Assistive Technology at the Department of Occupational Therapy, Coventry University. Darren has a strong interest in assistive technology, home adaptations, research methods and applied research. Darren is currently leading a project to develop an online Assistive Technology Learning Tool to assist students and practitioners to gain understanding of the range of assistive technology and its potential to enhance the lives of service users, patients and carers.

Bernie Davies

Bernie Davies is Senior Lecturer in Adult Nursing at Coventry University. She teaches pre- and post-registration students across modules including long-term conditions, evidence-based practice, continence promotion and wound care. She has a particular interest in interprofessional education and is a lead for the online interprofessional learning pathway delivered across health and social care courses at Coventry University and Warwick medical school. She has worked as a sister and then clinical teacher in older adult rehabilitation and in acute medicine.

Helen Ford

Helen Ford is Senior Lecturer at Coventry University, whose predominant responsibility is pre-registration teaching. Helen trained in the West Midlands and worked in clinical practice for 10 years, specialising in medical admissions. The poor nutritional state of many of the patients sparked her interest in patient nutrition, and though nutrition has gained much interest in recent times, she feels that there is scope for more education to help those working with people with long-term conditions adopt a multiprofessional approach.

Jo Galloway

Jo Galloway is Deputy Director of Nursing, Quality and Safety at NHS Warwickshire. Her career spans acute care, commissioning and education, and she has a wealth of experience in managerial, clinical and educational roles in a number of senior posts, both within the NHS and higher education institutions. Her clinical expertise is within rehabilitation and the care of older people. Jo has also co-authored a book on leadership and management in healthcare.

Gay James

Gay James started her nursing career with RGN training at Westminster Hospital, London, followed by experience in general medicine and surgery at Westminster and Kings College Hospital, then Intensive Care course at Guys hospital. Following an MSc in Pain Management, Gay came to realise that the subject of pain is an important priority for patient care, and that learning about it should start in pre-registration education. She hopes that her enthusiasm for improving recognition and appropriate management for pain inspires students to make it a priority for patients.

Jill Main

Jill undertook her nursing training at Edinburgh University and qualified in 1978. She has extensive experience in the fields of both elderly and generalist palliative care. Her academic qualifications include a BSc (Social Science/Nursing) and an MSc (Health Sciences Research). She currently works in South Birmingham Community Health in the Safeguarding Vulnerable Adults team, and also has a remit for end-of-life care in the Trust.

Sue Randall

Sue Randall is Senior Lecturer and Pathway Leader for Long-term Conditions in the Department of Nursing, Midwifery and Health Care at Coventry University, where she teaches across foundation degree, pre-registration, undergraduate and postgraduate nursing. In addition, Sue has an applied research portfolio which includes workforce transformation around the long-term conditions agenda, and evaluations of community matron services. Sue trained at The Middlesex Hospital in London, specialising in orthopaedics and working in elective, trauma and at the supraregional bone tumour unit. From there, she worked as a Health Visitor with a generic caseload of young families and housebound elderly, before establishing the Stop Smoking in Pregnancy Service in South Warwickshire. All of these eclectic experiences have built up a knowledge base which promotes the skills required in current healthcare to support individuals with long-term conditions.

Annette Roebuck

Annette Roebuck is an occupational therapist with experience in a wide range of health and social care settings. Her interest in risk assessment and management was initially sparked when undertaking home visits. The debates that occurred between the multidisciplinary team, clients and family members when attempting to meet clients' wishes underlined the complexity of this issue. Experience in a low secure unit for people with challenging behaviour added a new dimension to her perspectives on risk and empowerment. She now lectures at Coventry University and uses risk management knowledge to empower service users to be members of the module team.

Andrew R Thompson

Dr Andrew R Thompson is Senior Clinical Lecturer and Chartered Clinical & Chartered Health Psychologist. He is employed on the Sheffield NHS/University of Sheffield Clinical Psychology Training Programme as Director of Research Training. In addition, he provides two clinical sessions per week at Rotherham NHS Foundation Trust providing a Clinical Health Psychology service focusing on assisting adjustment to LTCs. He has a long-standing research interest in adaptation to disfigurement.

Robert Tummey

Robert has been working in mental health nursing for over 20 years as both a clinician and an academic. He has worked on hospital wards, in the community setting, and has been a nurse specialist in three separate fields of mental health and a Nurse Consultant. As a psychotherapist, he has worked in both the NHS and the independent sector, providing an integrative approach to counselling and psychotherapy. Publications include *Planning Care in Mental Health Nursing* and *Critical Issues in Mental Health*. Currently, he is Course Director of Mental Health Nursing at Coventry University and in the midst of PhD study.

Andy Turner

Dr Andy Turner is a Senior Research Fellow and the Lead for the Self Management of Long-term Health Conditions research group in the Applied Research Centre in Health & Lifestyle Interventions at Coventry University. He has been evaluating health coaching and self-management programmes for patients and their carers for over 10 years and has published over 30 self-management papers and book chapters. He is trained in motivational interviewing and psychological coaching and is a personal trainer. He has recently developed the Help to Overcome Problems Effectively (HOPE) health coaching and support programme for people living with long-term health conditions and their carers.

Gillian Ward

Dr Gillian Ward is an occupational therapist and a principal lecturer in assistive technology at Coventry University, lecturing on undergraduate and postgraduate courses. She has a keen interest in the use of assistive technology to support older people and those with LTCs. She also works with the Health Design and Technology Institute at Coventry University to support workforce development needs in relation to assistive technology and provide academic leadership, governance and ethical advice on usability studies of assistive technology products.

Claire Whittle

Claire qualified as an RGN in 1982 at the Queen Elizabeth School of Nursing. After two staff nurse posts, she specialised in Intensive Care Nursing where she became a sister and clinical teacher. Claire lectured in nursing at the University of Birmingham from 1995–2009. For the past 10 years, she has developed a special interest in the development of Integrated Care Pathways, and is working with clinical staff to develop care pathways across a variety of care settings. Claire has been involved with the development and leading the evaluation of the Supportive Care Pathway, a pathway for patients with life-limiting illness with supportive care needs irrespective of diagnosis. Claire is the chairperson for the Midlands Care Pathways network (PACE, Pathways Association of Central England) and a board member of the European Pathways Association. Claire is now at Heart of England NHS Foundation Trust as a Faculty of Education Quality Manager.

Introduction – Rationale and Ethos of the Book

This book is intended to place individuals with a long-term condition (LTC) at the heart of healthcare practice. There is currently considerable discussion around the management of individuals with LTCs. The demographic make-up of society is changing with the proportion of older people growing and living longer. A fifth of the population is over 60 and the over-85s are the fastest growing sector (DH 2008). Currently, 15.4 million people in England report living with an LTC and this is projected to rise to 18 million by 2025 (DH 2008).

Social attitudes are also changing. The Darzi Report (DH 2008) highlights growing expectations of healthcare within the general public. Other policy (DH 2006) recommends changes in the way services are delivered, with patients and service users having more control, as well as closer links between health and social care. Emphasis is now on managing and living with an LTC with 'co-production' of health and care outcomes which are supportive and enabling of care closer to home (DH 2008).

Enabling the workforce to reflect on and improve practice is a key focus of this book. Rather than being disease-focused, it aims to break down key issues and concepts which unify many different LTCs. This will include psychological and social issues that make up a considerable part of living with an LTC. The use of care studies will link the concepts to specific diseases, allowing the reader to build their own knowledge and link theory to practice.

The major difference with this book is a move away from a disease-focused medical model. It aims to consider key elements of living with an LTC based on a partnership approach, to marry the needs of individuals with those of future and current health professionals.

The book is split into 3 sections:

- Section 1: Living with a Long-term Condition
- Section 2: Empowerment
- Section 3: Care management

Within each of the chapters, issues of policy, culture and ethics are intertwined. Learning objectives will assist the reader. Resources and areas of further reading are also outlined for potential exploration. Links to specific LTCs are made through the case studies, where appropriate. These, often moving examples, are followed by points for reflection through which readers can consider their own practice.

Section 1: Living with a Long-term condition

Chapter 1: **Nutrition**: Helen Ford
This chapter considers one of the most fundamental aspects of life, that of nutrition. Although the subject of much current research, nutrition is still a factor that is easily overlooked in clinical practice, perhaps because it can appear to be a complex subject. The chapter by Helen Ford aims to demystify the subject, and demonstrates through the use of case studies how knowledge about nutrition can be incorporated into the practice of caring for individuals with an LTC.

Chapter 2: **Chronic Pain: Living with Chronic Pain:** Gay James
Gay James's comprehensive chapter on the management of pain is written around the central theme that chronic pain is, in itself, an LTC. Starting with a useful examination of the physiology of pain, the chapter continues with the prevalence of chronic pain and strategies for effective assessment of chronic pain, including assessing pain in those with cognitive impairment. Using the WHO pain ladder, appropriate treatment modes are explored.

Chapter 3: **Depression and Long-term Conditions**: Robert Tummey
Robert Tummey's chapter addresses some of the key issues and themes around the acknowledge-ment, impact and subsequent treatment of depression in individuals living with an LTC. Depression as a cause or consequence of an LTC and the resulting experience are examined. Prevalence of depression, terms and definitions help to promote understanding of depression.

Section 2: Empowerment

Chapter 4: **Adaptation in Long-Term Conditions: The Role of Stigma Particularly in Conditions that Affect Appearance**: Dr Andrew R Thompson
Critical to the way that individuals meet the challenge of an LTC diagnosis is adaptation to a new, often challenging way of life. In Andrew Thompson's chapter, psychosocial impacts are explored and the variation found in individuals of these impacts. The chapter demonstrates how interventions can facilitate adaptation and reduce stigmatisation, with an emphasis on empowerment. Finally, the chapter makes practical suggestions for clinical practice.

Chapter 5: **Self-management in Long-term Conditions**: Sue Randall and Andrew Turner
This chapter by Sue Randall and Andrew Turner considers the move in relationships between health-care professionals (HCPs) and patients. It defines self-care and self-management and discusses the context of self-management for those individuals living with an LTC. It considers underpinning theo-ries on which models to empower individuals in self-management are based. Through the use of case studies, examples of the effectiveness of self-management as a cornerstone of the management of LTCs are examined.

Chapter 6: **Assistive technology – A Means of Empowerment**: Darren Awang and Dr Gillian Ward
In this exciting chapter, Darren Awang and Gill Ward consider what is meant by the term 'assistive technology' and how this is empowering individuals with LTCs to be partners in care. It also considers the impact of technology on healthcare professional's management of care. It gives consideration to training needs of HCPs, as well as a glimpse at future developments.

Chapter 7: **Risk and empowerment in Long-term Conditions**: Annette Roebuck
Annette Roebuck's chapter explores the challenges for HCPs of managing risk in a meaningful way, which does not prevent individuals with LTCs from living their lives. Empowering individuals with LTCs and the role this plays in the patient/HCP relationship and in managing risk is also examined.

Section 3: Care management

Chapter 8: **Care coordination for Effective Long-term Condition Management**: Sue Randall
The context of the LTC agenda is explored in this chapter. Sue Randall considers care coordination in its broadest sense across many boundaries, and then brings this into focus in the way everyday services are managed to promote effective and quality care for individuals with LTCs by HCPs.

Chapter 9: **Rehabilitation in Long-term Conditions**: Bernie Davies and Jo Galloway
Rehabilitation is no longer solely carried out in wards, and this chapter by Bernie Davies and Jo Galloway brings the subject of rehabilitation up-to-date. Care closer to home is explored, as well as other settings for effective rehabilitation. The factors influencing patient choice are discussed, balanced with the need to manage a diversity of providers. With this in mind, co-ordination of care becomes ever more important, cutting across the boundaries with social care.

Chapter 10: **Palliative care in Long-term Conditions: Pathways to Care**: Claire Whittle and Jill Main
As this chapter by Claire Whittle and Jill Main shows, though palliative care is a concept tied with cancer, it also applies to those dying with an LTC. The principles of symptom control and family care are entirely relevant to LTCs, and the chapter explores various frameworks and models that can be used to assist those whose practice involves caring for the dying. Very often, however, disease trajectories for those with LTCs are not linear, and the chapter also examines when palliative care should start.

Consideration of what constitutes an LTC

In recent times, there has been a move away from the term 'chronic illness' to a more positive term: that of long-term conditions. When undertaking a literature search, it is sensible to use both terms to ensure a comprehensive literature base is uncovered. In the USA, and indeed the World Health Organisation typically use the term 'chronic illness' or 'disease'. However, it can be argued that having a diagnosis of a chronic health problem does not mean ill health as such. LTCs can be seen on a continuum. There are many individuals with hypertension or asthma who, through taking appropriate medication and altering lifestyle where appropriate, are continuing life in their usual way. Of course, both these disease processes carry the risk of extreme consequences: stroke may result from hypertension, whereas a person with asthma suffering a severe attack may require ventilation. Both diseases can result in death.

At the other end of the spectrum, a progressive and aggressive LTC, such as motor neurone disease, can affect an individual's ability to carry out activities of daily living from soon after diagnosis. It is this complexity which makes a patient-centred approach to care so imperative in ensuring that life is of good quality for individuals with an LTC and for their carers. In addition then, to being aware of disease processes, good quality care results from healthcare professionals working together across boundaries for the good of patients. After all, without patients healthcare professionals (HCPs) are redundant!

It is not unusual for HCPs to feel anxious when they lack knowledge about a disease. However, everyone cannot know everything about all things. The key is partly to know where to find the information required – colleagues, both in your organisation and outside, patients and carers, third-sector organisations, books, internet, etc. – can all be valuable sources.

Equally important is the ability to think outside the box and to think in terms of the skills and knowledge you do have. A patient may be admitted who has advanced Multiple Sclerosis. You may not be familiar with this disease, but have a lot of experience caring for people with stroke. Certain difficulties experienced by both patients will be the same: communication difficulties, swallowing difficulties, mobility difficulties, issues around toileting, and so on. So start with what you know, and seek help to build up the specialist knowledge required for every new situation. We hope that this book will be a useful starting point to empower you to do this.

Sue Randall and Helen Ford
May 2010
The editors are happy to be contacted by email:
s.randall@coventry.ac.uk
h.ford@coventry.ac.uk

Every effort has been made to contact all the copyright-holders for permission to reproduce images. However, in some cases we have been unable to reach copyright holders, despite strenuous efforts. We would be pleased to acknowledge any such diagrams in the first instance.

References

Department of Health (DH) (2006) *Our Health, Our Care, Our Say*. London: The Stationery Office.
DH (2008) *High Quality Care for All (The Darzi Report)*. London: The Stationery Office.

Section 1

Living with a Long-term Condition

Chapter 1
Nutrition

Helen Ford

Learning objectives

After reading this chapter, the reader will have:

- Gained an understanding of how nutrition is a factor both in the cause of LTCs and as a treatment of LTCs
- Developed their understanding of the components of a healthy diet, and be able to demystify dietary advice for patients/clients
- A greater knowledge of obesity, its aetiology, link to LTCs, and current treatment recommendations
- Enhanced their understanding of undernutrition in LTCs, and how this can be identified and treated effectively

---

Introduction

This chapter explores the importance of good nutrition in both the prevention and management of long-term conditions (LTCs). The impact of poor diet and nutrition on individuals will be discussed, including obesity and, at the other extreme, undernutrition. In particular, the reasons why people with LTCs are at risk of poor nutrition will be examined, including both the effects of hospitalisation and exacerbations of disease. By the end of the chapter, it is hoped that the reader will have a solid foundation of knowledge about nutrition, and that they will be able to use this knowledge in improved assessment and care of their patients.

Nutrition in context

The Department of Health (DH) (2008a) state that 15. 4 million people (almost one in three of those living in England) have an LTC. This statistic includes people across the age continuum, yet of those over 60, the proportion with an LTC increases to three out of five people. As has been identified

---

Long-term Conditions: A Guide for Nurses and Healthcare Professionals, First Edition. Edited by S. Randall and H. Ford.
© 2011 Blackwell Publishing Ltd. Published 2011 by Blackwell Publishing Ltd.

elsewhere in this book, LTCs do not necessarily occur singly as people may have more than one LTC, and again this incidence rises as age increases. For example, to look at some common conditions:

- In England, 6.7 million people have clinically identified hypertension.
- Diabetes (Types 1 and 2) affects 174, 000 or 6% of the Welsh population.
- 864, 000 people will experience a stroke at some point in their lives across England and Northern Ireland.
- Coronary heart disease affects almost 2 million people in England, from a population of approximately 61 million. This equates to 3.3% of the population, whereas in Scotland this percentage rises to 4.2%.
  Sources: Department of Health 2008b, The Scottish Executive 2003, Welsh Assembly Government 2008, Northern Ireland Executive 2009.

For conditions such as these, diet has been identified as one of the main factors influencing whether someone will develop them or not. Demographic data from the DH suggest that there is wide variation in prevalence of these diseases across the United Kingdom and access to the right kinds of foods to maintain a healthy diet is undoubtedly important. For example, the White Paper 'Towards a Healthier Scotland' (The Scottish Office 1999) stated that Scotland's diet is a major cause of poor health, and that the Scottish diet is traditionally high in fat, salt and sugar, and low in fruit and vegetables. In addition, households that include someone with an LTC are more likely to be low earners, and those on low wages are less likely to be able to afford or have access to healthy food. The World Health Organisation (WHO 2002: 30) in their consultation document 'Diet, Nutrition and the Prevention of Chronic Disease' argue that in fact, events during the life-course of an individual are as important when considering good nutrition as focusing on snapshots in time, and that

such factors are also being recognized as happening further and further 'upstream' in the chain of events predisposing humans to chronic disease.

However, it must be recognised that some LTCs are not precipitated by diet and other lifestyle factors. For individuals with conditions such as chronic obstructive pulmonary disease (COPD), rheumatoid arthritis (RA) or osteoarthritis, neurological conditions such as epilepsy, motor-neurone disease or multiple sclerosis, or mental health problems such as depression or dementia, poor diet may not have been a factor in the cause of the disease. However, as the reader will see, research into the role of good nutrition and health is showing that interventions to ensure that malnutrition is prevented, detected and managed can positively affect the outcome of a disease, modify symptoms, and reduce morbidity and mortality. This idea, of promoting nutrition to the forefront of a care programme, can be known as 'nutrition as treatment' and it recognises the power of carefully planned nutrition interventions to maintain positive health. However, nutrition does not happen in a vacuum, and the social, cultural, political and economic environment in which a person lives will all affect their eating habits.

How nutrition fits into the management of LTCs

As the number of people with one or more LTCs continues to grow over the next 20 years, the DH (2005) argue that health and social care services will need to focus on improving health outcomes through better detection and prevention of health problems. Promoting the benefits of a healthy lifestyle, including diet, can improve a person's quality of life and allow them to lead as full a life as they choose rather than becoming isolated and defined solely by their disease. An example of this is hypertension. The Health Survey for England (Office for National Statistics 2005) found that among people with no LTC, approximately 9% had a blood pressure (BP) above 150/ 90. However, this figure rose to 50% for people with one or more LTCs. The DASH (Dietary Approaches to Hypertension) study (Harsha et al. 1999) is a famous study that showed after eight weeks of a diet rich in fruit and vegetables and low fat dairy products, an 11.4 mm Hg drop in systolic BP and a 5.5 mm Hg drop in diastolic BP was observed in hypertensive subjects, compared with those eating a standard American diet. Gaining control of blood pressure alone would reduce the risks of further health problems and may also mean fewer tablets to take in the morning! For the person with an LTC, well-being would be improved as their confidence increased in their ability to manage the disease, rather than the disease managing them, and this could in turn lead to further positive changes in lifestyle.

Promoting health

The DH has identified four levels of care for LTCs (DH 2005). The first level is that of *promoting health*, both in the population as a whole to prevent LTCs from developing in the first place, and for those already with an LTC. For those working in health and social care, supporting people to make healthy choices is as important as other more clinical roles. Good knowledge of what constitutes a healthy diet is important here, as is being able to empower people to manage obesity and stabilise weight. Hydration must be included within this; for example, adequate hydration reduces risk of falls among the elderly (American Geriatrics Society, British Geriatrics Society and American Academy of Orthopaedic Surgeons Panel on Falls Prevention 2001). An example of a visually appealing tool to promote healthy hydration has been produced by the British Nutrition Foundation (2010b) and can be seen in Figure 1.1.

Supported self-care

The second level is *supported self-care* and aims to empower people with LTCs to manage their condition effectively by improving skills and knowledge. The Expert Patients Programme (EPP), for example, is one initiative where individuals are trained by others with an LTC in how to best help themselves to cope with their condition. How to improve diet and maintain optimum health is one of the possible training sessions available in the EPP.

Disease management

The third level of care delivery is that of *disease management*. Here, proactive disease management to diagnose problems and work actively with patients who have a single LTC or range of problems can make a difference to their health and well-being. An example would be a patient with Type 1 diabetes mellitus, who has a designated contact such as a Diabetes Nurse Specialist to help advise on what to do in the event of illness that might impact upon good glycaemic control.

Case management

Finally, for the most complex cases or patients with high-intensity needs, *case-management* is used. Here, a community matron, for example, works as a single point of contact to look holistically at a person's needs and prevent, where possible, unplanned hospital admissions. As will be seen later in this chapter, prevention of undernutrition for people with high-intensity needs will reduce the downward spiral of decline that can lead to hospitalisation or long-term institutionalisation.

With these thoughts in mind, it is now time to think about what nutrition is.

Section 1

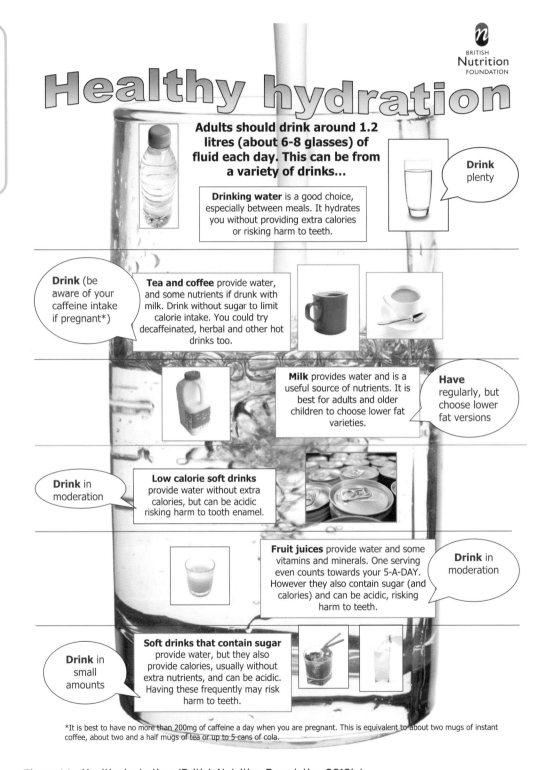

Figure 1.1 Healthy hydration. (British Nutrition Foundation 2010b.)

What is nutrition?

Definitions of nutrition vary, depending on the source. The Wellness Community (2009) is an American non-profit organisation that provides support for people with cancer. They define nutrition as:

> A three-part process that gives the body the nutrients it needs. First, you eat or drink food. Second, the body breaks the food down into nutrients. Third, the nutrients travel through the bloodstream to different parts of the body where they are used as 'fuel' and for many other purposes. To give your body proper nutrition, you have to eat and drink enough of the foods that contain key nutrients.

This definition is useful in that it gives lay people a simplified version of what nutrition is, yet from a biological perspective. It emphasises the physiological processes that enable the body to extract the nutrients it needs from the food or liquid consumed. However, it must be obvious to the reader that nutrition is not just about the acquisition of nutrients. Another definition of nutrition is:

> the study of the relationship between people and their food.

> (Barasi 2003: 4)

This definition is somewhat different, as it introduces the notion that food is not simply fuel, but a part of people's everyday lives in the same way that a partner or a child may be. It acknowledges that although food is a necessity, it is also part of a complex web of social and psychological processes, and as such has been the subject of much research by social scientists. An illustrative example of this can be found in the Food Standard Agency's (FSA) (2002) survey on 'Food Fundamentals'. The FSA interviewed adults from different social groups in order to understand their attitudes and approaches towards food, including food trends and food scares. They found that the people interviewed could be divided into the following three broad groups:

- *Enthusiasts:* These were a minority of the sample who were deeply involved with food, who enjoyed all aspects of its preparation and consumption, and were confident they knew what was good or bad.
- *Functional eaters:* The other minority, at the opposite end of the spectrum from the enthusiasts, who looked upon food as fuel, and were mainly concerned with value and cost.
- *Consumers:* The largest group, who enjoyed and consumed food and its associated products and media, and were receptive to food fashion and marketing.

Habits and attitudes

The habits of these broad groups of people are just one way of identifying attitudes of people towards their diet. The implications of groupings such as this are that they can contribute to a deeper understanding of the factors that shape food choices, from among the many different choices that can be made. The survey above showed that eating habits differ between age groups: convenience foods were believed to be becoming increasingly popular, particularly in those aged 20-30. The older respondents, however, felt that convenience foods encouraged lazy eating habits, and on occasion criticised their own children for taking grandchildren to fast-food outlets. This type of information is useful because in understanding how people make choices regarding food, healthcare interventions on diet and nutrition can be more closely tailored to the values and needs of the individual. However, the very word 'choices' here may be misleading, as for some people their choice is severely limited by the money or time available to them. The DH (2008a), for example, state that households that contain someone with an LTC are more likely to have a low income and that this will have a measurable effect on the quality of food purchased and eaten.

In order to effectively engage with people about nutrition, healthcare professionals need to recognise that attitudes about food are fundamental, particularly when exploring strategies for change as in LTC management. Telford et al. (2007) conducted a qualitative study into the meaning of nutrition for people living with a chronic disease. They found that, for those who took part in the study:

- Nutrition is more than eating; it 'nourished the soul'.
- Having an LTC could disrupt family routines as the individual could not bear the thought of eating or food preparation, for example.
- Having an LTC such as diabetes meant constantly having to think about food; eating was not done when hungry, instead it was done for 'blood sugars'.
- Indulging in certain foods (such as chocolate for a person with diabetes) caused the person to feel 'bad', 'irresponsible', and led to feelings of reduced personal effectiveness and self-esteem.

How food is produced, where raw materials come from, where food is obtained, how it is cooked, how it is served and the very purpose of diet can be, in the developed world, a matter of individual preference. By understanding this, it is possible to engage with patients or clients in a meaningful way and enable care that takes these factors into account.

Summary

Gaining adequate nutrition is complex, and is not just about getting enough calories. Attitudes to food can shape how people, including those with LTCs, make food choices.

Basics of nutrition

At a very basic level, nutrition can be seen to form a balance between the requirements of the body and the nutrients necessary to keep it functioning. However, the term 'nutrients' does not provide much information in itself, and so can be further divided into micro- and macro-nutrients. Before reading about nutrients, a read of Case study 1.1 should help illustrate why it is important for health professionals to understand about the basic building blocks of nutrition.

Case study 1.1 Ray

Aby Taylor works in a GP practice as a Practice Nurse. She is responsible for diagnosing and managing diabetes, in partnership with patients. Today, she is seeing a 72-year-old man called Ray, who has been diagnosed with Type 2 diabetes a year ago. As well as this, Ray has hypertension, high blood cholesterol and has a body mass index of 31, making him obese. He has been prescribed a range of medications to treat his conditions but Aby feels that Ray could be supported to take a more active role in his disease management, including that of his diet. By his own admission, Ray has never really taken much interest in food, and as a life-long single man has not needed to cook for himself. Instead, he would and still does eat his main evening meal at the local pub, along with a few pints of beer. Since his diagnosis, Ray has developed some of the symptoms of complications of diabetes, in particular, a lack of feeling in his toes and legs. This is a result of persistently high blood sugar. Although Ray realises the seriousness of this, he still does not entirely see the need to manage his diet more carefully. He has tried to eat more fruit and vegetables, but finds this hard because he does not like vegetables. Ray enjoys curries and 'meat and two veg' type meals, without the vegetables. Ray has stated that he would rather 'live his life as he wants' as opposed to conforming to someone else's idea of a healthy lifestyle.

Points for reflection

- What impact is Ray's diet having upon his glycaemic control?
- What knowledge does Aby need to have about the role of specific nutrients in Ray's diet?
- What are the good and bad aspects of Ray's diet?
- How can Aby work with Ray to help him have a healthier diet?

Ray's attitude to food is, in part, shaping his attitude to the diabetes. Ray has viewed food as fuel, as a means to an end, rather than something to take a great interest in. Having not had a family, Ray has only had to please himself with regard to what he eats, and views shopping as a chore. Currently, he is aware that he needs to make changes to his diet and think more about 'healthy eating'. However, it is likely that his understanding of what makes a diet healthy is sketchy, and he may lack the practical skills needed to turn knowledge of this into actual meals.

Ray's diet is likely to be too high in saturated fat and salt. Pub meals are often made up by catering companies and reheated in the kitchen so Ray cannot know the nutrition content of his meals. Similarly, ready meals, which Ray may be tempted to eat for ease of use can contain 40% of the recommended daily intake of salt (FSA 2003). High salt intake could worsen Ray's hypertension. His efforts to increase his intake of fruit and vegetables are to be commended; though making a substantial change to an aspect of lifestyle is often better done in small steps. In addition, although he does not need to stop drinking alcohol altogether, a high intake, over the current recommended guidelines, will also be adversely affecting his blood sugar.

Aby may need to go back to basics with Ray, to assess his understanding of diabetes, diet, and the development of secondary complications such as neuropathy. Ray may not clearly understand how these all link to each other. Once Aby has established Ray's level of understanding, she will find it easier to select the correct information to educate Ray. Aby should also establish what Ray's priorities are in relation to his health. If Ray does indeed not wish to alter his diet and lifestyle, although this will be frustrating to Aby, she will need to respect that it is his choice. Making changes to lifestyle does not happen in a linear fashion for most people, and they may not be ready to make a change, or may relapse after having made that change. Aby must not allow herself to become judgemental as this will reduce the trust that Ray has in their partnership.

Macronutrients

These are the broad food groups that most people are familiar with: carbohydrates, fats, and proteins.

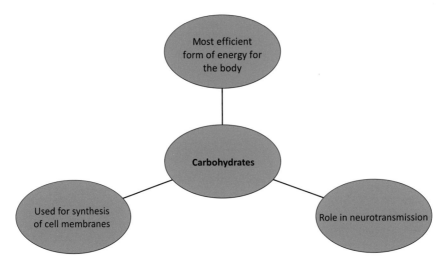

Figure 1.2 Why are carbohydrates necessary?

Carbohydrates
Carbohydrates can be in simple or complex form, yet they are all made up of carbon, hydrogen and oxygen molecules. In their simplest form, carbohydrates are monosaccharides such as glucose, galactose or fructose. Glucose is the most common carbohydrate in the body, and is the primary fuel for organs such as the brain and nervous system. Because of its necessity, glucose is closely controlled within the body by hormones such as insulin and glucagon. Available from sweets, cakes, biscuits, ice creams and honey, intake of refined glucose should be limited; however, plant sources such as fruit and vegetables are encouraged for the other essential components of a healthy diet that they provide. For people with diabetes, intake of fruit and vegetables, and complex carbohydrates is recommended as the cornerstone of an appropriate diet. The reasons why carbohydrates are necessary are illustrated in Figure 1.2.

Disaccharides
Disaccharides are formed when monosaccharides pair up into sucrose, galactose and lactose. Lactose is milk sugar, and apart from milk, it is also present in any food containing milk powder such as some breakfast cereals, chocolate, instant mashed potato and creamed soups. Sucrose is what most people will recognise as sugar, the white crystalline form of which has been the subject of much discussion for its 'bad' properties. The idea that sugar is bad for health originated from thoughts that it provides no nutrition apart from energy, i.e. 'empty calories'. People whose diet is high in sugary foods may consume many calories but will not gain much else nutritionally. However, this statement assumes that sugar is eaten in isolation from the rest of diet, yet studies have shown that where overall energy intake is high, a high intake of sugar may not lead to poor intake of other nutrients (Food and Agriculture Organisation of the United Nations (FAO) 1998). The problem arises for those whose overall energy intake is not so high, so overconsumption of sugar may well lead to imbalance and poor intake of other nutrients. However, the FAO (1998) state that there appears to be no direct link between consumption of sucrose and the development of heart disease. Current advice on sugar consumption favours more complex carbohydrates because of the stability they bring to blood sugar levels, but simple sugars such as sucrose are not necessarily banned, even for people with diabetes.

Oligosaccharides

Oligosaccharides are carbohydrates that are formed from fewer than ten monosaccharides. They are probably the least well known form of carbohydrate by name, yet are present in foods such as onions, leeks, garlic, artichokes, lentils and beans. Oligosaccharides are resistant to digestion in the upper gastrointestinal tract so once they reach the colon undigested, they can ferment. This causes the familiar problem of flatulence and bloating, which may cause some people to avoid these foods altogether. For people with bowel conditions such as Crohn's disease or diverticulitis, a low residue diet may be recommended. This diet aims to reduce the amount of undigested food in the digestive tract and, therefore, reduces the painful symptoms of abdominal cramps, bloating and flatulence. People on a low residue diet will try to avoid foods rich in oligosaccharides wherever possible.

Polysaccharides

Polysaccharides can be either starches or non-starch polysaccharides (NSPs). Obtained from plant sources, starches are the energy contained within the plant cells, whilst the NSPs are from the cell walls that make up the structure of the plant – also known as fibre. Familiar to all, carbohydrates can be found in bread, chapattis, potatoes, yams, beans – indeed anything of plant origin. NSPs have been of interest over the past 30 years due to evidence showing that a diet high in fibre may help prevent certain diseases of the gastrointestinal tract such as cancer (FAO 1998), and diverticular disease is treated with a high-fibre diet. Because there are many different forms of NSPs, Barasi (2003) argues that the term 'high-fibre diet' has no meaning scientifically; however, people seem to have an understanding of 'high fibre', and so it can be a useful way of encouraging a greater intake of fruit and vegetables.

Glycaemic index (GI)

Another term related to carbohydrates is 'glycaemic index' (GI). This index ranks carbohydrate-containing foods according to how quickly they cause the blood sugar level to rise. Foods with a high glycaemic index will cause blood sugar levels to rise rapidly, and include white bread, potatoes, soft drinks and bananas. Apples, beans, peaches and milk are digested and absorbed more slowly, and do not usually cause such a rapid rise in blood sugar. There is a lot of interest in low GI foods as it appears they can promote effective glucose and lipid control in people with diabetes. A recent Cochrane review (Thomas and Elliott 2009) of low GI (or low GI load) diets compared to high GI (or high GI load) diets, or other diets, found that among the 402 participants included in the review, those on the low GI diet showed a significant decrease in HbA1C with no increase in hypoglycaemic episodes. However, Diabetes UK, the leading organisation promoting information and resources for people with diabetes, does not currently recommend focusing exclusively on low GI diets as a way of managing carbohydrate, as there is not sufficient evidence of a long-term benefit (Nutrition Subcommittee of the Diabetes Care Advisory Committee of Diabetes UK 2003). Difficulties include the fact that GI values can vary even in the same food: for example, a banana will have a different GI depending on how ripe it is. Also, combining foods can alter their GI value, and most of us eat meals where foods are combined together in some sort of recipe!

Fats

Current dietary recommendations promote a low fat diet, both to maintain optimum health and as a method of weight loss in obesity. Consequently, there is much confusion over the role of fats in the diet, and this is compounded by terms such as saturated fat, Omega-3, fish oils, and so on. At its simplest, fat does not dissolve in water, and can be obtained as a hard fat or an oil. A diet that did not include any fat at all would not be healthy, as fats are essential elements in many functions of

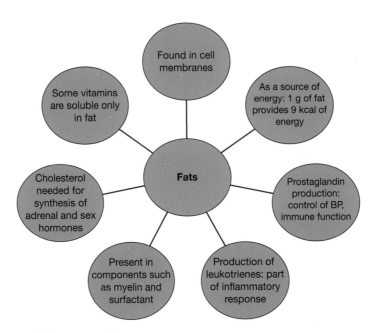

Figure 1.3   Why are fats necessary?

the human body.See 'why are fats necessary' below (Figure 1.3). The most basic form of fat is called a triglyceride and there are many different types of triglycerides, yet they are all formed from a backbone of glycerol with three fatty acids attached. The fatty acids that form the triglyceride are further divided into the following categories that will be familiar to the reader:

- Saturated fatty acids
- Monounsaturated fatty acids
- Polyunsaturated fatty acids (PUFAs)

What makes a fat saturated?

Whilst most people will have heard of this term, not everyone will know what it means. All fats are made up of carbon, hydrogen and oxygen atoms, and all fatty acids have a carbon atom to which the other atoms are arranged in combination. Different combinations will form different fatty acids. Olive oil, for example, is mainly made up of three different fatty acids. A saturated fat is one where each carbon atom is attached to as many hydrogen atoms as is possible, hence, the carbon is 'saturated' with hydrogen. See Figure 1.4 for an example.

In a monounsaturated fat such as olive oil, two of the hydrogens are missing, so two carbons must form a double bond with each other instead. One double bond means that the fat is unsaturated in one place, i.e. 'mono'. See Figure 1.5 for an example.

Stearic acid, a saturated fatty acid

Figure 1.4   Saturated fat.

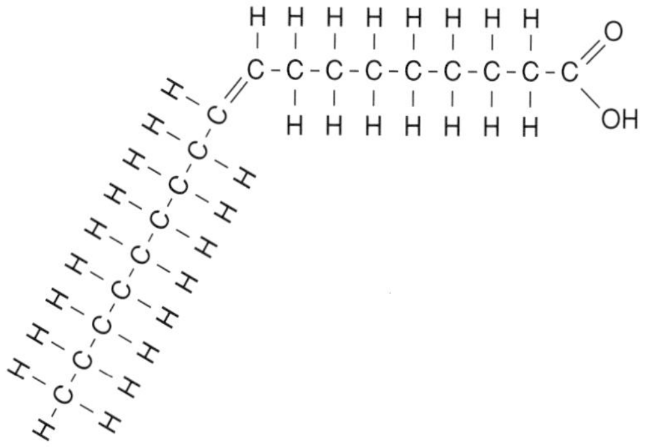

Oleic acid, a monounsaturated fatty acid

Figure 1.5 **Monounsaturated fatty acid.**

A polyunsaturated fat like sunflower oil, therefore, has more than one double bond between carbons along its main carbon chain. See Figure 1.6 for an example.

Omega fatty acids

These double bonds are in very specific places, and the Omega system classifies fatty acids according to where the first double bond is. Omega fatty acids 3, 6 and 9, therefore, have their first double bond in a different place. Omega fatty acids are a hot health topic, with diets high in Omega-3 making claim to improve concentration and mental processing in children, as a natural cure for attention-deficit hyperactivity disorder (ADHD), and as an effective way of reducing the risk of heart attacks and strokes, for example. However, though fish oils may benefit people with known heart disease, there is little convincing evidence that it will prevent heart disease among those not already known to have this problem (NHS Choices 2009).

Trans fats

Trans-fatty acids appear to compromise health by raising blood cholesterol (FSA 2007). It is the processing of the food that produces the trans-fats, present in some margarines, pastry, cakes, crisps and meat products. The processing adds hydrogen to polyunsaturated fats, which changes the shape of the molecule. In this way, the fat becomes 'hydrogenated'. Some trans-fats can also occur naturally in the meat and dairy products of ruminants. Trans-fats are useful to the food industry as they tend to be hard at room temperature so make margarine less liquid. Also, hydrogenated fats tend to spoil more slowly, increasing the shelf-life of products. Current population-wide intakes of trans-fats do not exceed recommended maximum intakes in the United Kingdom (FSA 2007); however,

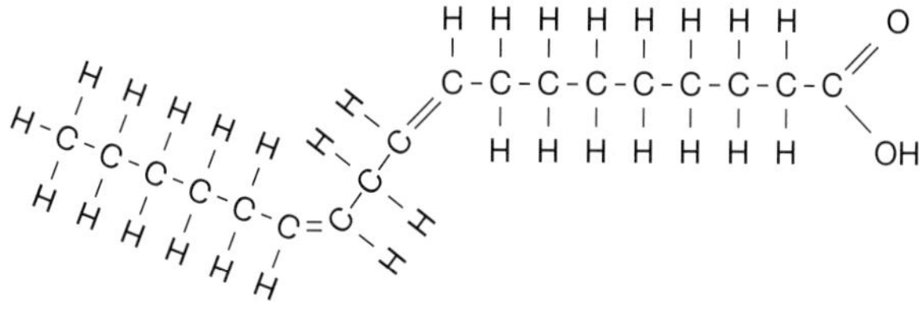

Linoleic acid, a polyunsaturated fatty acid

Figure 1.6 **Polyunsaturated fatty acid.**

among certain sectors of the population, for example the economically disadvantaged, reliance on heavily processed foods may increase their intake to unhealthy levels. As food producers in the United Kingdom appear to be eliminating trans-fats from their products, the FSA (2007) argue that attention should be on total intake of saturated fat, which far exceeds recommended maximum intakes.

The role of fats in health

The role of fats in the diet, as mentioned, causes much debate and confusion. What is clear is that some polyunsaturated fatty acids are necessary for humans as they cannot be manufactured in the body from other dietary components. These essential fatty acids are linoleic acid (an Omega-6) and alpha-linoleic acid (an Omega-3). The current recommendations to ensure that diet contains enough of *both* of these are based on the fact that levels of Omega-3 in the diet appear to be declining at the expense of Omega-6 acids (British Nutrition Foundation 2010a). Omega-3 acids are important in the early stages of development of the child's retina and nervous system, and for its subsequent healthy functioning. The current recommendations are based, therefore, on obtaining sufficient amounts of both to provide a balance. Omega-3 polyunsaturated fatty acids are found in dark green leafy vegetables, meat from grass-fed sheep and cows, and nuts and seeds. These provide short-chain fatty acids and the body will create the more useful long-chain ones from these; however, benefits from vegetable sources may not be as great as from fish. Oily fish such as mackerel, salmon and fresh tuna provide long-chain fatty acids that the body can easily use. Omega-6 polyunsaturated fatty acids can be found in meat, eggs, nuts, and oils such as sunflower, soya or sesame (Barasi 2003).

Cholesterol

Non-essential fats that can be made in the body are phospholipids and sterols. Phospholipids can be found in surfactants in the lung and in the myelin sheath around neurones. The most well-known sterol is cholesterol which has been the subject of an enormous amount of research due to its implications in cardiovascular disease. Cholesterol is obtained from meat and animal products, and a small amount is necessary in the diet as it has a role in cell membranes, ion transport, and the synthesis of hormones such as oestrogen and testosterone. Detailed discussion of cholesterol and its metabolism and regulation can be found in a text such as Barasi (2003).

Fats and coronary heart disease

The link between fats and coronary heart disease (CHD) has also been the subject of much research. The latest thinking on this indicates that the relationship between saturated/polyunsaturated fats and heart disease is too simplistic. Some saturated fatty acids have greater effects than others, while monounsaturated fatty acids may contribute to a lowering of cholesterol. The transport of cholesterol in the body also allows the introduction of two more terms that the reader may have encountered – low-density lipoproteins (LDLs) and high-density lipoproteins (HDLs). LDLs are responsible for carrying cholesterol to the tissues, while HDLs remove surplus cholesterol. Thus, lowering LDL cholesterol and raising HDL cholesterol has been the subject of much research, in order to prevent incidence of CHD. This includes the use of statins to lower LDL cholesterol (DH 2000). It also appears (Kris-Etherton and Yu 1997) that intake of cholesterol in food is not the main factor that leads to an increase in cholesterol in the blood. Rather, total intake of saturated fat from the diet is more closely linked to raised blood cholesterol, so general dietary advice would be to reduce total saturated fat intake.

Proteins

The basic building blocks of proteins are amino acids. Although there are only 20 different amino acids, they can be combined in thousands of different ways to create the millions of proteins found in nature. Proteins can be obtained from plant or animal sources. For the humans, eight proteins

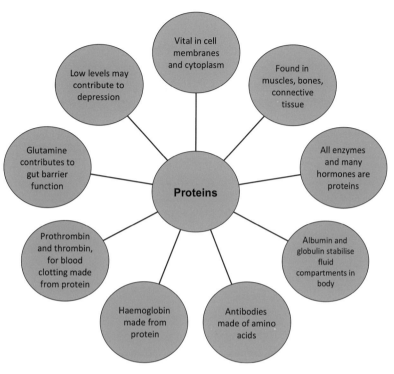

Figure 1.7   **Why are proteins necessary?**

are termed 'essential' because they must be eaten and cannot be produced in the body from plant sources. The total amino acids in the body are termed the 'amino acid pool', as amino acids can either be used as they are in the case of essential, or dismantled and recycled to make others as required. Where insufficient amounts of a particular amino acid is available from the pool to the cells, the cell can either make less of the protein it requires or it can break down some of its own protein stores for the amino acids contained within. Neither of these situations is ideal though, and reduced protein intake over the long term can result in a deterioration of body function and chronic protein deficiency, which is one form of malnutrition. The reasons why proteins are essential are summarised in Figure 1.7.

Protein and renal disease

People with chronic kidney disease used to be advised to eat a reduced protein diet in order to slow deterioration of kidney function. However, this is not the case now. Improved treatments for blood pressure, for example, have reduced the effect low-protein diets can have, and the concern that malnutrition can result from many years of diets low in protein presents an unacceptable risk. People with chronic kidney disease are advised to eat a diet that is neither too low nor too high in protein, while those on peritoneal dialysis or haemodialysis may need a diet that provides a slightly higher protein intake to offset treatment effects (EdREN 2010).

Diet and mental health

The link between diet and mental health has also been the subject of investigation. A meta-analysis by Van der Does (2001) looked into the effects of tryptophan depletion on mood state. Tryptophan is an essential amino acid. People who had recovered from depression, were otherwise healthy but vulnerable or those who had seasonal affective disorder were found to respond to a tryptophan depletion challenge by showing low mood states. Van der Does (2001) hypothesised that dietary habits may affect tryptophan levels, but further research is needed. This has led to a number of claims encouraging people to eat foods containing tryptophan to boost mood; however, the link has not yet been demonstrated clearly.

Micronutrients

Micronutrients include vitamins and minerals. They are needed in very small quantities but are essential for normal functioning of the body and to maintain health. Many people take vitamins and minerals in the form of supplements; however, the Government argues that a healthy, balanced diet will provide all the micronutrients necessary. In fact, overdose of vitamins such as vitamin A can potentially be harmful in the long term as some research suggests that doses in excess of 1.5 mg daily, taken over many years, can mean bones may be more likely to fracture in old age (FSA 2009).

Vitamins

Vitamins can be divided up into fat or water soluble. Fat-soluble vitamins do not need to be eaten every day as they will be stored in body fat for use when needed. Water-soluble vitamins cannot be stored and so ideally should be eaten every day. Tables 1.1 and 1.2 summarise sources and functions of fat- and water-soluble vitamins, respectively.

Minerals

These are only required in very small amounts. Current guidelines for salt intake, for example, stand at 6 g per day (FSA 2010). There are many minerals needed by the body. Table 1.3 presents a summary of the most common ones.

How much do we need to eat?

In essence, the different macro- and micronutrients necessary for the body to function has led to recommendations in the United Kingdom about estimated average requirements. As no one type of food or food group can provide all the essential nutrients needed, a 'balanced' diet is important. A balanced diet means that no food will be excluded, even cakes or biscuits, because as long as they

Table 1.1   Fat-soluble vitamins

Vitamin and name	Dietary source	Functions
Vitamin A (retinol)	Milk, butter, cheese, egg yolk, fish, liver, green and yellow vegetables	Maintains healthy skin Vision in dim light Strengthens immune system
Vitamin D (calciferol)	Fish, liver, oils, milk, cheese, egg yolk and sunlight	Healthy bones and teeth
Vitamin E (tocopherol)	Egg yolk, milk, butter, green vegetables and nuts	Good immune function
Vitamin K (Phylloquinone)	Fish, liver, fruit and green vegetables	Necessary for normal blood clotting

Source: Waugh and Grant (2006). Copyright Elsevier.

Table 1.2 Water-soluble vitamins

Vitamin and name	Dietary source	Functions
B$_1$ (thiamine)	Yeast, liver, nuts, pulses, legumes and egg yolk	Carbohydrate metabolism and nerve cell health
B$_2$ (riboflavine)	Yeast, liver, eggs, green vegetables and milk	Carbohydrate and protein metabolism, and healthy skin
B$_6$ (pyridoxine)	Meat, liver, beans, egg yolk and vegetables	Protein metabolism
B$_{12}$ (cobalamin)	Milk, liver and egg	DNA synthesis
B (folic acid)	Liver, dark green vegetables and eggs	DNA synthesis Haemoglobin production
B (niacin)	Pulses, yeast, fish and wholemeal products	Cell function
B (pantothenic acid)	Liver, yeast, egg yolk and vegetables	Metabolism of amino acids
B (biotin)	Liver, yeast, kidney, pulses and nuts	Metabolism of carbohydrates and fats
C (ascorbic acid)	Citrus fruits, berries, green vegetables, liver and potatoes	Healthy red blood cells Collagen formation

Source: Waugh and Grant (2006). Copyright Elsevier.

are eaten in the context of an otherwise varied diet, they pose no risk. Problems arise of course when one food group becomes more dominant in the diet, such as energy-dense foods like those provided by fast food which tends to be high in fat. Conversely, elimination of a particular food group can also pose a short- or long-term risk such as that illustrated by vegan diets low in protein. The term 'balanced' can also be applied to the balance needed between energy input (howsoever derived) and energy expenditure, in order to maintain a stable weight.

Table 1.3 Common dietary minerals

Mineral	Source	Function
Calcium	Dairy products, eggs and green vegetables	Component of bones Normal blood clotting Muscle contraction
Iron	Liver, beef, egg yolk, wholemeal bread and green vegetables	Formation of haemoglobin
Potassium	Most foods	Muscle contraction Transmission of nerve impulses Electrolyte balance
Sodium	Fish, meat, eggs, milk and added as salt	Muscle contraction Transmission of nerve impulses Electrolyte balance

Source: Waugh and Grant (2006). Copyright Elsevier.

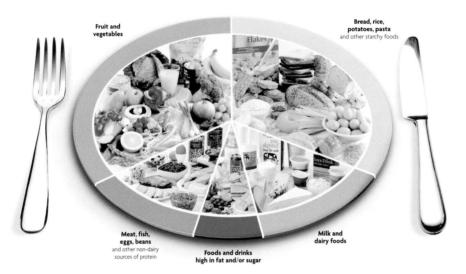

The eatwell plate
Use the eatwell plate to help you get the balance right. It shows how much of what you eat should come from each food group.

Fruit and vegetables

Bread, rice, potatoes, pasta and other starchy foods

Meat, fish, eggs, beans and other non-dairy sources of protein

Foods and drinks high in fat and/or sugar

Milk and dairy foods

The eatwell plate shows how much of what you eat should come from each food group. This includes everything you eat during the day, including snacks.

So, try to eat:

▶ plenty of fruit and vegetables

▶ plenty of bread, rice, potatoes, pasta and other starchy foods – choose wholegrain varieties when you can

▶ some milk and dairy foods

▶ some meat, fish, eggs, beans and other non-dairy sources of protein

▶ just a small amount of foods and drinks high in fat and/or sugar

Look at the eatwell plate to see how much of a whole day's food should come from each food group and try to match this in your own diet.

Try to choose options that are lower in fat, salt and sugar when you can.

For more information on eating a healthy diet, visit: eatwell.gov.uk

Published by the Food Standards Agency. food.gov.uk Design by Bell. Print by Taurus Print & Design Ltd.
Printed in the UK on paper comprising a minimum 75% recycled fibre. © Crown copyright 2007. FSA /1198/0907

Figure 1.8   The eatwell plate. (http://www.food.gov.uk/multimedia/pdfs/publication/ eatwellplate0210.pdf.)

The Eatwell Plate

The Eatwell Plate (Food Standards Agency 2001) (see Figure 1.8 and Table 1.4) was devised after extensive consumer research to illustrate in a clear manner how a healthy diet could be envisaged. The diagram of the plate with the food groups divided up into proportions can be used by anyone involved in promoting a healthy diet. Its positive points include the following:

● It provides visually instant information on the proportions of various foods that make up a healthy diet.

Table 1.4   Proportions of the Eatwell Plate

Food group	Recommended proportion of diet (%)
Bread, rice, potatoes and pasta	33
Fruit and vegetables	33
Meat, fish and alternatives	12
Milk and dairy foods	15
Fatty and sugary foods	8

- It can help all those involved in giving nutritional advice to send out a consistent message.
- It can be tailored to individual preferences of diet, cultural norms, availability of foods and cost of providing a flexible educational tool.

Using the Eatwell Plate

One method of assessing the balance of a person's diet is to find out what he eats on a typical day, or to be more accurate, a typical week. An example of a single day's intake for a 40-year-old woman is shown in Table 1.5. In the left-hand column all the food eaten that day has been listed. In the right-hand column each food has been matched to its main group. This information can then be used to provide a rough total of each food group to see if the diet follows the FSA (2001) recommendations.

Table 1.5   Using the Eatwell Plate

Daily intake	Food group from the Eatwell Plate
Breakfast	
Two pieces of wholemeal toast with butter and marmalade	Bread × 2
	Fat and sugar
Cup of tea	
Glass of orange juice	Fruit
Snack	
One banana	Fruit
Two chocolate biscuits	Fat and sugar
Lunch	
A salmon sandwich made with two slices of wholemeal bread, canned salmon and cucumber	Bread × 2 Fish
One pot of low-fat yoghurt	Dairy
Tea	
Homemade Thai curry made with lean chicken, fresh herbs and coconut milk, tomato and cucumber salsa	Meat Vegetable × 2
Chocolate mousse	Fat and sugar
Four additional cups of tea throughout the day made with semi-skimmed milk	Small amount dairy

To calculate the proportions of each food group eaten, add up the total portions of all foods eaten from the right-hand column. In this case, it is 15 (4 + 3 + 4 + 2 + 2). Then, divide each individual portion per food group by 15:

4 × bread/cereal (4 ÷ 15) = 27%
3 × fat and sugar (3 ÷ 15) = 20%
4 × fruit or vegetables (4 ÷ 15) = 27%
2 × dairy (2 ÷ 15) = 13%
2 × meat or fish (2 ÷ 15) = 13%

As can be seen, compared with the Eatwell Plate, the fat and sugar intake is too high, and the fruit and vegetable intake is too low. Nutritional advice to this woman would, therefore, include tips on how to alter these proportions in favour of a more healthy balance. Self-reporting is notoriously unreliable, however; people can tend to over- or under-estimate what they eat in terms of individual food groups or total intake, so other methods of assessment may be needed to supplement a food diary.

Healthy lifestyle

In addition to the Eatwell Plate, the FSA (2010) suggest the following guidelines that place a balanced diet into a healthy lifestyle:

- Base your meals on starchy foods.
- Eat lots of fruit and vegetables.
- Eat more fish.
- Cut down on saturated fat and sugar.
- Try to eat less salt - no more than 6 g per day.
- Get active and try to be a healthy weight.
- Drink plenty of water.
- Don't skip breakfast.

Summary

Each nutrient has a specific role within the body. A balanced diet, therefore, is one that provides all these nutrients in sufficient quantity to meet an individual's needs.

Assessing dietary intake

Before planning any dietary changes, it is necessary to try to assess what an individual is eating. This can be done in a number of ways, but as can be seen each method will have its own advantages and disadvantages. The choice of method will depend on several factors, such as the clinical setting. For example, an in-depth weighed inventory would not be appropriate for screening risk of nutritional deficiency due to the need to balance time and resource constraints with the sensitivity of the test in detecting those at risk. In an obesity clinic however, a detailed food intake assessment together with information on exercise history and any co-morbidities would be needed, in order to pinpoint eating habits and establish where dietary changes may need to occur.

The weighed inventory

This method involves the individual patient/client weighing and recording all they have eaten in a week. The total intake of nutrients can then be calculated. The weighed inventory is considered to be the most accurate way of calculating nutrient intake, yet it can be subject to problems. Individuals need a good level of motivation to complete the task of weighing everything they have eaten over a week. Also, the method relies very much on the accuracy of reporting by the individual – they may not report the total of everything they have eaten either to hide intake of fat or sugar or because of forgetfulness. Lafay et al. (2000) found in a study of 1034 men and women using a three-day food record that the energy percentage of fat and carbohydrate was lower in under-reporters than in those that reported accurately, in contrast to protein intakes. Lafay et al. (2000) speculated that this was due to the perception of foods as being 'good' or 'bad', 'healthy' or 'unhealthy'. The weighed inventory is used mainly for assessing nutritional intake in order to manage obesity. The DH (2008a) show that obesity levels among people with no LTC is around 20% – this rises to over 30% in those with two or more LTCs. However, this method of would not be suitable for those without the necessary cognitive or physical capabilities to weigh and record their food intake. For example, people with dementia or acquired brain injury may not realise that their diet may be detrimental to their health, yet accurately assessing it can pose challenges if a clear picture of exactly what they are eating is hard to obtain.

Food diaries

Here, individuals are required to write down everything they consume over a week. Additional information such as portion sizes, recipes, makes of bought food and cooking methods will also be needed. From this information, the nutrient intakes can be calculated. Ways of increasing the accuracy of food diaries have been sought; for example, photographs of each meal can be taken. To make the task of calculating the nutrients easier, databases of portion sizes and information on common foods have been developed, including the DINER (Data Into Nutrients for Epidemiological Research) database (Welch et al. 2001). Again, however, food diaries can be subject to under- or over-reporting by the individual concerned with consequent loss of accuracy. Also, assuming accurate reporting, a seven day diary will be able to calculate energy intake to within 15–20% of the actual intake (Black 2001), whereas for some micronutrients such as vitamin C this figure is much lower due to it being found in fewer foods that may not be consumed as frequently.

Food frequency questionnaires

These are useful for studying the food intakes of a large number of people in a relatively inexpensive way. People are asked to remember what they have eaten and record this in a questionnaire. This can be difficult – can you remember how many times, for example, you have eaten fried food in the last week? Rather than looking at a person's whole diet, these questionnaires may focus on a specific subset of foods, which will be less time consuming to undertake. Results may not be very accurate however, and as such are not the best method for estimating intake.

Table 1.6   Calculating BMI

The BMI calculation: BMI = weight (kg) × height (m)

The dietary interview

This is commonly used by dieticians and nutrition specialists, and requires a good level of skill to be able to elicit helpful information. The individual being interviewed must respond to questions about their intake during a particular time frame, for example one day, yesterday or over a week. The interviewer must also establish portion sizes, though this carries the same risks for under- or over-reporting as the previous methods. Remembering intake for one day may also be inaccurate as that day may not have been a usual day, representative of the diet as a whole.

Assessing nutritional status

Body Mass Index (BMI)

This is a method that most readers will be familiar with. How to calculate it is shown in Table 1.6. Rather than focussing on diet, it establishes a figure based on a person's weight and height. The result shows whether or not a person has an appropriate weight for their height. GP practices are required to maintain a register of adults over 16 who have a BMI of 30 or more as part of the Quality and Outcomes Framework (DH 2004). The classifications of BMI are shown in Table 1.7.

The BMI is not without its problems however. Very muscular individuals would obtain a high BMI, but could not be termed 'obese'. The BMI, therefore, does not give an accurate idea of body composition. Also, it has been argued that this calculation does not take into account the different body composition of people from ethnic groups other than the white Europeans upon whom the BMI tables are based (Deurenberg and Deurenberg-Yap 2001). It also makes the assumption that people who are obese are unfit and unhealthy while people who have a lower BMI (in the 'normal' category) are naturally healthier. Of course, this may not be the case. Difficulties can occur too with obtaining the measurements needed. Where it is difficult to obtain an accurate weight or height, the mid-arm circumference or upper arm bone length can be used to establish muscle wasting or fat instead.

Table 1.7   Classifications of BMI

BMI	
40 +	Morbidly obese
35-39.99	Obese class 2
30-34.99	Obese class 1
25-29.99	Overweight
18. 5-24.99	Normal
<18.5	Underweight

Source: NHS 2006.

Skinfold thickness measurements

When done by a trained person, these measurements can provide reasonably accurate estimates of body fat. By pinching up and measuring body fat at the mid-biceps, mid-triceps, subscapular or supra-iliac sites, the skinfold thickness, three measurements are taken and the results averaged.

Waist-hip ratio

This is becoming increasingly popular as a method that anyone can do, so can be used by people at home. It is recommended by the NHS (2006) for primary care clinicians in conjunction with other assessments of body weight and shape. Tape measures for this have been issued by the British Diabetes Association, for example. The measurement of waist around the umbilicus is divided by the measurement around the hips at the widest part of the buttocks. This central fat deposition has been shown by Yusuf et al. (2005) to be a more accurate predictor of myocardial infarction than BMI in a case-control study of 27, 000 subjects from 52 different countries. This method accounts for different distributions of body fat and more muscular physiques, unlike the BMI.

Biochemical markers

Albumin levels have been used for assessing overall nutritional status. However, it is not a particularly reliable method as many other factors can affect albumin levels, for example liver disease and severe illness.

Summary

Nutritional status of patients/clients can be assessed by a variety of methods. Each has its advantages and disadvantages, and choice will depend on the client and location of use.

Nutrition problems in long-term conditions

Now that we have looked at what nutrition is and how a healthy diet is made up, the next part of this chapter will look at disorders of nutrition, specifically obesity and undernutrition. As will be seen, both can be defined as states of malnutrition yet have very different aetiologies. Both states, however, are interlinked with LTCs either as a *cause* of disease in the case of obesity and poor diet, for example, or *caused* by disease in the case of undernutrition.

Obesity

Obesity is the public health issue that is currently dominating policy and research. Case study 1.2 illustrates some of these issues surrounding obesity.

Section 1

Case study 1.2 John

John is a 34-year-old man who is in a rehabilitation unit after sustaining a head injury in a motorbike accident. John now has acquired brain injury (ABI) and, as a result, he is wheelchair bound. John becomes easily frustrated, has a short attention span and becomes easily tired. He also becomes argumentative at times. John can swallow normally and has good upper body strength. Prior to the accident, John had bouts of depression for which he was prescribed fluoxetine. John is not married but has a girlfriend with whom he lives in a flat. His parents live nearby and visit every day. John worked in an office in a desk job, and played rugby every Saturday until a minor knee injury forced him to give it up. According to his girlfriend, John had intended joining a local gym but somehow never got round to it. Accordingly, John was roughly four kilograms overweight at the time of the motorbike accident. However, since the brain injury John's weight is now such that his weight is 95 kg and his height is 1.75 m. For the staff of the unit, his food appears to have become a bit of a battleground. John's family insists on bringing him chocolates and biscuits, which he loves. They do this because they feel helpless in the face of John's injury and this is something they feel they can do to make him happy. The staff, however, can see that this is contributing to John's weight gain as he eats these foods in preference to proper cooked meals. John's weight gain is starting to hinder his rehabilitation programme, in particular work on mobility.

Points for reflection

- What is John's BMI?
- What factors are contributing to John's weight gain?
- How could staff manage the situation to establish a healthier diet?
- How would a healthier diet benefit John?

John's weight gain is not a new phenomenon, but had started before his accident. However, since the accident John has a cluster of factors that are making him gain more weight. His mobility is reduced at the moment, and unfortunately this is getting progressively worse as he puts further weight on. Additionally, John's temperament is labile due to the ABI, and this makes communication with him difficult at times, particularly for the family. They will need support and information on how to deal with this, as John's rehabilitation continues. Because the family don't wish to upset John, they continue to bring him the biscuits, sweets and cakes that he loves, yet as these foods are high in fat and sugar they will contribute not only to further weight gain but to reduced intake of other nutrients by displacing other food groups from John's diet.

Staff looking after John needed to agree on a new approach to managing his diet. This would involve two things: agreeing with the multidisciplinary team about a common approach to understanding John and his family's views about nutrition, and its role in John's recovery. When people are ill, it is common for relatives to provide treats to stimulate a jaded appetite; however, John's family need to see that John is not 'ill' per se, but needs to undergo rehabilitation to be able to live as independently as possible.

After discussion with John's family and girlfriend about how they view his accident and rehabilitation, John's named nurse was able to establish that indeed, they believed they were showing their love for him by providing food that he enjoyed. Through careful listening to their concerns, the named nurse was able to agree to a shared understanding about the role of nutrition in John's recovery. The family agreed that they would limit their provision of cakes and biscuits to John, and that they could instead provide carefully and attractively prepared fruit instead, to tempt John.

As John was not filling up on fatty, sugary foods, he became hungry and this was a chance to encourage him to choose a variety of foods. John's weight loss was gradual; however, as he was able to mobilise more with the help of the physiotherapists, his self-care abilities improved and this had a positive effect on John overall.

Why is obesity a public health issue?

The reasons for the current policy and research into obesity are the following:

- The effects on the obese individual in terms of development of obesity-related disease, mortality and psychosocial problems leading to reduced quality of life.
- *The cost of treating obesity and its related problems in an NHS that has finite resources:* Peters et al. (2002) suggest that the cost may overwhelm the healthcare systems of some countries. (This thinking, of placing a cost on a disease is controversial to some, as it implies blame. For example, such figures are not so often encountered for other conditions, for example cancer or mental health illnesses).

The decision by the WHO to classify obesity as a disease has generated much controversy. However, moving obesity away from a purely aesthetic concern to one that has clinical implications is a deliberate strategy that is intended to underline the serious consequences of rising weight, both for the individual and society as a whole.

Prevalence of obesity

Taking all age groups together, overall a quarter of adults in England in 2007 were obese, though clearly differences can be seen between different age groups. Two-thirds of men and just over half of women were classified as overweight, including obese (Figure 1.9).

Trends in obesity

Although the overall trend is towards rising levels of obesity, there are demographic variations. In 2007, the Health Survey for England (HSE) (NHS Information Centre 2007) used equivalised household income, where the number of people in the household is taken into account. They found the following:

- No difference in mean BMI by equivalised income was found among men.
- Among women, those in the lowest income households were more likely to have a higher BMI.
- However, there was no clear relationship between income and BMI for men.
- Prevalence of high BMI was lower for women in managerial, professional and intermediate households compared with routine and manual households.
- Men who were married or cohabiting were more likely to be obese than single men.
- Bangladeshi and Chinese men were least likely to be obese.
- Among women, Chinese women had the lowest levels of obesity.

Section 1

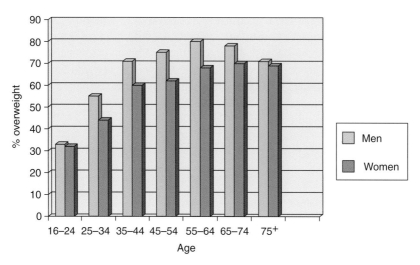

Figure 1.9 Proportion of adults in England who are overweight including obese, by age and gender, 2007. (NHS Information Centre 2007.)

Why do people become obese?

Current thinking into the reasons for rising obesity levels has moved away from blaming the failure of biological mechanisms within the body. In previous times, the availability of food was not as assured as it is now. Human physiology developed in response to a need for high levels of physical exercise to find food and of periodic famine. It has been suggested that the usual diet of pre-agricultural people was made up of berries, some meat and fish, and wild plants and was, by comparison with today's diet, low in carbohydrates (Westman et al. 2007). Because of the need to ensure a sufficient energy intake for survival and reproduction, human physiology developed the ability to slow down the metabolism during periods of famine. Additionally, Peters et al. (2002) state that when physical activity was not needed, the body probably developed a bias towards conserving energy. If we transpose these innate states, developed as humans evolved, into the environment of today, then we can easily see how obesity can occur. Dietary intake no longer relies on foods relatively low in energy. Because of the easy and cheap availability of high-energy foods laden with fat, sugar and processed carbohydrate, it is not hard to consume much more than what is required physiologically. Levels of activity have also plummeted; the use of labour-saving devices and dominance of motorised transport, for example, have meant that useful levels of daily activity are not needed. Whereas before the main driver of appetite was to ensure that energy intake matched physical activity, now we find that energy intake can be very high and that the body does not have a mechanism that makes us engage in greater levels of activity to counterbalance the high-energy intake. Nearly every aspect of the modern lifestyle predisposes us to obesity – this is termed the 'obesogenic environment' (Foresight 2007). Maintaining a healthy body weight is no longer driven instinctively by physiology; rather it has become an activity that has to be thought about and planned.

Health risks associated with obesity

To what extent does obesity present a risk factor in the development of chronic disease? There is an increasing body of evidence linking obesity to many non-communicable diseases. Research into obesity has shown that fat cells have an endocrine function, and that the release of free fatty acids may be the most important factor in disease development (Bray 2004). However, there is also much evidence exploring the links between poor diet and disease, and it must be remembered that although obesity would appear to be a very visual indicator that a person's diet is poor, there are many people who are not obese whose poor diet can predispose them to disease. Conversely, it must not be assumed that because someone is obese they must necessarily be unhealthy. Nonetheless, Bray (2004) shows that evidence finds the following:

- Type 2 diabetes is strongly associated with obesity in both genders across all ethnic groups (Bray 2004). Insulin resistance occurs when body cells do not respond to its action and this can result in Type 2 diabetes. Syndrome X or metabolic syndrome is characterised by a combination of obesity, insulin resistance, abnormal blood fats and hypertension. People with Syndrome X are three times more likely to die from cardiovascular disease than those without (British Nutrition Foundation 2005).
- Obese people are estimated to be five times more likely to develop hypertension.
- Obesity appears to be correlated with raised incidence of gall bladder disease, particularly gall stones.
- Coronary artery disease and stroke are strongly linked to obesity. Adipose tissue has been found to secrete substances linked with a number of processes that contribute to the development of cardiovascular disease (British Nutrition Foundation 2005).
- Cancer risk is increased, though for individual cancers this is variable. 10% of deaths from all cancers are associated with obesity; this rises to 30% for endometrial cancer. The relative risk of developing colon cancer increases by 2.7 times in those who are obese.
- There is association between obesity and the development of osteoarthritis, though it is possible that the lack of mobility caused by arthritis may contribute to the obesity.
- Reproductive function is reduced: 6% of infertility in females has been attributed to obesity.
- Liver disease and obesity are linked: 40% of non-alcoholic steatohepatitis (fatty liver) is found in obese people.
- Obese people are more likely to have mental health problems such as depression, and suffer stigmatisation and discrimination.

The cost of obesity
The cost of obesity in terms of treatment and secondary effects is illustrated in Table 1.8.

Table 1.8   The cost of obesity: now and projected (£ billion/year)

Total NHS cost of:	2007	2015	2025	2050
Diabetes	2.0	2.2	2.6	3.5
Coronary heart disease	3.9	4.7	5.5	6.1
Stroke	4.7	5.2	5.6	5.5
Other related diseases	6.8	7.4	7.8	7.8
Total	17.4	19.5	21.5	22.9
Percentage of NHS budget	6.0%	9.1%	11.9%	13.9%

Source: Foresight 2007.

Interventions

Because the problem of obesity is rooted in many factors, any Government strategy to improve health has to be multifactorial, and a summary of such interventions is outlined below (NICE 2006a). For clinicians working in practice, a care pathway has also been developed to aid clinicians in managing obesity. See Figure 1.10.

Community-based interventions

These are aimed at empowering people to be able to make healthy choices in an otherwise obesogenic environment. The following are some of these interventions:

- *Raising awareness of obesity by promoting health:* The NHS Change4Life campaign, for example, is aimed at families (http://www.nhs.uk/change4life/Pages/Default.aspx). A website is available for families to register with, and it contains such tips as 'five a day', 'me-sized meals', 'snack check' and 'sugar swaps'. Leaflets are distributed to children via schools, and posters are displayed in public places. The effectiveness of such campaigns, however, remains to be seen.
- *Improving access to healthier foods:* These local initiatives involve multi-agency working, including primary care trusts, trade and retail associations, local residents and community organisations. Food mapping can be part of this, and it involves pinpointing everywhere within a certain locality that a particular food can be obtained from. This gives valuable information on the types of food available locally, its cost, distance to residential areas, transport links, and so on. For those with LTCs, transport and relative poverty may be issues, and an awareness of where people purchase food can help understand the difficulties they face when trying to eat healthily.
- *Restricting the promotion of unhealthy foods to children and improving nutrition in schools:* The aim here is to prevent the 'upstream' effects of poor diet on health.

Organisational interventions

These are aimed at getting organisations such as workplaces or local councils to explore how they can promote a healthier lifestyle. These measures can include the following:

- Promoting healthy foods in canteens or healthy food for meetings.
- Encouraging employees to cycle or walk to work by offering support for purchase of bicycles or providing showers at work.
- Where employee health checks are offered, weight, diet and activity should be addressed. The occupational health nurse clearly has a role here.
- Making available time for physical activity or work on healthy eating.

Social networking

Here, opportunity is provided for people to be healthy and perhaps learn with other people:

- Walking clubs
- Healthy lifestyle self-help groups, for example meal preparation

Individual interventions

These are aimed at reducing a person's overall BMI. It is not necessary to try to get weight within the normal range, and in practice this is rarely achieved (Wilding 2007). Even relatively small reductions

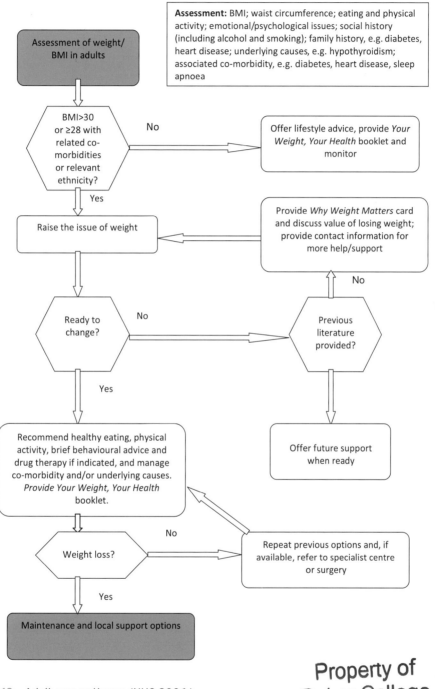

Assessment of weight/ BMI in adults

Assessment: BMI; waist circumference; eating and physical activity; emotional/psychological issues; social history (including alcohol and smoking); family history, e.g. diabetes, heart disease; underlying causes, e.g. hypothyroidism; associated co-morbidity, e.g. diabetes, heart disease, sleep apnoea

BMI>30 or ≥28 with related co-morbidities or relevant ethnicity?

No → Offer lifestyle advice, provide *Your Weight, Your Health* booklet and monitor

Yes

Raise the issue of weight

Provide *Why Weight Matters* card and discuss value of losing weight; provide contact information for more help/support

Ready to change?

No → Previous literature provided?

No

Yes

Recommend healthy eating, physical activity, brief behavioural advice and drug therapy if indicated, and manage co-morbidity and/or underlying causes. *Provide Your Weight, Your Health* booklet.

Offer future support when ready

Weight loss?

No → Repeat previous options and, if available, refer to specialist centre or surgery

Yes

Maintenance and local support options

Figure 1.10   Adult care pathway. (NHS 2006.)

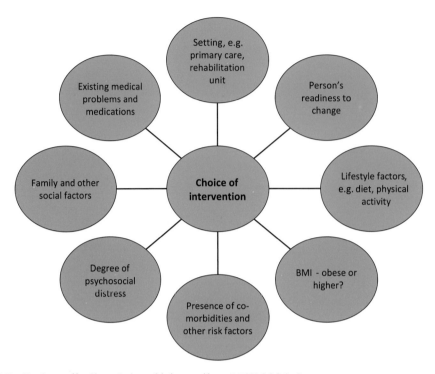

Figure 1.11   Factors affecting choice of intervention. (NICE 2006a.)

of 5–10% in weight can bring about measurable health benefits. It is thought that this is due to loss of visceral fat which is found around the heart, lungs, liver, pancreas and intestines. Loss of visceral fat improves a person's metabolic profile as a whole (remember that this fatty tissue is thought to have an endocrine function of its own), regardless of ideal body weight, and as such can improve health by reducing the risk of developing the non-communicable diseases indicated earlier.

Choice of intervention is dependent on several factors, as illustrated in Figure 1.11.

Dietary advice

Current NICE (2006a) guidelines recommend that weight loss should be sustainable using a 600 kcal per day deficit. This will provide a diet that is not too restrictive in terms of variety of foods eaten. Low calorie (1000–1600 kcal/day) and very low calorie diets (VLCDs) (<1000 kcal/day), whilst not forbidden, are not felt to be sustainable as they could be limited nutritionally and are difficult for the individual to maintain unless highly motivated. Ayyad and Andersen (2000) conducted a systematic review of research into the long-term efficacy of diets and found that VLCDs were associated with only a 15% median success rate after at least 3 years follow-up. Given a figure such as this, it is questionable whether it is ethical to recommend VLCDs. Weight cycling, where individuals lose weight initially then put it back on in an up-and-down cycle, can lead to feelings of frustration and lack of motivation to lose weight in future. Perhaps a more useful approach would be to encourage healthy eating overall, with a healthy attitude to food and appetite rather than encouraging individuals to develop a fetishistic approach to eating.

Commercial/community/self-help weight management programmes

If these are to be effective, they should offer not just dietary advice but also more holistic approaches, including exercise and lifestyle factors. Techniques for managing difficult situations should also be discussed, for example how to manage when eating out, or how to deal with temptation or lapses. For example, in a randomised, unblinded controlled trial of four commercial weight loss programmes in the United Kingdom, Truby et al. (2006) compared Dr Atkins' New Diet Revolution, Slim-Fast Plan, Weight-Watchers Pure Points Programme, Rosemary Conley's Eat Yourself Slim Diet and Fitness Plan to see how effective they were. All four diets resulted in weight loss over a six-month period, with the Atkins' Diet showing the greatest weight loss in the first four weeks. By the end of the trial period however, it was no more or less effective than the other three. One of the challenges of weight loss, however, is maintaining it and so healthy eating rather than dieting is argued to be better. People become used to the pleasurable taste of commercially sweetened or fattened foods, and diet products can do nothing to undo this.

Diet and exercise

The NICE (2006a) guidelines recommend increasing levels of exercise for overweight people even if this does not result in weight loss. Exercise has been found to increase levels of high-density lipoproteins, and irrespective of weight, has been shown to confer a relative reduction in risk of hypertension and cardiovascular events. Release of endorphins during exercise may also promote a sense of well-being. Shaw et al. (2006) conducted a review of exercise for overweight and obesity for the Cochrane Database, and they concluded that exercise is associated with reduced cardiovascular disease risk even if no weight was lost. When combined with a weight loss intervention, exercise was shown to be effective particularly when combined with dietary intervention. They also found that of the trials included in their review, the type of exercise (high or low intensity) was not important.

Exercise that can be easily included in everyday life, such as using the stairs instead of the lift, walking or cycling instead of driving where possible, can be a good starting point for increasing activity levels. Clearly, for people with LTCs current activity and physical fitness levels need to be taken into account before any programme of exercise can be recommended. However, exercise has been shown to have positive psychological as well as physical outcomes for people with LTCs. For example, Neuberger et al. (2007) found that compared with a control group, a sample of 220 adults with RA showed a decrease in symptoms of pain, fatigue and depression following a low-impact aerobic exercise programme. Although this is a small study, there is a growing body of evidence in the value of exercise for other conditions as well as RA. Even adults with LTCs that appear to mitigate against any form of exercise can benefit; for example, pulmonary rehabilitation programmes are designed to improve exercise tolerance through exercise training in people with chronic lung disease. Improved exercise tolerance will mean that those with chronic lung disease can manage their own activities of daily living more independently, and a positive cycle may improve feelings of self-efficacy. In turn, this may encourage people to improve other aspects of their lifestyle including nutrition. Exercise can now be prescribed as part of a range of interventions to help people maintain healthy weight.

Behavioural approaches

These include behaviour and cognitive behavioural therapy. These aim to increase the ability of the person to show restraint in their eating patterns and to be motivated to be more physically active. They can also help develop coping skills to manage temptation such as emotionally laden situations that would normally send the individual to overeat. Such approaches can also help the individual to sustain a healthy lifestyle once the initial period of euphoria has worn off. In contrast, group therapies are widely used in commercial diet programmes and self-help groups, and their purpose is to provide social support, problem solving and encouragement to continue. Generally, behavioural approaches such as these can be successful when combined with other approaches such as dietary management. Dansiger et al. (2007), in a meta-analysis of dietary counselling (advice to limit fat or calorie intake) compared to a control intervention of no or minimal input found that modest weight loss could be achieved.

Medications

There are now a number of medications that can promote significant weight loss, such as Orlistat and Sibutramine. Orlistat works by reducing the amount of fat absorbed in the gut, and as such have side effects of fat in the stools, abdominal discomfort, and potentially embarrassing uncontrolled loss of loose stool. Sibutramine acts centrally to decrease appetite. These medications are controversial however. In promoting the idea that weight loss is the primary goal in a healthy lifestyle, and that a taking a pill can help this, it can be argued that they are unhelpful in prevention and treatment of obesity. The issue of how pervasive the notion of weight loss is, particularly among women, is reflected in the fact that of 33, 000 women polled in an American survey, 75% reporting feeling too fat. The Centres for Disease Control (Berg 1993) found that 62% of women who were trying to lose weight were not overweight to begin with. Larger people are now subject to discrimination. Gortmaker et al. (1993) compared indicators of socio-economic status between women who were overweight, of average size and those who had chronic disease. Of the three groups, the women who were overweight were less likely to be married, have completed fewer years of school, and had lower household incomes than the women from the other two groups. Obesity is also associated with blame. In a study of medical students and physicians, obese people were felt to be ugly, sad, lacking in self-control, bad and difficult to manage (Rothblum 1992). The concept of an ideal weight may itself be flawed, as weight cycling with its unhealthy consequences and the negative health consequences of some diets (loss of bone mass, obsession with food) continue to promote poor health. Many now feel that focus should now be on a person's overall health behaviours including plenty of fresh fruit and vegetables, exercise, low salt, low sugar and a positive self-image. The taking of a tablet to reduce weight, therefore, can continue in this destructive cycle of poor self-image and lack of attention to healthy behaviours. These medications can have a positive role however, for example to promote rapid weight-loss before surgery.

Bariatric surgery

This can include such measures as gastric banding, gastric balloons or stomach stapling to reduce the volume of the stomach, and promote a feeling of fullness on very small amounts of liquid food. They are only recommended for treatment of severe obesity in the United Kingdom. Studies have shown that surgery can have significant effects in terms of weight loss, yet quality of life after treatment remains to be adequately explored. O'Brien et al. (2006) conducted a study comparing surgery with non-surgical methods of weight control in mild to moderately obese people. The non-surgical intervention comprised an intensive period of very low calorie diet (500 to 550 kcal/day) of one to three packets of Optifast (Novartis, Fremont, MI, USA) per day for three months, followed by a combination of some very-low-calorie meals and 120 mg of Orlistat before higher-calorie meals for one month, and 120 mg of Orlistat before all meals for the next two months. After the intensive period, patients continued to take very-low-calorie meals or Orlistat as tolerated. All patients were encouraged to follow good eating habits and exercise for ≥200 min/week. O'Brien et al. (2006)

found that the surgical intervention was most effective in producing weight loss at the end of the trial period. However, the following questions can be raised about the philosophy of such a study, in comparing surgical methods of weight loss with very restrictive diets:

- Were the non-surgical interventions in the control arm likely to produce a sustainable weight loss?
- What might the long-term effects of such a restrictive diet be on physical, psychological and social outcomes?
- Were the patients on low-calorie diets likely to become hungry?
- How can patients on low-calorie diets be motivated to continue?

Summary

Obesity is a condition that has clear links to a variety of diseases. Management of obesity has to take into account many factors, not just diet, and the overall aim of any management plan has to be to improve lifestyle as a whole.

Having explored obesity and its links to chronic disease, the final section of this chapter examines undernutrition and its treatment.

Undernutrition

For most people, the term 'malnutrition' conjures up images of undernutrition. The British Association for Parenteral and Enteral Nutrition (2009: 4) define malnutrition as:

> ...a state of nutrition in which a deficiency or excess (or imbalance) of energy, protein, and other nutrients causes measureable adverse effects on tissue/body form (body shape, size and composition and function, and clinical outcome.

This definition is broad, and includes obesity as well as states of undernutrition. Within this section on undernutrition, malnutrition will be the term used to be consistent with BAPEN, however the meaning should be taken to be undernutrition rather than obesity. Malnutrition can occur in two forms:

- where the diet provides enough energy from carbohydrate but lacks protein, or
- where there is a deficiency in both energy and protein.

Both of these states imply that a diet is not healthy, and with loss of these vital macronutrients a consequent lack of micronutrients is also highly likely. A BMI of <18 kg/m^2 is used as a measurable parameter for undernutrition (BAPEN 2009).

Who becomes malnourished?

BAPEN (2009) estimate that over three million adults in the United Kingdom are undernourished or at risk of malnutrition. The majority of these people (93%), perhaps surprisingly, are living at home in the community, with 2–3% of these in sheltered housing, 5% in care homes and just 2% in hospital. Those most vulnerable to become undernourished are the elderly, those with LTCs, those recently discharged from hospital, and those who are poor and socially isolated. The population is set to age over forthcoming decades. Because of this, the number of people likely to have an LTC in England alone will rise by 23% over the next 25 years (DH 2008a).

Factors leading to malnutrition

As with obesity, the factors that contribute to malnutrition are varied. Eating is not just about the acquisition of nutrients, and for many with LTCs a combination of both the disease process itself and social variables will affect the diet eaten. These are summarised in Figure 1.12. Case study 1.3 illustrates some of the difficulties faced by people with LTCs, in particular the elderly.

Case study 1.3 Mrs James

Mrs James is a 72-year-old lady who has been admitted to hospital from a nursing home. Mrs James has had COPD for 10 years for which she takes inhalers. Her last exacerbation was 8 months ago following a severe cold. She was in hospital for three weeks, during which she ate little, according to her relatives. Mrs James also had a fall 18 months ago and has mobilised little since. She now has a pressure sore on her sacrum and appears very thin. After a thorough assessment, her BMI is found to be 14. The nursing home states that Mrs James's dietary intake is non-existent apart from ice cream, a Vanilla Build-Up and a few spoons of soup per day.

Prior to the fall, Mrs James was living at home with the help of her two daughters. Having COPD made it difficult for her to get to the supermarket as it involved catching a bus or relying on her daughters to take her. As she valued her independence, she did not like being a burden to her daughters. She began to shop at the local corner shop more and more as this was easier to manage. Gradually, however, her disease state worsened and she became more and more apathetic, preferring to stay in and watch television. Her daughters tried to ensure that Mrs James had at least one decent meal a day by cooking something for her and taking it round. However, as both daughters had young families of their own, this became increasingly difficult to manage.

Points for reflection

- How does having COPD predispose people to undernourished states?
- What are the early signs of malnutrition?
- What other co-factors are there that will alter Mrs James' nutritional requirements?
- What is the safest way for Mrs James to gain weight?

Mrs James started with one LTC that affected her ability to obtain adequate nutrition. Having COPD, for example, can predispose people to malnutrition for the following reasons:

- Food intake can be limited to avoid a stifling feeling of fullness that makes it difficult to breathe.
- As it is difficult to eat and breathe at the same time, food intake can be low.
- Treatment effects, such as taking steroids, which alter appetite, or antibiotics that can induce nausea may cause food intake to be limited.
- Mucus production can alter taste and be off-putting.

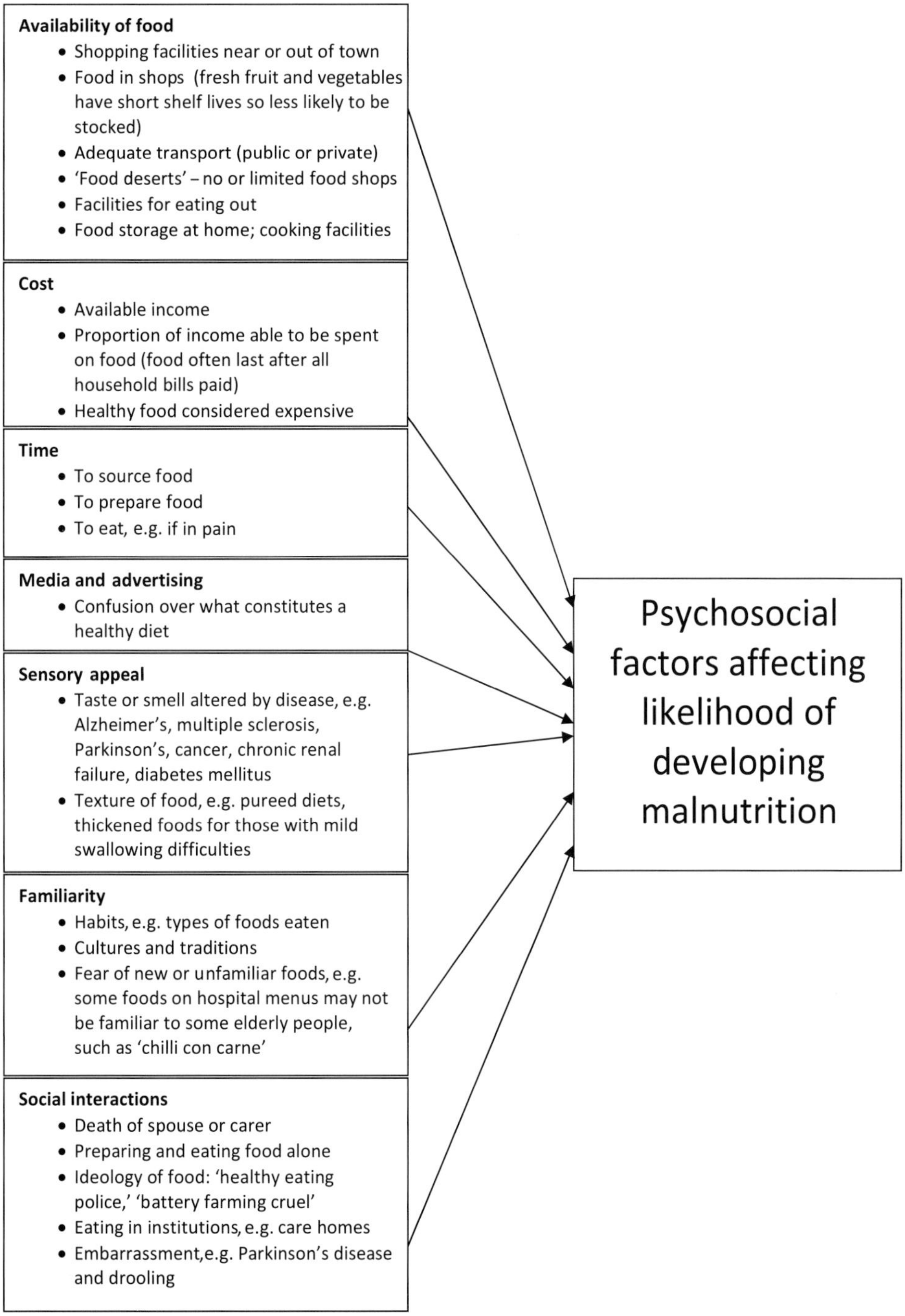

Availability of food
- Shopping facilities near or out of town
- Food in shops (fresh fruit and vegetables have short shelf lives so less likely to be stocked)
- Adequate transport (public or private)
- 'Food deserts' – no or limited food shops
- Facilities for eating out
- Food storage at home; cooking facilities

Cost
- Available income
- Proportion of income able to be spent on food (food often last after all household bills paid)
- Healthy food considered expensive

Time
- To source food
- To prepare food
- To eat, e.g. if in pain

Media and advertising
- Confusion over what constitutes a healthy diet

Sensory appeal
- Taste or smell altered by disease, e.g. Alzheimer's, multiple sclerosis, Parkinson's, cancer, chronic renal failure, diabetes mellitus
- Texture of food, e.g. pureed diets, thickened foods for those with mild swallowing difficulties

Familiarity
- Habits, e.g. types of foods eaten
- Cultures and traditions
- Fear of new or unfamiliar foods, e.g. some foods on hospital menus may not be familiar to some elderly people, such as 'chilli con carne'

Social interactions
- Death of spouse or carer
- Preparing and eating food alone
- Ideology of food: 'healthy eating police,' 'battery farming cruel'
- Eating in institutions, e.g. care homes
- Embarrassment, e.g. Parkinson's disease and drooling

Psychosocial factors affecting likelihood of developing malnutrition

Figure 1.12   Factors leading to malnutrition. (Adapted from Pollard et al. (2002).)

As malnutrition becomes established, apathy takes hold and a spiral of decline follows that is hard for the individual to reverse alone. The good news is that malnutrition can be halted at any point in its development. However, carers, both formal and informal, need to know how to spot the early signs of malnutrition.

Like many who start off with one LTC, age can tend to mean that others become superimposed. The effects of multiple LTCs are compounded – Mrs James pressure sore will also be altering her nutritional requirements as the body attempts to heal the chronic wound. Her energy needs will increase slightly, and she needs adequate intake of protein, vitamins A, B, and C, and essential fatty acids too.

Due to the chronic nature of Mrs James malnutrition, she will need to be reintroduced to feeding very slowly, beginning with enteral feeding. The risk of refeeding syndrome (see below) is very real, yet the temptation is to provide a full range of nutrients and energy to improve her condition quickly.

Gradually, the nutrition team were able to increase Mrs James feeding regime and she started to gain weight. With careful attention from the nursing staff, her wound also began to heal. Mrs James is now able to take diet orally. This is carefully planned to accommodate her COPD, and she also has sip feeds to complement her diet as needed. Her daughters are delighted that their mother is now able to take an interest in her surroundings, and hold a conversation with them, as she is now strong enough to sit up in bed.

Disease-related malnutrition

In addition to psychosocial factors that affect people's food intake, the presence of disease itself can affect nutrition. McLaren (2009) helpfully divides these disease-related factors up into the following:

- Those causing decreased dietary intake
- Impaired gastrointestinal function
- Altered metabolism

Decreased dietary intake

Neurological disorders such as stroke, dementia, and Parkinson's disease can cause a variety of problems for the individual including loss of taste, progressive dysphagia, taste changes and depression. Anorexia (loss of appetite) is a common feature of many LTCs, and may be related to pain from arthritis, cancer, renal disease, or mental health problems such as depression, alcoholism or drug addiction. Poor dentition and presence of mouth ulcers can affect dietary intake too. People with COPD or cardiac failure may fear eating meals that are too large as the feeling of fullness affects their ability to breathe. Drugs such as digoxin and fluoxetine can reduce appetite.

Impaired gastrointestinal function

Conditions such as Crohn's disease or ulcerative colitis can reduce absorption of nutrients. Ulcerative colitis and coeliac disease can cause protein to be lost from the bowel, whereas liver disease and the presence of fistulas can cause losses of various nutrients from the gut. Periods of diarrhoea and pain will also reduce food intake.

Altered metabolism

This can be due to the presence of infection, which raises metabolic rate. COPD is known to increase energy requirements because of the increased respiratory muscle activity. People with Parkinson's disease also have increased energy requirements particularly in the early stages of the disease.

Table 1.9 Drug–nutrient interactions

Drug	Effect
Antacids	Reduced absorption of iron
Sulphasalazine	Reduced folic acid absorption
Anti-convulsants	Disturbed vitamin D metabolism
Phenytoin	Folic acid antagonist
Long-acting antibiotics	Destruction of gut flora
Short-acting antibiotics	Nausea
H2 antagonists	Reduced vitamin B_{12} absorption
Vitamin E supplements	Increased bleeding tendency
Fish oil supplements (not oily fish)	Increase effects of anticoagulants

Source: Mason 2002a.
Note: The opinion of a pharmacist should always be sought before recommending any supplements if a patient is on any medication, prescribed or otherwise.

Serious insults to the body such as major surgery, sepsis, trauma or pressure ulcers alter nutritional requirements towards needing more energy to enable the body to repair and for the various metabolic processes involved in maintaining homeostasis.

For those with LTCs, the presence of a disease may predispose them to malnutrition, as seen above. The disease itself may require treatment with drugs which may in turn affect acquisition, absorption or metabolism of nutrients. This is a 'double-whammy' effect that means people with LTCs may be especially prone to malnutrition. Some examples of drug effects are presented in Table 1.9.

Conversely, some drugs are dependent on limiting or elimination of certain foods from the diet in order to work properly (Mason 2002b). Absorption of biphosphonates, used for osteoporosis, can be markedly altered by any food, even mineral water, and so must be taken with plain water half to one hour before anything is consumed. Foods high in vitamin K such as broccoli, kale, spinach and sprouts can decrease clotting times in those taking warfarin. Grapefruit juice inhibits enzymes that metabolise many drugs including triazolam, calcium channel blockers, cyclosporine, oral contraceptives, and certain statins such as atorvastatin, lovastatin and simvastatin. Severe headaches and a potentially fatal increase in blood pressure can occur in people taking MAO inhibitors if they eat foods containing tyramines. These are found in many cheeses, yoghurt, cured meat products (for example salami), avocados, bananas, marmite, soy sauce, red wine and caffeinated products. Finally, for those with Parkinson's disease, levodopa absorption can be affected by protein, and so must be taken 45 minutes before consuming such foods.

What are the effects of malnutrition?
The effects of malnutrition are many and varied. It is a progressive condition and at first may go unnoticed. However, it is closely entwined with LTCs and care must be taken **not** to consider malnutrition as an unavoidable side effect of disease or of ageing. The effects of malnutrition, according to BAPEN (2009), are shown in Figure 1.13.

Apathy can be the first effect of malnutrition but because it is hard to separate the problems associated with the burden of disease from poor diet it can easily go unnoticed. Once apathy sets in then a gradual spiral of decline can occur with multiple disease states existing simultaneously.

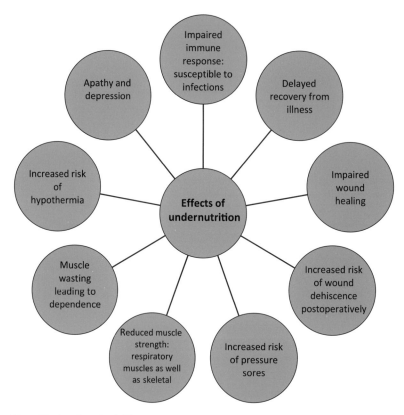

Figure 1.13   The effects of malnutrition.

The hospital experience

Many people with LTCs experience varying disease trajectories. A smooth trajectory, whereby the course of the disease is predictable, is not always possible particularly for conditions such as COPD or cardiac failure. These diseases are characterised by periods of quiet, where the symptoms appear to be manageable and under control. However, exacerbations of the disease can mean sudden hospital admission and treatment, often as an emergency. This leads to a further opportunity for malnutrition, and the experience of people in hospital has led to high-profile campaigns such as the Royal College of Nursing's Nutrition Now or the Age Concern's Hungry to be Heard. Reasons for worsening of malnutrition in hospital can be seen in Table 1.10.

Hospitals now have an obligation to improve nutrition for patients, as set out in the Essence of Care (DH 2001). This provides benchmarks against which standards of care can be set, and encourages sharing of best practice. However, a recent report (Health Service Journal 2009) suggested that despite these initiatives, nutrition in hospital is still fragmented and patchy, and that not all services are compliant with requirements to screen patients for malnutrition on admission, for example.

Metabolic stress

Clearly, people must go into hospital for treatment of serious conditions that could not otherwise be managed at home. Sepsis, trauma (including burns) and surgery are such problems; however, they are serious in that they can lead to a state of metabolic stress. This is a state whereby the

Table 1.10   Why do people become malnourished in hospital?

- Effects of the disease itself. For example, severe breathlessness and lack of appetite
- Poor mealtime practices where activities like tests, visits from staff and so on interrupt eating or may mean meals are missed altogether
- Practical issues such as food being placed out of patients reach
- Unpleasant sights or smells
- Anxiety related to diagnosis or treatments
- Treatment-related factors that may cause nausea, vomiting or other unpleasant symptoms
- Failure of staff to identify malnutrition
- Failure of staff to treat identified malnutrition

body tries to adapt to the insult it has experienced and it enters a protective mode that involves most of its metabolic pathways. The process of metabolic stress is divided into two phases - the ebb and flow. The ebb phase lasts about 12-24 hours, and is followed by the flow phase where the body starts to fight back and, among other things, mobilise nutrients to cope with the insult. The metabolic characteristics of each phase are shown in Table 1.11.

What are the implications of metabolic stress for the patient?

This metabolic stress state and starvation are not the same, and have different responses within the body. Undernourished states are characterised by decreased energy expenditure, and use of body protein and fat for energy. In stress states, the body enters a hypermetabolic state, and the stress causes accelerated energy expenditure and glucose production. Hyperglycemia can occur either from insulin resistance or excess glucose production via gluconeogenesis, and muscle breakdown is also increased. The aim of nutritional support in hypermetabolic states is to provide enough energy but not too much, and to prevent catabolism if possible. Enteral nutrition may well be required as nutrients and fluids can be controlled to respond to the patient's needs. For those caring for patients with LTCs, transfer of relevant information on discharge to those continuing care is essential, as is provision of information to the patient and relatives on how best to maintain adequate nutrition in the recovery phase. Advice from nurse specialists and community dieticians would be useful here.

Table 1.11   The phases of metabolic stress

Ebb phase	Flow phase
- Hypovolaemia - Shock - Tissue hypoxia - Decreased cardiac output - Decreased oxygen consumption - Lowered body temperature - Insulin levels drop and glucagon is elevated leading to hyperglycaemia	- Increased cardiac output begins - Increased body temperature - Increased energy expenditure - Total body protein catabolism begins - Marked increase in glucose production, circulating insulin/glucagon/cortisol - Sodium and fluid retention

Table 1.12   Who should be screened for malnutrition?

- All hospital inpatients on admission
- All outpatients at their first appointment
- All people in care homes on admission
- All people on registration at GP surgeries
- All people where there is clinical concern, for example unintentional weight loss, fragile skin, poor wound healing, wasted muscles and impaired swallowing

Screening for malnutrition

In addition to the methods of establishing dietary intake mentioned above, BAPEN recommend that *risk* of malnutrition should be calculated. They argue that this should not just be for people traditionally considered to be high risk such as those in hospital. Care homes, sheltered housing schemes and GPs all have a responsibility to screen for malnutrition – remember that most people with it are free-living in the community. Table 1.12 summarises who should be screened according to NICE Guidelines (2006b).

The Malnutrition Universal Screening Tool (MUST)

The Malnutrition Universal Screening Tool (Elia 2003) is a validated tool that screens for risk of impaired nutritional status using the following three questions:

1. BMI calculation
2. Recent unplanned weight loss
3. Presence of acute illness

These questions are used because they are felt to be the most useful indicators of potential for malnutrition, and can be combined to produce a tool that is quick and easy to use. Each of these questions is given a score depending on the severity of the risk and so overall risk can be calculated. See Table 1.13 for actions to take depending on risk (Elia 2003).

Local guidelines on how to address the malnutrition risk can then be implemented in the care plan. The MUST is available for download from the BAPEN website, along with further advice on how to use it effectively.

There are other tools available to calculate risk for malnutrition; for example, the Mini Nutritional Assessment Short Form (Rubenstein et al. 2001) or the Nutrition Risk Score (Reilly et al. 1995). To use these effectively, staff need to be trained in how to use them, and clear policies and plans should

Table 1.13   Actions to take after assessment with the MUST

Low risk	Repeat screening. Hospital weekly, care homes monthly, community annually for those aged 75 or over.
Medium risk	Observe and record dietary intake for three days if patient is in hospital or care home. If there is improvement or adequate intake, then follow local policy and repeat screen. If concern, then follow local policy.
High risk	Treat unless detrimental to do so. Refer to dietician. Improve and increase dietary intake. Repeat screening.

be available to help provide the nutritional support needed by the client. Any tool used for screening nutritional status must be validated for its ability to recognise abnormalities, and must also be reliable so that the same score would be obtained by different users on the same client (inter-rater reliability).

Risk of malnutrition: whose responsibility is it?

For the best assessment of risk of malnutrition, communication needs to be improved between carers, clients and healthcare staff. Some individuals may be at risk of malnutrition and not be aware of it, for example those with cognitive impairment such as dementia. Communicating a need for nutritional support can also be impaired. Simple questions from carers or relatives such as 'what did you eat today?' or a quick look in the cupboards or fridge can reveal a lot about how a person is managing their diet. Each member of the multidisciplinary team shares responsibility to assess, plan and implement care related to malnutrition.

Treating malnutrition

The aim here is firstly, where possible, to promote increased intake through healthy eating. Confusion around healthy eating can be a problem though; for example, the standard messages about low fat diets may not apply to someone who is undernourished, and they need to be reassured that it is OK to add energy to their diet. Initial management to maximise energy and protein in food may include steps such as those found in Table 1.14.

Sip feeds

If oral intake remains low, and improvement in the patients nutritional status does not appear to have improved when rescreened, then sip feeds can be introduced. These are for patients who come into one or other of the following ACBS (Advisory Committee on Borderline Substances) categories (NICE 2006b), and they must be prescribed:

- Short bowel syndrome
- Intractable malabsorption
- Preoperative preparation of patients who are malnourished
- Proven inflammatory bowel disease
- Total gastrectomy

Table 1.14 Ways of increasing energy and protein intake

- Each day have three meals and two to three nourishing snacks.
- Use at least one pint of full cream milk daily (silver top, sterilised or UHT), with food or as milky drinks.
- Have at least six to eight cups of fluid each day; try water, fruit juice, fruit squash, soups, milky drinks, tea and coffee.
- Try not to drink too much liquid before meals, since this may reduce appetite.
- Include a serving of meat, chicken, fish, eggs, cheese, yoghurt, nuts, beans or lentils, at least twice a day.
- Have at least one helping of bread, potatoes, rice, pasta, cereal or chapattis at breakfast, lunch and evening meal.
- Aim for at least five portions of fruit and vegetables daily (i.e. two portions of fruit and three servings of vegetables).
- If you can only manage small serving of vegetable or fruit, include a glass of fruit juice or squash which has added vitamin C.

- Dysphagia
- Disease-related malnutrition (this can incorporate a range of conditions and is open to interpretation)

Sip feeds are designed to complement oral food intake, and cannot be used to replace food entirely. They come in various flavours and may be juice or milkshake in style. The use of sip feeds needs to be monitored, however, as patients can become reliant on them. Patients need to be advised to continue to try to eat as healthily as possible regularly, and not rely on these sip feeds for all their nutrition. Nutritionally complete sip feeds are available, and these can be used in place of diet in short term.

Once an agreed target has been reached, for example a certain amount of weight gain, then the feeds can be stopped. Monitoring of the patient must continue however, to avoid relapse.

Enteral nutrition

For some patients, taking adequate nutrition orally is not possible. In the management of LTCs, the reasons for this are shown in Figure 1.14.

If no nutrition intake is likely for more than 5 days, then enteral feeding should be considered.

Enteral feeding provides nutrition either via a nasogastric or nasojejunal tubes, or via percutaneous gastrostomy (PEG) or jejunostomy (PEJ) tubes. This type of feeding uses the bowel rather than feeding directly into a vein; this has benefits as rates of infection are lower and using the bowel maintains its health. Where feeding is likely to be prolonged (more than four to six weeks), PEG

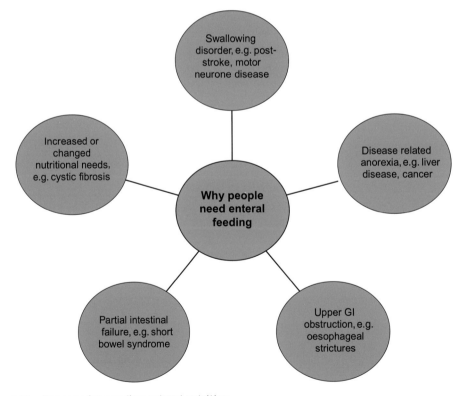

Figure 1.14   Reasons for needing enteral nutrition.

feeding is recommended as this is generally tolerated better then nasal tubes – they don't fall out, cannot be seen and are more comfortable. Any decision to feed a patient enterally must be taken with involvement of the multidisciplinary team, and of course must be acceptable to the patient and their carers. Many patients now continue with enteral feeding at home – in 2007, 21,858 people were registered with the British Artificial Nutrition Survey (BAPEN 2008) as having this treatment. Discharge plans must include involvement of the patient, carers, community nurses, community dieticians and GPs. Training in pump use, infection control, feeding, stoma care, management of complications, and lists of who to contact must be available and reinforced with written information. Also, it must be noted that enteral administration of drugs may not be straightforward: elixirs or solutions are preferred as the crushing of tablets or breaking open capsules means that the drug is not being used according to its license. Responsibility for the actions of the drug administered under these conditions then becomes that of the prescriber and person administering it.

Complications of enteral feeding

Enteral feeding is considered to be a medical intervention, and enabling a person to take in adequate nutrition and hydration is a basic duty for healthcare staff. However, as with any intervention informed consent must be obtained and it must be understood that the procedure is not without risks.

These can include the following:

- *Nasal insertion problems:* Nasal damage, intracranial insertion, bronchial placement.
- *PEG/PEJ insertion problems:* Bleeding, intestinal perforation.
- *Post-insertion trauma:* Discomfort, erosions, fistulae, strictures.
- *Displacement:* Tube falling out, bronchial placement of feed.
- *Reflux:* Oesophagitis, aspiration.
- *GI intolerance:* Nausea, bloating, pain, and diarrhoea related to the feed used.
- *Metabolic problems:* Refeeding syndrome, hyperglycaemia, fluid overload, electrolyte disturbance.
- *Administration problems:* Tube blockage, infection via sets and feeds.
  Source: Stroud et al. 2003.

Aside from the physical complications, the ethical concerns of any type of artificial feeding must be taken into account. Case study 1.4, about Mr Patel, vividly highlights some of the dilemmas surrounding enteral feeding; these can also be applied to parenteral feeding.

Refeeding syndrome

This is a potentially fatal disorder of metabolism, and appears to be related to adaptations made by the body when in a state of malnutrition. In this syndrome, cells leak electrolytes such as potassium and calcium and water leaks into the cell. If feed is administered too quickly these processes are suddenly reversed, and insulin, secreted again after an absence, causes movement of these electrolytes into the cells. Consequent falls in circulating levels and alterations in extracellular and circulating fluid levels can precipitate respiratory failure, cardiac arrest, lethargy, confusion, coma and death. For this reason, feeding after a period of no or very little nutritional intake (more than 5 days) must be commenced very slowly and gradually increased.

Parenteral feeding

For those unable to take nutrition via the gut, either orally or enterally, parenteral nutrition (PN) can be considered. This is where predigested food is given via an intravenous line. Candidates for

PN include those whose illness is severe, who have a poor tolerance of long-term enteral feeding, or who have gastrointestinal disorders such as Crohn's disease or short bowel syndrome (NICE 2006b). Parenteral feeding, like enteral feeding, can be done at home and this is becoming increasingly common as support networks become established. There are various solutions available for PN, and the choice of which to use depends on the exact needs of the individual. PN is not without complications however, and catheter-related infection is common. Because of the high concentration of the solutions used, PN must be given into a large vein such as the vena cava. Metabolic complications can also occur, such as fluid or electrolyte shifts as nutrients are introduced (see 'Refeeding syndrome').

Case study 1.4   Mr Patel

Mr Patel has had an anterior cerebral haemorrhage two weeks ago, which has left him with a right-sided hemiplegia, hemianopia, dysphasia and dysphagia. Because of this, he is being fed via a PEG tube. Mr Patel appears depressed and wants the tube removed. He has pulled one PEG tube out, despite the stitch keeping it in place. However, his family are keen for him to continue with the feeding via the tube.

Points for reflection

- Who decides whether the PEG tube should remain in situ?
- What other clinical factors need to be taken into account when considering artificial feeding?
- How might Mr Patel feel about not being able to eat?
- What ethical issues might arise should Mr Patel's condition deteriorate?

The insertion of the tube should have been carried out after full discussion of the implications of the treatment with Mr Patel and the family. However, research by Brotherton et al. (2007) suggests that where patients lack capacity to give informed consent, the views of the family may not closely represent those of the patient. In this small study, there appeared to be disagreement between patients and carers as to whether they had a choice to have PEG feeding or not. Interestingly, there seemed to be greater agreement between nurses and patients than relatives and patients on aspects of PEG feeding.

After one month, only 2% of people will experience dysphagia following a stroke. It may be beneficial for Mr Patel to continue the PEG feeding in order to prevent malnutrition during this period. Mr Patel may express his dissatisfaction with the PEG tube by puling it out. If he is deemed competent to make decisions then this action is a clear statement of intent and should be respected. However, the emotional and cognitive effects of the stroke may mean that he is not deemed competent at this time and so any care given must be in his best interests. Once malnutrition becomes established, Mr Patel will enter the spiral of decline and his condition will further deteriorate.

Mr Patel may not accept that he will have a quality of life with a PEG feed. Ability to eat forms part of a person's body image and is inextricably linked to their perceptions of their mind, body and life itself. Mr Patel may wish to take in nutrition orally despite the risks of aspiration pneumonia; if he is competent then his wishes must be respected after ensuring that he does understand the risks of doing this.

If Mr Patel's condition deteriorates and he is dying, then the presence of the PEG feed raises other ethical problems about prolonging survival and withdrawal of treatment. In this case, under English law, relatives cannot make decisions on behalf of an adult patient and so cannot override the decisions of the doctor in charge of the care.

Summary

Malnutrition is of great concern, and its causes are many. Treatment depends on assessment of risk and consequent active management.

Conclusion

This chapter has been presented in three sections. The first section explored what nutrition is and the building blocks of a healthy diet. For people with LTCs, a healthy lifestyle, including diet, can promote well-being and empower them to look after themselves to maximize health. Healthcare staff can use this information to enhance their own understanding of nutrition and so counsel patients/clients effectively.

The section on obesity provides a summary of the latest guidelines and research in its treatment, again to enable the healthcare practitioner to deliver care that is accepting of different sizes while at the same time helping patients to lose weight.

Finally, the section on malnutrition allows healthcare staff to reflect on how easily it can occur in people with LTCs, and how their disease trajectory may cause still further opportunities for weight loss and altered metabolism.

References

American Geriatrics Society, British Geriatrics Society and American Academy of Orthopaedic Surgeons Panel on Falls Prevention (2001) Guidelines for the prevention of falls in older persons. *Journal of the American Geriatrics Society* **49** (5), 664-672.

Ayyad, C. and Andersen, T. (2000) Long-term efficacy of dietary treatment of obesity: a systematic review of studies published between 1931 and 1999. *Obesity Reviews* **1**, 113-119.

Barasi, M. (2003) *Human Nutrition: A Health Perspective*. 2nd edn. London: Hodder Arnold.

Berg, E.M. (1993) *Health Risks of Weight Loss*. Hettinger, ND: Obesity and Health

Black, A.E. (2001) Dietary assessment for sports dietetics. *British Nutrition Foundation Nutrition Bulletin* **26**, 29-42.

Bray, G. (2004) Medical consequences of obesity. *The Journal of Endocrinology and Metabolism* **89** (6), 2583-2589.

British Association for Parenteral and Enteral Nutrition (BAPEN) (2008) *Annual BANS Report, 2008. Artificial Nutrition Support in the UK 2000-2007*. Redditch: BAPEN.

British Association for Parenteral and Enteral Nutrition (BAPEN) (2009) *Improving Nutritional Care and Treatment. Perspectives and Recommendations from Population Groups, Patients and Carers*. Redditch: BAPEN.

British Nutrition Foundation (2005) *Cardiovascular Disease: Diet, Nutrition and Emerging Risk Factors*. London: Blackwell.

British Nutrition Foundation (2010a) Fat. Available at: http://www.nutrition.org.uk/nutritionscience/nutrients/fat?start=2 (accessed 11 May 2010).

British Nutrition Foundation (2010b) Healthy Hydration Guide. Available at: http://www.nutrition.org.uk/nutritioninthenews/hydration/healthy-hydration-guide (accessed 13 May 2010).

Brotherton, A., Abbott, J., Hurley, M. and Aggett, P. (2007) Home percutaneous endoscopic gastrostomy feeding: perceptions of patients, carers, nurses and dieticians. *Journal of Advanced Nursing.* **59** (4), 388-397.

Dansiger, M.L., Tatsioni, A. and Wong, J.B. (2007) *Annals of Internal Medicine* **147**, 41-50.

Department of Health (2000) *National Service Framework for Coronary Heart Disease.* London: The Stationery Office.

Department of Health (DH) (2001) *The Essence of Care: Patient Focused Benchmarking for Healthcare Practitioners.* London: The Stationery Office.

Department of Health (DH) (2004) *Quality and Outcomes Framework (QOF).* London: The Stationery Office.

Department of Health (DH) (2005) *Supporting People with Long-Term Conditions: An NHS and Social Care Model to Support Local Innovation and Integration.* London: The Stationery Office.

Department of Health (DH) (2008a) *Raising the Profile of Long-Term Conditions Care: A Compendium of Information.* London: The Stationery Office.

Department of Health (DH) (2008b) *Ten Things You Need to Know About Long-Term Conditions.* Available at: http://www.dh.gov.uk/en/Healthcare/Longtermconditions/DH_084294 (accessed 12 August 2009).

Deurenberg, P. and Deurenberg-Yap, M. (2001) Differences in body-composition assumptions across ethnic groups: practical consequences. *Current Opinion in Clinical Nutrition and Metabolic Care* **4** (5), 377-383.

EdREN: Edinburgh Renal Unit (2010) Available at: http://www.edren.org/pages/edreninfo/diet-in-renal-disease.php (accessed 11 May 2010).

Elia, M. for the Malnutrition Advisory Group (2003) *The 'MUST' Report. Nutritional Screening of Adults: A Multidisciplinary Responsibility.* Redditch: British Association for Parenteral and Enteral Nutrition.

FAO (1998) *Carbohydrates in Human Nutrition. FAO Food and Nutrition Paper 66. A Joint FAO/ WHO Expert Consultation.* Rome: FAO.

Food Standards Agency (2001) The Eatwell Plate Available at: http://www.eatwell.gov.uk/ healthy-diet/eatwellplate/ (accessed 12 August 2009).

Food Standards Agency (2002) *Food Fundamentals. Qualitative Research Report.* London: FSA.

Food Standards Agency (2003) Ready Meals Salt Survey Tables – 'Healthy Options'. Available at: http://www.food.gov.uk/multimedia/webpage/readymealtablehealthy (accessed 12 August 2009).

Food Standards Agency (2009) Vitamin A Available at: http://www.eatwell.gov.uk/healthydiet/nutritionessentials/vitaminsandminerals/vitamina/ (accessed 12 August 2009).

Food Standards Agency (2007) Trans-fatty Acids. Report of the FSA Board to the Secretary of State for Health. Available at: http://www.food.gov.uk/multimedia/pdfs/board/fsa071207.pdf (accessed 11 May 2010).

Food Standards Agency (2010) 8 Tips for Eating Well. Available at: http://www.eatwell.gov.uk/healthydiet/eighttipssection/8tips/ (accessed 11 May 2010).

Foresight (2007) *Tackling Obesities: Future Choices – Modelling Future Trends in Obesity and their Impact on Health.* London, Government Office for Science.

Gortmaker, S.L., Must, A., Perrin, J.M., Sobol, A.M. and Dietz, W.H. (1993) Social and economic consequences of overweight in adolescence and young adulthood. *New England Journal of Medicine* **329**, 1008-1012.

Harsha, D.W., Lin, P.H., Obarzanek, E., Karanja, N.M., Moore, T.J. and Caballero, B. (1999) Dietary approaches to stop hypertension: a summary of study results. DASH Collaborative Research Group. *Journal of the American Dietetic Association* **99** (8 suppl), S35-9.

Health Service Journal (2009) Action Plan Fails to Leave a Mark on Malnutrition Rate in NHS Hospitals. Available at: http://www.hsj.co.uk/5001052.article (accessed 2 June 2009).

Kris-Etherton, P.M. and Yu, S. (1997) Individual fatty acid effects on plasma lipid and lipoproteins: human studies. *American Journal of Clinical Nutrition* **65**, S1628-S1644.

Lafay, L., Mennen, L., Basdevant, A., Charles, M.A., Borys, J.M., Eschwège, E., Romon, M. and the FLVS Study Group (2000) Does energy intake underreporting involve all kinds of food or only specific food items? Results from the Fleurbaix Laventie Ville Santé (FLVS) Study. *International Journal of Obesity* **24**, 1500-1507.

Mason, P. (2002a) Nutritional supplements and drugs. *The Pharmaceutical Journal* **269**, 609-611.

Mason, P. (2002b) Food and medicines. *The Pharmaceutical Journal* **269**, 571-573.

McLaren, S. (2009) Disease-Related Malnutrition in Hospital and the Community. Available at: *Nursing Times Net* http://www.nursingtimes.net/nursing-practice-clinical-research/disease-related-malnutrition-in-hospital-and-the-community/1958371.article (accessed 12 August 2009).

National Institute for Health and Clinical Excellence (NICE) (2006a) *Obesity: Guidance on the Prevention, Identification, Assessment and Management of Overweight and Obesity in Adults and Children.* London: NICE.

National Institute for Health and Clinical Excellence (NICE) (2006b) *Nutrition Support in Adults: Oral Nutrition Support, Enteral tube Feeding and Parenteral Nutrition.* London: NICE.

Neuberger, G., Aaronson, L., Gajewski, B., Embretson, S., Cagle, P., Loudon, J. and Miller, P. (2007) Predictors of exercise and effects of exercise on symptoms, function, aerobic fitness, and disease outcomes of rheumatoid arthritis. *Arthritis and Rheumatism (Arthritis Care and Research)* **57** (6), 943-952.

NHS (2006) *Care Pathway for the Management of Overweight and Obesity.* London: NHS.

NHS Choices (2009) Fish Oil Not Secret to Long Life. Available at: http://www.nhs.uk/news/ 2009/08August/Pages/Fishoilnotsecrettolonglife.aspx(accessed 12 August 2009).

NHS Information Centre (2007) *Health Survey for England 2007.* London: The NHS Information Centre.

Northern Ireland Executive (2009) New Standards Promise: Equal Care for Heart Disease Patients Across Northern Ireland Available at: http://www.northernireland.gov.uk/news/news-dhssps/news-dhssps-june-2009/news-dhssps-17062009-new-standards-promise.htm (accessed 19 October 2009).

Nutrition Subcommittee of the Diabetes Care Advisory Committee of Diabetes UK (2003) Implementation of nutritional advice for people with diabetes. *Diabetic Medicine* **20**, 786-807.

O'Brien, P., Dison, J., Laurie, C., Skinner, S., Proletto, J., McNeil, J., Strauss, B., Marks, S., Schachter, L., Chapman, L. and Anderson, M. (2006) Treatment of mild to moderate obesity with laparoscopic adjustable gastric banding or an intensive medical program: a randomised trial. *Annals of Internal Medicine* **144**, 625–633.

Office for National Statistics (2005) General Household Survey. Available at: http://www.statistics.gov.uk/ (accessed 12 August 2009).

Peters, J.C., Wyatt, H.R., Donahoo, W.T. and Hill, J.O. (2002) From instinct to intellect: the challenge of maintaining healthy weight in the modern world. *Obesity Reviews* **3**, 69-74.

Pollard, J., Kirk, S.F.L. and Cade, J.E. (2002) Factors affecting food choice in relation to fruit and vegetable intake: a review. *Nutrition Research Reviews* **15**, 373-387.

Reilly, H.M. et al. (1995) Nutritional screening–evaluation and implementation of a simple nutrition risk score. *Clinical Nutrition* **14**, 269-273.

Rothblum, E. (1992) The stigma of women's weight: social and economic realities. *Feminism and Psychology* **2**, 61-73.

Rubenstein, L.Z. et al. (2001) Screening for undernutrition in geriatric practice: developing the short-form mini nutritional assessment. *Journals of Gerontology Series A: Biological Sciences and Medical Sciences* **56** (6), M366-372.

Shaw, K.A., Gennat, H.C., O'Rourke, P. and Del Mar, C. (2006) Exercise for overweight or obesity. *Cochrane Database of Systematic Reviews* (4), CD003817.

Stroud, M., Duncan, H. and Nightingale, J. (2003) Guidelines for enteral feeding in adult hospital patients. *Gut* **52** (suppl VII), vii1-vii12.

Telford et al. (2007) Constructions of nutrition for community dwelling people with chronic disease. *Contemporary Nurse* **23** (2), 202-215.

The Scottish Executive (2003) *The Scottish Health Survey: Summary of Key Findings.* Edinburgh: The Scottish Executive.

The Scottish Office (1999) *Towards a Healthier Scotland: A White Paper on Health.* London: The Stationary Office.

The Wellness Community (2009) What is Nutrition? Available at: www.thewellnesscommunity.org (accessed 28 July 2009).

Thomas, D. and Elliott, E.J. (2009) Low glycaemic index, or low glycaemic load, diets for diabetes el-litus. *Cochrane Database of Systematic Reviews Issue 1.* Art. No.: CD006296. DOI 10.1002/14651858. CD006296.pub2.

Truby, H., Baic, S., deLooy, A., Fox, K.R., Livingstone, M.B., Logan, C.M., Macdonald, I.A., Morgan, L.M., Taylor, M.A. and Millward, D.J. (2006) Randomised controlled trial of four commercial weight loss programmes in the UK: initial findings from the BBC diet trials. *British Medical Journal* **332** (7553), 1309-1314.

Van der Does, A.J.W. (2001) The effects of tryptophan depletion on mood and psychiatric symptoms. *Journal of Affective Disorders* **64** (2), 107-119.

Waugh, A. and Grant, A. (2006) *Ross and Wilson: Anatomy and Physiology in Health and Illness.* Edinburgh: Elsevier-Churchill Livingstone.

Welch, A.A., McTaggart, A., Mulligan, A.A., Luben, R., Walker, N., Khaw, K.T., Day, N.E. and Bingham, S.A. (2001) DINER (Data Into Nutrients for Epidemiological Research)–a new data entry program for nutritional analysis in the EPIC-Norfolk cohort and the 7-day diary method. *Public Health Nutrition* **4** (6), 1253-1265.

Welsh Assembly Government (2008) *Key Health Statistics for Wales 2008.* Cardiff: Welsh Assembly Government.

Westman, E.C., Feinman, R.D., Mavropoulos, J.C., Vernon, M., Volek, J.S., Wortman, J.A., Yancy, W.S., Phinney, S.D. (2007) Low-Carbohydrate Nutrition and Metabolism. *American Journal of Clinical Nutrition* **86**, 276-284.

Wilding, J.P.H. (2007) Treatment strategies for obesity. *Obesity Reviews* **8**(suppl 1), 137-144.

World Health Organisation (WHO)/ Food and Agriculture Organisation (FAO) of the United Nations (2002) Diet, nutrition and the prevention of chronic diseases: report of a joint WHO/FAO expert consultation. *WHO Technical Report Series 916* Geneva: World Health Organisation/FAO.

Yusuf, S., Hawken, S., Ounpuu, S., Bautista, L., Franzosi, M., Commerford, P., Lang, C., Rumboldt, Z., Onen, C. and Lisheng, L. (2005) Obesity and the risk of myocardial infarction in 27, 000 participants from 52 countries: a case-control study. *The Lancet* **366** (9497), 1640-1649.

Resources

In addition to the references provided throughout, the following websites are worth visiting for more specific information on nutritional needs of patients with various LTCs. These are by no means exhaustive, and the reader is encouraged to seek out more information from other sites as required.

Alzheimer's Society Available at: www.alzheimers.org.uk
British Association for Parenteral and Enteral Nutrition Available at: www.bapen.org.uk
British Dietetic Association Available at: www.bda.uk.com
British Nutrition Foundation Available at: http://www.nutrition.org.uk/
British Lung Foundation Available at: http://www.lunguk.org
Food Standards Agency Available at: www.fsa.gov.uk
Parkinson's Disease Society Available at: www.parkinsons.org.uk

Further reading

Germov, J. and Williams, L. (eds.) (2008) *A Sociology of Food and Nutrition: The Social Appetite.* 2nd edn. Melbourne: Oxford University Press.

Ogden, J. (2003) *The Psychology of Eating: From Healthy to Disordered Eating.* Oxford: Blackwell.

Chapter 2
Chronic Pain: Living with Chronic Pain

Gay James

Learning objectives

By the end of this chapter, the reader will be able to:

- Describe the concept of chronic non-malignant pain, identifying possible patient conditions and problems that can lead to pain of this type
- Identify the incidence of chronic non-malignant pain in the community
- Examine the implications of chronic pain on healthcare requirements for an ageing population
- Discuss the importance of psychology and the impact of this on an individual's ability to cope with chronic pain
- Describe the impact of chronic pain on biological, psychological and social aspects of an individual's life and the importance of these factors for pain assessment
- Identify biological, psychological and social interventions for managing chronic non-malignant pain, including pharmacological and non-pharmacological approaches
- Empower individuals to cope with ongoing pain

Introduction

Pain is generally accepted as a normal part of life: as we develop from childhood we learn to recognise the significance of pain and injury. Through learned behaviour, influenced by our socio-cultural setting, we generally conform to the accepted behaviour for pain. Pain is generally viewed as an unpleasant, undesirable symptom, warning the individual that something is wrong. It is identified as one of the most frequent reasons for seeking medical care (Field and Swarm 2008). This chapter focuses on the impact that living with chronic non-malignant pain has on an individual, and the

---

Long-term Conditions: A Guide for Nurses and Healthcare Professionals, First Edition. Edited by S. Randall and H. Ford.
© 2011 Blackwell Publishing Ltd. Published 2011 by Blackwell Publishing Ltd.

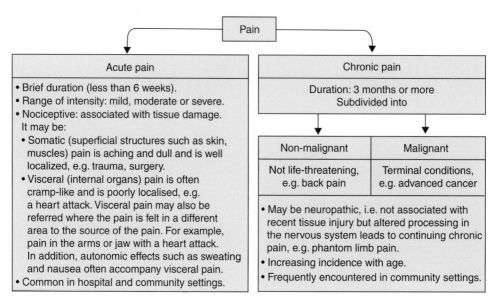

Figure 2.1   Types of pain.

interventions that can support people to manage this significant challenge to their health and well-being. Pain has been defined as:

> an unpleasant sensory and emotional experience associated with actual or potential tissue damage or described in terms of such damage.
>
> International Association for the Study of Pain 1994: 3

Pain is generally thought of as acute or chronic; however, this usually describes the duration of the pain, but not its intensity. Figure 2.1 shows the differences between acute and chronic pain.

Acute pain is characterised by its short duration and foreseeable end, and frequently the injury or pathology that activates it resolves as healing takes place, for example a bone fracture. Acute pain raises awareness of the disorder and behaviour is adjusted, causing a reduction in activity which helps the healing process. By contrast, chronic pain is:

> Pain without apparent biological value that has persisted beyond normal tissue healing time (usually taken to be 3 months).
>
> International Association for the Study of Pain 1994: 1

Such persistent pain frequently restricts even normal activities of living, leading to disability and causing a negative impact on quality of life. Because of this, the chronic pain itself becomes a long-term condition (LTC) requiring support to minimise the harmful effects on health and well-being. In fact, Cousins (2007) identifies that acceptance of persistent pain as a disease entity is an important step towards improving its management. This chapter explores the causes of pain, and effective strategies for assessment and treatment of chronic pain. The first section, therefore, examines what causes pain and the physical processes through which pain is felt.

Causes and pathology of pain

The differences between acute and chronic pain

Acute pain is generally caused by tissue injury which activates inflammatory chemicals: this activates pain transmission, and is known as *nociceptive* pain. Treatment interventions may be focused on recognition of the cause of injury, and pharmacologically on reduction of inflammatory mediators of pain.

The causes of chronic pain are varied and are further subdivided by McCaffery and Pasero (1999) into the following two main types:

1. Chronic malignant pain
2. Non-malignant pain

This chapter primarily focuses on chronic non-malignant pain as it is frequently experienced by patients associated with a range of LTCs.

Biology of pain

Sensitivity to pain is clearly an important biological function which allows us to recognise and respond to tissue injury. MaCaffery and Pasero (1999) explain the four basic processes involved in normal pain transmission. These are represented in Figure 2.2.

Transduction
Commonly the process starts with *transduction* where many inflammatory chemicals are released by damaged tissues. These sensitising substances (bradykinin, prostaglandins, substance P, serotonin and adenosine) initiate nerve conduction along sensory pain neurons.

Transmission
Then, transmission involves impulse conduction within fast (A-delta) and slower, unmyelinated (C fibres) neurons from the peripheral nervous system towards the spinal cord. These signals then enter the spinal cord at the dorsal horn or *pain gate* region of the central nervous system.

The pain gate
The gate control theory of pain is an important concept, first explained by Melzack and Wall in 1965 (Melzack and Wall 1996: 165–193), and it explains how pain can be modulated in the spinal cord (see Figure 2.3). Peripheral neurons to central neurons within the spine allow the impulse to cross over the spinal cord and ascend to the brain stem, and many areas are believed to be involved within the brain for conscious appreciation of pain. This transmission is influenced by the balance of activity taking place within the pain gate. The pain gate is believed to involve processing of neurotransmitters which may result in both modulation and inhibition of pain transmission, or excitation (Godfrey 2005, Chamley and James 2007). For example, activation of fast non-pain, touch-temperature neurons can inhibit pain transmission in the pain gate. This is the basis of some peripheral non-pharmacological interventions that can reduce pain perception by using ice, heat or transcutaneous nerve stimulation (TENS). There are also mechanisms that modulate and inhibit pain transmission from the pain gate by

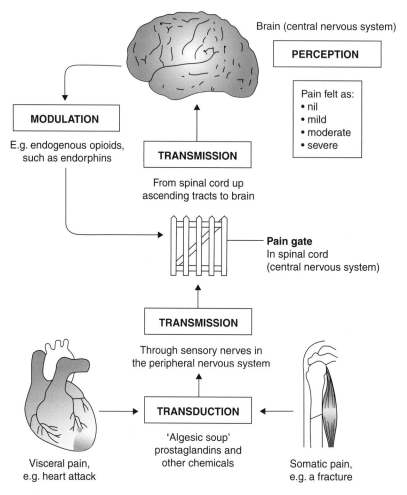

Figure 2.2 Pain physiology.

descending neuronal pathways from the brain; this inhibition involves natural endogenous endorphins and serotonin.

It is recognised that psychological factors influence pain perception due to their influence on pain modulation. Transmission of pain from the periphery depends, therefore, on the balance of activity in peripheral sensory neurons and modulation from descending inhibitory pathways.

Neuroplasticity

The recognition that pain mechanisms and pathways are responsive and, therefore, alter their activity and sensitivity in response to persistent activation (unrelieved pain) and nerve injury is described as neuroplasticity (Godfrey 2005, Cousins 2007), where the pain pathway may become dysfunctional leading to persistent pain. Awareness of this enables us to appreciate the existence of chronic pain as a disease entity. The neuromatrix model of pain (Melzack 1999) acknowledges the importance of the brain in pain processes. This model embraces many aspects of the pain gate (Godfrey 2005).

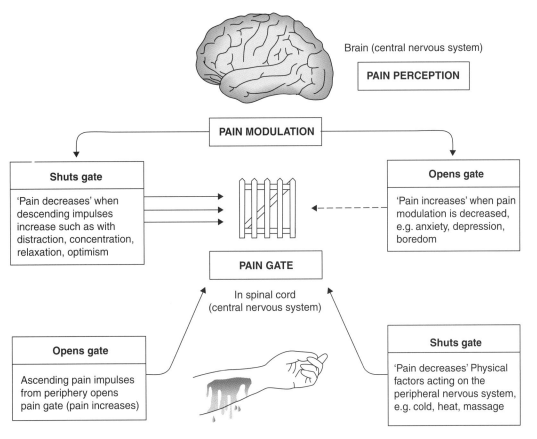

Figure 2.3   Gate control theory.

It also includes the impact of past experiences, cultural factors, emotional state sensory inputs and modulation by endogenous opioids, and the endocrine and immune systems.

The complexity of pain mechanisms can help nurses to appreciate why pain is such a unique individual experience. The same condition does not lead to the same experience of pain for all individuals, as the factors which influence the pain gate, pain modulation and possible adaptation with neuroplasticity are quite individual. Horn and Mufano (1997) suggest that endorphin production is influenced by age and activity. This explains why the emphasis in pain management is to assess *with* the patient, as pain is unique to that individual influenced by the situation at that time. Many conditions can damage the peripheral or central nervous system, and may produce neuropathic pain in an area caused by the dysfunctional pathway (Greener 2009).

Types of chronic pain

Chronic pain may originate from nociceptive or neuropathic pain mechanisms, and Table 2.1 illustrates the characteristics and possible causes of each. Accurate assessment to identify the nature of chronic pain is important, as suitable analgesia is likely to differ for the two different pain types.

As indicated above, chronic pain may originate from nociceptive or neuropathic pain mechanisms.

Table 2.1   Chronic non-malignant pain

Nociceptive pathology	Neuropathic pathology
Pain originating from inflammatory chemicals released by damaged tissues.	Pain signals originating within peripheral or central nervous system; indicate abnormal altered processing of sensory nerves.
Normal processing of stimuli by sensory nerves. **Somatic pain** – originates from bone, joints, muscle, skin, and connective tissue.	Follows injury to nervous system and may also involve dysregulation of the autonomic nervous system.
Visceral Pain – originates from internal organs. **Examples of conditions associated with nociceptive pain include many caused by degenerative disease:**	**Examples of conditions associated with neuropathic pain include:**
Rheumatoid arthritis, osteoarthritis, peripheral vascular disease due to ischaemia, and simple low back pain.	Phantom limb pain following amputation, diabetic neuropathy, trigeminal neuralgia, postherpetic neuralgia, human-immunodeficiency virus (HIV) associated neuropathy, multiple sclerosis, stroke, and epilepsy.

Source: Greener 2009, McCaffery and Pasero 1999.

Careful pain assessment can identify the presence of neuropathic pain, and some conditions may have both types; for example, low back pain can have nociceptive qualities due to muscular sprain and also be associated with sciatica due to prolapsed intervertebral discs which can lead to neuropathic pain. Greener (2009) states nurses should suspect neuropathic pain when a patient reports a severity or extent of pain that seems out of proportion for the tissue injury. A characteristic of this neuropathic pain is abnormal sensitivity known as *allodynia* (pain resulting from a stimulus that would not normally produce pain, such as light touch or a breeze). Case studies 2.1 and 2.2 illustrate the differences between the two types of pain.

Case study 2.1   Mrs Smith

Mrs Smith is a 54-year-old teacher who developed rheumatoid arthritis aged 40 following the birth of her daughter. It started with painful swollen finger joints. Diagnosis was confirmed following blood test for the rheumatoid factor.

Treatment over the last 14 years has focused on the use of various complex disease- modifying anti-rheumatoid drugs (DMARDs) which reduce the inflammatory response, regularly reviewed by the rheumatologist. Over time, treatments become less effective which leads to exacerbations of symptoms and increased pain and stiffness. However, as the disease cannot be cured, pain management is an important part of coping with this lifelong condition (Oliver 2009). Pain management with appropriate simple analgesics has made an important contribution to maintaining normal activity and lifestyle.

Points for reflection

- What type of chronic non-malignant pain is Mrs Smith experiencing?
- Thinking about the disease process rheumatoid arthritis, what is the cause of this pain?
- Looking at her history, what factors do you think will open or close the pain gate for Mrs Smith?

Case study 2.2 Mrs Jones

Mrs Jones is a 62-year-old woman who has had persistent pain and allodynia around her left flank. Even the weight of clothing on her skin causes pain, which feels like a burning sensation. She has had this for the last 2 years following an episode of shingles (herpes zoster), and has a diagnosis of postherpetic neuralgia (PHN). The persistent pain has had a negative impact on her previously normal activity and lifestyle leading to sleep deprivation and social withdrawal. She recognises that few people understand this chronic pain. The pain was unresponsive to the usual analgesics, so at present she has been prescribed Amitriptyline (an antidepressant) which enhances pain modulation. This has resulted in reduced burning allodynia and improved sleep.

Post herpetic neuralgia (PHN) is a specific pain syndrome which may arise for 10-20% of people following an episode of shingles, where the varicella-zoster virus (chicken pox) is reactivated. This can be years or even decades after the initial chickenpox infection. Acute pain is the most common presenting feature of shingles; however, if the pain persists long after the rash has gone it would then be categorised as chronic pain due to dysfunctional pain mechanisms (Hawksley 2006). The cause of the pain and diagnosis following shingles is an important part of medical history. However, the emphasis for care is management of the persisting pain and the impact it has on an individual's life.

Points for reflection

- What type of chronic non-malignant pain does Mrs Jones have?
- What characteristics would alert you to the presence of this type of pain?
- Why would the usual analgesics not work for Mrs Jones?
- How does the neuroplasticity concept explain this persistent pain?

As will be seen throughout this chapter, there are many different problems which may lead to chronic pain and the chronic pain itself should be focused upon as an LTC. The emphasis should, therefore, be on assessment of the impact that chronic pain has on the individual and identification of best management to minimise disruption on lifestyle. Here, the nurse can play an important role in partnership with the patient.

Incidence of chronic non-malignant pain

The Chronic Pain Policy Coalition (CPPC 2006) has collated evidence from several studies and estimates that around 7.8 million people in the United Kingdom live with chronic pain. This represents one-third of all households in the United Kingdom having at least one adult in pain. The Pain in Europe survey into prevalence of chronic, non-malignant pain embraced 16 countries and 46,000 people (Fricker 2003, Breivik et al. 2006). The survey revealed the following:

- Nearly 'one in five' Europeans have chronic pain (19%).
- Individuals were living with chronic pain for an average of seven years.
- Two-thirds of chronic pain sufferers experience moderate pain.
- One-third experienced severe pain.
- 'One in five' chronic pain sufferers had been diagnosed with depression as a result of their pain.

As can be seen, not only does chronic pain have a negative impact on quality of life, it is also a massive socio-economic burden for the health services and society at large. See Figures 2.4 and 2.5 for causes and location of pain according to the respondents of the survey.

Field and Swarm (2008: 7) identify that 70–85% of adults experience at least one episode of back pain in their lifetime. Most, however, will recover within a month; with 80–90% of people recovering within 12 weeks. However, if disability from back pain persists for longer than 6 months, fewer than half return to work. In the majority of cases, the cause of pain is identified as unknown.

It would appear that in some neurodegenerative disorders such as Parkinson's disease and multiple sclerosis, pain can become prominent at an early stage; Scherder et al. (2005) argue that this may be explained by the fact that the location of the neuropathology and degeneration involve key areas involved in the normal inhibition of nociceptive stimuli. Scherder argues for more research in this area and advocates that people who care for individuals with these disorders should be alert to pain.

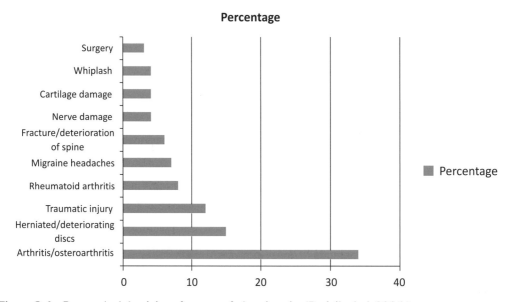

Figure 2.4 Respondents' opinion of causes of chronic pain. (Breivik et al. 2006.)

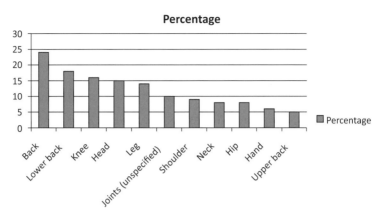

Figure 2.5 Respondents' opinion of location of chronic pain. (Breivik et al. 2006.)

Incidence of pain in specific populations

Ageing and pain

The Survey of Chronic Pain in Europe (Fricker 2003, Breivik et al. 2006) reveals that the proportion of individuals who reported chronic pain increased with age. The 41–60 age group appeared more likely than younger or older groups to suffer chronic pain. However, the survey acknowledges that it did not attempt to reach the elderly in residential nursing homes so this may not give an accurate picture. Elliott et al. (1999) also identified that chronic pain was associated with older age, living in rented or council accommodation and being retired or unable to work. The frequency of more severe pain increased with age. From a biological perspective, it is clear that common causes of chronic pain from degenerative musculoskeletal and neurological origins have increasing incidence as we age. Schofield et al. (2008) identify that a number of different pain problems are more prevalent in older people, including osteoarthritis, osteoporotic fractures, central post-stroke pain, PHN and peripheral vascular disease.

Gibson (2006) explored older peoples' pain and explained that it is a challenging area as the aging process is a complex and non-uniform area. By 2050 it is estimated that in developed countries, around 36% of the population will be over 65 years old, and this age group is recognised as having the highest incidence of painful diseases. Acute pain is less frequent among the presenting symptoms in older patients for a range of medical complaints. Gibson (2006) describes how some studies appear to indicate a reduced sensitivity to mild noxious pain. This is clinically important as it may lead to underreporting of mild pain and the risk of undiagnosed disease; for example, the recognition and reporting of pain associated with myocardial infarction (MI) is desirable as it prompts appropriate management and care. In older persons, 35–42% may experience a painless MI, known as a silent heart attack. This is an obvious disadvantage as prompt recognition attracts appropriate timely interventions to preserve myocardium, and absence of pain may delay diagnosis and treatment.

Of clinical significance to chronic pain, Gibson (2006) identifies that evidence from experimental and clinical studies indicates there may be increased vulnerability to severe or persistent pain, as it appears that the effectiveness of the natural descending pain-inhibitory mechanisms (especially the endogenous opioid mechanisms) deteriorate with advancing age. Gibson (2006: 2) states:

We must be aware of the increased risk of and susceptibility to severe or persistent pain in older adults and make strenuous efforts to provide adequate pain relief for this vulnerable group.

Section 1

Dementia and pain

An example of the challenge of providing adequate pain relief is for people with dementia. Dementia is recognised as a problem which will affect a considerable proportion of the over 65-year-olds in the future. According to Alzheimer's Society UK (2010) it is estimated that there will be over one million people in the United Kingdom with dementia in 2025. At present, 64% of people living in care homes have a form of dementia, two-thirds of sufferers live in the community, while one-third live in a care home. This represents a large, vulnerable group from a pain management perspective. The vulnerability of these individuals is compounded as cognitive impairment reduces effective communication of their pain as the condition progresses. Scherder et al. (2005) explored developments in pain in dementia and identified studies that reveal undertreatment and reduced use of analgesics in this group. He advocates the need to improve our knowledge of pain recognition in this group; this is considered further in the 'Pain Assessment' section.

Psychology and social considerations in chronic pain

The gate control theory, described above, allows the influence of psychological factors on pain to be considered. It allows identification of a greater complexity in pain perception involving three dimensions (Mann and Carr 2009: 10). These dimensions are illustrated in Table 2.2.

When thinking about chronic pain, the pain gate model can be useful as it aids the appreciation of conditions or factors that may open or close the pain gate. These may be used to explain which factors make pain better or worse, and these factors can also be used as pain management interventions. Factors that influence individual perception of pain are summarised in Table 2.3.

Individual characteristics which influence chronic pain responses: self-efficacy, locus of control and coping style

Self-efficacy

Horn and Munafo (1997) explore several factors which may influence an individual's experience of chronic pain, in particular self-efficacy (Bandura 1990) which is described as similar to confidence. It can be thought of as the belief by a person that they can achieve goals and tasks in everyday life. This attribute is not thought to be static, and can be influenced by time and circumstances such as presence of chronic pain. For example, in an individual with persistent back pain, the presence of the pain can reduce their self-efficacy. This, in turn, may cause them to feel more anxious when carrying out certain activities such as exercise or socialising, and ultimately may lead to avoidance of these situations. Some treatment interventions, for example cognitive behavioural pain management programmes, use measurement of self-efficacy as an outcome measure to evaluate the benefit of treatment on an individual's confidence.

Table 2.2 Dimensions of pain perception

- Physical:Sensory – discriminative *location, duration, intensity*
- Emotional: Motivational – *how the body reacts*
- Mental: Cognitive evaluative – *making sense of pain from past experience beliefs*

Table 2.3   Conditions that influence perception of pain

Conditions that open the gate and increase pain perception	Conditions that close the gate and decrease pain perception
Physical conditions	Physical conditions
Size of injury	Drugs
Low activity levels	Counter stimulation (cold, heat, massage)
Emotional conditions	Emotional conditions
Anxiety, fear	Positive emotions
Tension	Rest
Depression	Relaxation
Mental conditions	Mental conditions
Concentrating on the pain	Distraction
Boredom	Involvement in activities, hobbies, interests

Source: Adapted from Sarafino 2008.

Locus of control

Locus of control is a concept that relates to self-efficacy. It is described by Horn and Munafo (1997: 79), and was first proposed by Rotter in 1966. Individuals, shaped through their life experiences, are believed to have either an internal or an external locus of control. This will influence their beliefs about chronic pain and subsequent ability to accept their condition and plan coping strategies (internal locus of control), or continue to seek the answer in others providing appropriate treatments (external locus of control). With an internal locus of control an individual believes events relate more to personal effort and hard work, and, therefore, may be more motivated to take up recommended advice and coping strategies. This can be described as more 'problem-focused' or 'active coping'. The coping style an individual uses in response to chronic pain will clearly be an important area for review as the individual with chronic pain is at the centre of care, and interventions are focused around enabling the individual to use active coping strategies to manage their pain. Such approaches may particularly suit individuals who have an internal locus of control.

Table 2.4 identifies beliefs underlying learning and responses to pain. This illustrates how the nature of beliefs people hold about their pain can affect their day-to-day coping with the pain, and subsequent effect on their activities.

The impact of pain

On lifestyle

Many reports agree that chronic pain can lead to personal suffering which has a negative impact on lifestyle. With chronic pain, psychological factors become more dominant, and sleep deprivation, tiredness and depression are common (NHS Quality Improvement Scotland 2006, CPPC 2006, Field and Swarm 2008: 9). The impact of chronic pain has been described by Field and Swarm (2008: 3) as a chronic pain stress cycle, with the physical presence of pain leading to fear, anxiety, sleeplessness and heightened pain perception. The behavioural responses lead to reduced activity, subsequent functional disability and social withdrawal, which impacts on relationships with others. As pain may

Table 2.4 Beliefs underlying learning and responses to pain

BELIEF: Hurt and harm: 'pain means tissue injury'
FACT: Often chronic pain is no longer a useful indicator of tissue damage, particularly in neuropathic pain.
BELIEF: Cessation of activity is the correct response for pain
FACT: Reduction in normal activity and exercise leads to deconditioning and exacerbation of pain. Functional assessment and education by a physiotherapist is a valuable intervention.
BELIEF: Pain means I deserve a break, secondary gains reinforce this response
FACT: Social/environmental factors play a leading role in pain behaviours. If pain leads to increased attention from others and release from responsibilities this will reinforce pain-related behaviour.
Though these responses from others may be viewed as appropriate and supportive for acute pain, for example following bone fracture, in long term they can lead to dependence and reduced self-efficacy (confidence) and self-esteem. Cognitive behavioural approaches can be beneficial for this.

Source: Adapted from Field and Swarm (2008: 25).

limit the person's capacity for paid employment and social interactions, the financial impact also has a negative impact on self-esteem and further contributes to relationship stressors. Table 2.5 illustrates the impact of chronic pain on a person using Roper et al.'s (1996) activities of daily living model.

Clearly therefore pain causes stress, and the cycle of pain-stress is summarised in Figure 2.6.

On the older person

For the older person with chronic pain who lives alone, the opportunity to distract themselves with activities which focus away from the pain experience may be limited, which, in turn, increases perception of the pain and the impact it has on daily life. Field and Swarm (2008) explain that as pain becomes chronic, psychological factors have increased significance for pain perception and patient coping. There are many more factors that can influence the perception of pain by an elderly individual, and these are summarised in Table 2.6.

Table 2.5 Impact of pain on activities of daily living

Activity of daily living	Impact of chronic pain (CPPC 2006)
Communication	49% diagnosed with depression
Work and play	49% forced to take time off work
	48% impact on attending social activities
	30% impact on an independent lifestyle
	47% impact on driving
	61% negative impact on working outside the home
Mobility	73% report problems with exercising
	47% impact on walking
Rest and sleep	65% negative impact on sleeping
Sexuality	43% negative impact on sexual relations

Table 2.6 Factors which may increase pain perception in the older person

	Chronic pain	Ageing
Physical conditions	• Persistent pain • Possible reduced efficiency of moderating endorphins • Reduced activity levels	• Complex multiple pathology • Polypharmacy and contraindications reduce analgesic choices
Emotional conditions	• Sleep deprivation • Anxiety and relationship problems • Depression common	• Attitudes to retirement (positive or negative) • Opportunity for emotional expression and social interaction may be reduced
Mental conditions	• Persistent pain and fatigue leads to reduced concentration. • Catastrophising • Isolation	• Reduced social interaction can limit opportunities for distraction • Cognitive impairment associated with dementia

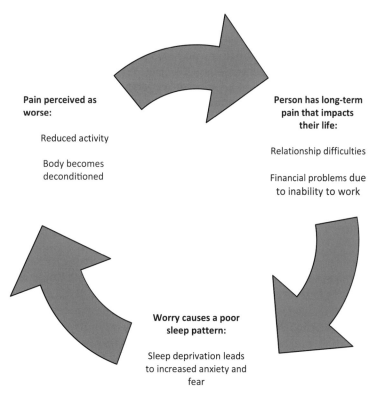

Pain perceived as worse:

Reduced activity

Body becomes deconditioned

Person has long-term pain that impacts their life:

Relationship difficulties

Financial problems due to inability to work

Worry causes a poor sleep pattern:

Sleep deprivation leads to increased anxiety and fear

Figure 2.6 The relationship between pain and stress.

Chronic pain syndrome

It must be recognised that many people with chronic pain do manage despite their pain, yet a small proportion of patients are known to show maladaptive behaviour which is referred to as chronic pain syndrome (CPS) (Shaw 2006). This is described as a psychosocial disorder where the pain has become the central focus of a patient's life. These individuals exhibit depression, anxiety and are not able to maintain responsibilities, and frequently seek radical interventions. Shaw (2006) explained that the features of CPS should not be used to define all patients with chronic pain. McHugh and Thoms (2001) undertook a small study of patients attending the pain specialist services in 11 UK hospitals. These patients reported that pain had profound effect on their lives: 33% were classified as medically disabled and 55% of patients had given up work because of chronic pain. A main concern identified was that the patients wanted a reason for their chronic pain. Shaw (2006) argues that there is evidence that those who manage their lives in spite of the chronic pain will have minimal contact with healthcare professionals, so the true impact of pain is not represented by those that attend chronic pain clinics.

Emotional impact

According to Field and Swarm (2008: 13), there appears to be general agreement that depression is common in patients with chronic pain, and many of the conditions causing chronic pain have a negative impact on normal activities of living and quality of life; for example, multiple sclerosis and rheumatoid arthritis. For further exploration of all aspects of depression in LTCs, see Chapter 3.

The CPPC (2006) identified 49 % of chronic pain patients as having a diagnosis of depression, and from a biological perspective pain and depression share neurochemical pathways. Treatment with antidepressants is argued by Field and Swarm (2008) to be desirable, with the recognition that the newer serotonin norepinephrine reuptake inhibitors (SNRIs) act better as antidepressants compared to Amytriptyline. However, Amytryptyline appears to be a more effective analgesic, which is why it is frequently used for neuropathic pain at a dose which is lower than that advocated for the management of depression (Bond and Simpson 2006: 233).

The impact of depression can have a negative effect on an individual's pain perception (pain gate more open) and reduces their ability to use active coping strategies. Therefore, its presence should be evaluated and appropriate treatment provided. The Pain in Europe report (Fricker 2003) identified that 27% of those surveyed said that they were less able or unable to maintain relationships with friends and family, and 19% were no longer able to have sexual relations. Clearly, these factors will have a profound negative impact on quality of life.

Summary

The holistic nature of chronic pain is that the chronic pain cycle can result in reduced activity and relationship problems. The elderly may have compounded multiple pathology and increased isolation. Individual issues influence confidence, locus of control and these influence pain impact.

Depression is very common and negatively impacts coping strategies

Chronic pain assessment

The Pain in Europe report (Fricker 2003) revealed that doctors are not sufficiently proactive with people suffering with pain. 71% of respondents said it was up to them to raise issues. Nearly a quarter felt they were not given enough time to discuss pain; furthermore, few doctors appeared to use recognised pain scales. The main issue of importance here is recognition of the presence of pain so that appropriate pain management interventions may be implemented and evaluated. Several reasons why pain is not effectively managed have been highlighted by McCaffery and Pasero (1999); these involve healthcare systems, healthcare professionals and patients. McCaffery and Pasero (1999) argue that practitioners commonly follow an acute pain model with the expectation of a particular physiological and behavioural response to pain. However, they explain that chronic pain rarely follows this pattern, as the body seeks homeostasis and equilibrium and so adapts or suppresses behaviour, while the patient values a stoic response (learnt response). One of the key points made by McCaffery and Pasero (1999) is that *verbal self-reporting of pain should be the gold standard for pain assessment*. This follows from the widely accepted statement by McCaffery (1968) following her early work on pain:

> Pain is whatever the experiencing person says it is, existing whenever the experiencing person says it is.

This simple statement contains the following key elements that healthcare staff should uphold:

- The individual nature of pain is emphasised.
- The authority and key person is identified as the patient themselves.

However, as Bird (2005) identifies, waiting for patients to report pain can result in poor management and, therefore, staff must be proactive and use appropriate tools which should suit the setting and the patient. The key message from the CPPC (2006) is recognition of pain; in fact, they advocate pain as the 5th vital sign. The purpose of this is to raise awareness and improve healthcare professionals' perception and responses to pain. In the author's view, this is particularly an issue for many chronic pain patients who may have come to accept pain as part of their life, with little opportunity to discuss this problem with health professionals. Most people with chronic pain are not in inpatient settings but trying to get on with life at home.

Assessment of pain in the older person

Bird (2005: 45) reviews assessment of pain in older people. She states:

> Everyone has a right to have their pain treated, and to perpetuate this myth (that pain is a part of growing old) constitutes a form of ageism.

Failure to recognise and assess pain can lead to poor pain management, impacting adversely quality of life. The British Pain Society and British Geriatrics Society have produced recent guidelines on the assessment of pain in older people (2007). These identify barriers to self-reporting indicating an age-related stoicism and reticence in reporting pain. The guidelines recommend a multidimensional approach including sensory dimensions, emotional components and impact on life. Observation of

Table 2.7   Summary of guidance for the assessment of pain in older people

Sensory dimension	• Words other than 'pain' that may be used; for example, *sore, hurting, aching* • Intensity scale is recommended: Either a simple descriptive '0 no pain, 1 mild pain, 2 moderate pain, 3 severe pain' or 0–10 numerical scale • *Location:* can use body map. • Nature and quality of pain, for example nociceptive and neuropathic allodynia • Stoicism and reticence can be a barrier to self-reporting; therefore, observation of facial expression and behaviour can be valuable. Also useful when cognitive impairment or communication difficulties arise
Emotional dimension	• How is pain perceived, for example dangerous, exhausting, frustrating, frightening • Mood, presence of depression
Impact on life	• This includes physical function and one indicator may be to use activities of daily living scales, reflecting dependency level, mood, sleep and mobility function • Assessment may also include the impact of pain as a barrier to diversional activities

Source: BPS 2007.

facial expression and behaviour are identified as an important component of assessing pain, particularly where patients have difficulty communicating. The guidelines also note that observation during movement enhances detection of pain. In addition, it identifies that with persistent chronic pain physiological cues including autonomic responses, for example pallor and tachycardia rarely occur and absence of these does not mean absence of pain. Table 2.7 outlines the guidance on assessment of pain in older people.

Key principles for chronic pain assessment

The NHS Quality Improvement Scotland (2006) identifies the following key principles for successful management of chronic pain:

• Accurate assessment
• Adequate intervention
• Frequent evaluation

Due to the complexity of chronic pain, a bio-psychosocial assessment using multidimensional pain tools is most effective. The commonly utilised categorical rating scales (0–3) frequently used for acute pain management in inpatient settings are unidimensional and focus on pain intensity. They are not suited to the assessment of chronic pain. Some examples of multidimensional tools are now presented.

Types of assessment tool

The CPPC (2006: 25) propose a basic ten-point scale that briefly explores biopsychosocial aspects of pain, focusing on the patients perception of pain intensity and pattern, emotional impact and social activities. It also explores perception of responses to treatment. See Figure 2.7.

PAIN RATING SCALE

(English)

Title:	Date: ....
First Name:...	Patient number: ....
Surname:	Clinic: ....

Please mark the scale below to show how intense your pain is.
A zero (0) means no pain, and ten (10) means extreme pain.

How **intense** is your pain **now**?

0	1	2	3	4	5	6	7	8	9	10
no pain										extreme pain

How **intense** was your pain **on average last week**?

0	1	2	3	4	5	6	7	8	9	10
no pain										extreme pain

Now please use the same method to describe how **distressing** your pain is.

How **distressing** is your pain **now**?

0	1	2	3	4	5	6	7	8	9	10
not at all distressing										extremely distressing

How **distressing** was your pain **on average last week**?

0	1	2	3	4	5	6	7	8	9	10
not at all distressing										extremely distressing

Now please use the same method to describe **how much your pain interferes** with your normal everyday activities.

0	1	2	3	4	5	6	7	8	9	10
does not interfere										interferes completely

If you have had treatment for your pain, how much has this relieved (taken away) the pain?

0%	10%	20%	30%	40%	50%	60%	70%	80%	90%	100%
no relief										complete relief

The British Pain Society
Facing the challenge of pain

© The British PainSociety 2006   www.britishpainsociety.org   Charity no. 1103260

Figure 2.7 CPPC scale. (Reproduced with kind permission of the British Pain Society.)

This clearly shows a patient-focused general assessment, but for a comprehensive assessment, once the existence of chronic pain is identified a more detailed tool may be required. The Brief Pain Inventory (short form) (Cleeland and Ryan 1994 in Mann and Carr 2006) is used in many pain clinics as a self-report pain rating scale for communicative patients. It is also noted as suitable for assessment of pain in older people by BPS (2007: 16). See Figure 2.8. This allows a more detailed assessment of pain intensity pattern and position, and asks the patient to consider the effects on mood and activities.

Pain assessment for people with dementia

Pain assessment for those with cognitive impairment is clearly an area of concern for nurses. These individuals will be in the community and residential nursing home settings and are potentially vulnerable; it is a high probability that these individuals will have pain due to degenerative conditions. Davies et al. (2004) studied 27 patients with cognitive impairment and 17 had three or more conditions. This raises concerns for nurses as self-reporting of this pain may be hampered by the dementia and the existence of a chronic pain problem may not be apparent to the carers. Davies (2004) undertook a review of literature in this area and devised a specific tool to facilitate pain assessment for this group. The multidimensional tool devised focuses on assessment of pre-existing painful conditions, physiological measures of pain, self-reports of pain, facial expression and changes from usual behaviour. It is recognised that behaviour in response to pain is not uniform; therefore, interpretation of behaviour requires skill. Bird (2005) explains that although facial expressions are common in many pain scales, 'they require validation cross culturally, with the older population and with cognitively impaired people' (p. 34). Schofield et al. (2008) identify that several facial expressions are acknowledged indicators of pain and may, therefore, be useful for assessment in the cognitively impaired. These are identified in Table 2.8. This assessment may involve informal carers, relatives as well as healthcare professionals.

Gibson (2006) states that it is possible for many with mild to moderate dementia to self-report pain and Davies et al.'s (2004) study found 59% of the 27 participants could self-report. Pain assessment for individuals who are non-communicative, for example those with advanced dementia, may require the use of appropriate observation scales. One example of this is the Abbey et al. (2004) pain scale, which is devised for pain assessment in residential care for advanced cognitive impairment. This is included in Figure 2.9.

Assessment of neuropathic pain

The nature or quality of pain experienced may reveal that it is neuropathic in origin, and identification is an essential step towards effective management. Neuropathic pain may require a specific tool;

Table 2.8　Facial indicators of pain

- Brow raising or lowering
- Cheek raising
- Eyelids tightening
- Nose wrinkling
- Lip corner pulling
- Chin raising
- Lip puckering

1903

PLEASE USE
BLACK INK PEN

Date: ☐☐ / ☐☐ / ☐☐
(month)   (day)   (year)

Subject's Initials : _____

Study Subject #: ☐☐☐

Study Name: _____

Protocol #: _____

PI: _____

Revision: 07/01/05

Section 1

Brief Pain Inventory (Short Form)

1. Throughout our lives, most of us have had pain from time to time (such as minor headaches, sprains, and toothaches). Have you had pain other than these everyday kinds of pain today?

☐ Yes   ☐ No

2. On the diagram, shade in the areas where you feel pain. Put an X on the area that hurts the most.

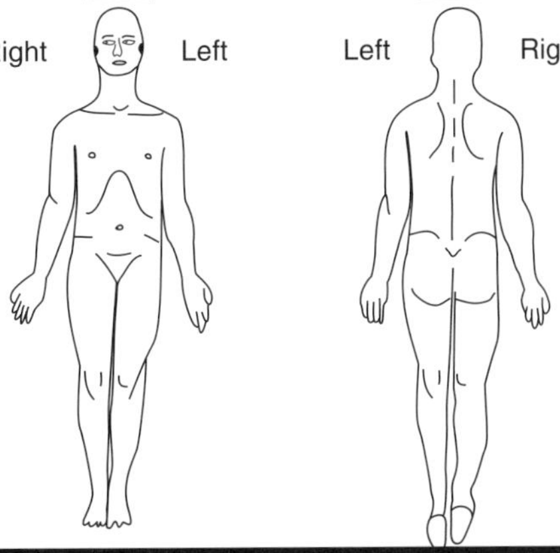

Front   Back

Right   Left   Left   Right

3. Please rate your pain by marking the box beside the number that best describes your pain at its worst **in the last 24 hours.**

☐ 0   ☐ 1   ☐ 2   ☐ 3   ☐ 4   ☐ 5   ☐ 6   ☐ 7   ☐ 8   ☐ 9   ☐ 10
No   Pain As Bad As
Pain   You Can Imagine

4. Please rate your pain by marking the box beside the number that best describes your pain at its least **in the last 24 hours.**

☐ 0   ☐ 1   ☐ 2   ☐ 3   ☐ 4   ☐ 5   ☐ 6   ☐ 7   ☐ 8   ☐ 9   ☐ 10
No   Pain As Bad As
Pain   You Can Imagine

5. Please rate your pain by marking the box beside the number that best describes your pain on the average.

☐ 0   ☐ 1   ☐ 2   ☐ 3   ☐ 4   ☐ 5   ☐ 6   ☐ 7   ☐ 8   ☐ 9   ☐ 10
No   Pain As Bad As
Pain   You Can Imagine

6. Please rate your pain by marking the box beside the number that tells how much pain you have right now.

☐ 0   ☐ 1   ☐ 2   ☐ 3   ☐ 4   ☐ 5   ☐ 6   ☐ 7   ☐ 8   ☐ 9   ☐ 10
No   Pain As Bad As
Pain   You Can Imagine

■ Page 1 of 2

Figure 2.8   Brief pain inventory.

Section 1

1903

PLEASE USE
BLACK INK PEN

Date: ☐☐ / ☐☐ / ☐☐
(month) (day) (year)

Subject's Initials : _____

Study Subject #: ☐☐☐

Study Name: _____
_____
Protocol #: _____
PI: _____
Revision: 07/01/05

7. What treatments or medications are you receiving for your pain?

[blank grid for text entry]

8. In the last 24 hours, how much relief have pain treatments or medications provided? Please mark the box below the percentage that most shows how much relief you have received.

0%	10%	20%	30%	40%	50%	60%	70%	80%	90%	100%
☐	☐	☐	☐	☐	☐	☐	☐	☐	☐	☐
No Relief										Complete Relief

9. Mark the box beside the number that describes how, during the past 24 hours, pain has interfered with your:

A. General Activity
☐0 Does Not Interfere ☐1 ☐2 ☐3 ☐4 ☐5 ☐6 ☐7 ☐8 ☐9 ☐10 Completely Interferes

B. Mood
☐0 Does Not Interfere ☐1 ☐2 ☐3 ☐4 ☐5 ☐6 ☐7 ☐8 ☐9 ☐10 Completely Interferes

C. Walking ability
☐0 Does Not Interfere ☐1 ☐2 ☐3 ☐4 ☐5 ☐6 ☐7 ☐8 ☐9 ☐10 Completely Interferes

D. Normal Work (includes both work outside the home and housework)
☐0 Does Not Interfere ☐1 ☐2 ☐3 ☐4 ☐5 ☐6 ☐7 ☐8 ☐9 ☐10 Completely Interferes

E. Relations with other people
☐0 Does Not Interfere ☐1 ☐2 ☐3 ☐4 ☐5 ☐6 ☐7 ☐8 ☐9 ☐10 Completely Interferes

F. Sleep
☐0 Does Not Interfere ☐1 ☐2 ☐3 ☐4 ☐5 ☐6 ☐7 ☐8 ☐9 ☐10 Completely Interferes

G. Enjoyment of life
☐0 Does Not Interfere ☐1 ☐2 ☐3 ☐4 ☐5 ☐6 ☐7 ☐8 ☐9 ☐10 Completely Interferes

Page 2 of 2

Figure 2.8 (*Continued*)

Karmarkar and Makin (2007) argue that an intensity tool is not useful for neuropathic pain. McCaffery and Pesaro (1999: 75) report on a tool developed specifically for neuropathic pain following a study of 288 patients by Galer Jensen in 1997. This explores eight common qualities of this pain as well as an overall unpleasantness scale, these are identified in Table 2.9.

However, White (2004) notes that a disadvantage of this specific neuropathic tool is that it fails to assess the impact the pain has on quality of life. This may be a valuable target for evaluation of treatment effects and so could be an important omission.

Diabetic neuropathy

Mann (2009) explores diabetic neuropathy and identifies that neuropathic pain is common but frequently underrecognised and misunderstood. Mann estimates that 10-20% of people with diabetes experience pain, with an incidence of 40-50% in those who develop diabetic neuropathy. Diabetic neuropathic pain appears in an area with altered sensitivity, strange or unpleasant sensations appear in an area that is usually numb (Mann 2009). Unfortunately, as the symptoms are difficult to describe, patients can fear they are imagined and think they will be disbelieved. The 2009 NICE Guidelines for Type Two Diabetes do advocate annual review with primary care so this should provide an opportunity to identify any neuropathic pain.

Assessment in the community

A pain diary may be advised for chronic pain of any type in order to promote effective communication about the pattern and impact of pain on an individual. A diary can also be useful for identifying if a pain is atypical which may indicate a change in condition. It may help to identify the relationship between pain and behaviours: for example, *what makes it better?* and *what makes it worse?*, or between pain and physiological conditions, for example menstrual cycle and pain may be linked. White (2004) also indicates that a diary used in the community rehabilitation setting can be valuable as daily assessment by healthcare professionals is not suitable in home setting. Moore (2007) has devised a pain toolkit which aims to provide support for self-management of pain, and he recommends keeping a diary to show positive evidence about self-management as a way of recognising how the coping strategies identified in the toolkit can lead to improvements. One disadvantage, however, is that a pain diary could lead an individual to focus too much attention on their pain and the negative impact it has on their lives. The purpose of the diary should, therefore, be clear, and it would not be useful for all individuals.

Summary

Effective assessment requires a multidimensional tool, for example CPPC, BPI and pain diary. Self-reporting may be less reliable and influenced by stoicism and reticence. Observations of facial expression and behaviour can enhance assessment. Specific tools exist for neuropathic pain and advanced dementia.

Use of the Abbey Pain Scale:

The pain scale is best used as part of an overall pain management plan. Some pain management strategies can be found in the web site below[i].

Objective
The pain scale is an instrument designed to assist in the assessment of pain in residents who are unable to clearly articulate their needs.

Ongoing assessment
The scale does not differentiate between distress and pain, therefore measuring the effectiveness of pain relieving interventions is essential.

Recent work by the Australian Pain Society[ii] recommends that the Abbey Pain Scale be used as a movement based assessment. The staff recording the scale should, therefore, observe the resident while they are being moved eg, during pressure area care, while showering etc.

Complete the scale immediately following the procedure and record the results in the resident's notes. Include the time of completion of the scale, the score, staff member's signature and action (if any) taken in response to results of the assessment, eg pain medication or other therapies.

A second evaluation should be conducted 1 hour after any intervention taken in response to the first assessment, to determine the effectiveness of any pain relieving intervention.

If, at this assessment, the score on the pain scale is the same, or worse, consider further intervention and act if appropriate. Complete the pain scale 4 hourly, meanwhile recording all the pain relieving interventions undertaken, until the resident appears comfortable. If pain/distress persists, undertake a comprehensive assessment of all facets of resident's care and monitor closely over a 24 hour period, including any further interventions undertaken. If there is no improvement during that time, notify the medical practitioner, of the pain scores and the action taken

---

[i] Australian Pain Society (2005) Residential Aged Care Pain Management Guidelines, August. **http://www.apsoc.org.au**
[ii] Gibson, S., Scherer, S and Goucke, R (2004) Final Report Australian Pain Society and the Australian Pain Relief Association Pain Management Guidelines for Residential Care: Stage 1. Preliminary field-testing and preparations for implementation. November
Further details re original validation can be found: Jennifer Abbey, Neil Piller, AnitaDe Bellis, Adrian Esterman, Deborah Parker, Lynne; Giles and Belinda Lowcay (2004) The Abbey pain scale: a 1-minute numerical indicator for people with end-stage dementia , *International Journal of Palliative Nursing*, Vol 10, No 1pp 6-13.

Jenny Abbey. April 2007.

Figure 2.9 Abbey pain scale. (Reproduced with kind permission of Jennifer Abbey on behalf of the Australian Pain Society.)

Interventions to manage chronic pain

The key issue for management of chronic pain is that the patient should be at the centre of any intervention, working in partnership with healthcare professions in order to improve their sense of control over pain. Shaw (2006) advocates a positive relationship with health professionals, stressing

Section 1

Abbey Pain Scale
For measurement of pain in people with dementia who cannot verbalise

How to use scale : While observing the resident, score questions 1 to 6.

Name of resident : ....

Name and designation of person completing the scale : ....

Date : .... **Time :** ....

Latest pain relief given was...**at**.........**hrs.**

Q1. **Vocalisation**
  eg whimpering, groaning, crying   Q1 ☐
  Absent 0   Mild 1   Moderate 2   Severe 3

Q2. **Facial expression**
  eg looking tense, frowning, grimacing, looking frightened   Q2 ☐
  Absent 0   Mild 1   Moderate 2   Severe 3

Q3. **Change in body language**
  eg fidgeting, rocking, guarding part of body, withdrawn   Q3 ☐
  Absent 0   Mild 1   Moderate 2   Severe 3

Q4. **Behavioural Change**
  eg increased confusion, refusing to eat, alteration in usual patterns Q4 ☐
  Absent 0   Mild 1   Moderate 2   Severe 3

Q5. **Physiological change**
  eg temperature, pulse or blood pressure outside normal limits,   Q5 ☐
  perspiring, flushing or pallor
  Absent 0   Mild 1   Moderate 2   Severe 3

Q6. **Physical changes**
  eg skin tears, pressure areas, arthritis, contractures,   Q6 ☐
  previous injuries
  Absent 0   Mild 1   Moderate 2   Severe 3

Add scores for 1 - 6 and record here ⟹ **Total Pain Score** ☐

Now tick the box that matches the
Total Pain Score ⟹

0 - 2	3 - 7	8 - 13	14 +
No pain	Mild	Moderate	Severe

Finally, tick the box which matches
the type of pain ⟹

Chronic	Acute	Acute on Chronic

Abbey, J., DeBellis, A., Piller, N., Esterman, A., Giles, L., Parker, D and Lowcay, B.
Funded by the JH&JD Gunn Medical Research Foundation 1998-2002
This document may be reproduced with this acknowledgement retained

Figure 2.9   *(Continued)*

Table 2.9   Descriptors and examples of neuropathic pain

Descriptors	Examples
Sharp	
Hot	
Dull	
Deep or superficial in intensity	Post-herpetic neuralgia is more likely to be described as sharp,
Cold	less cold and more itchy than other neuropathic pain
Sensitive	
Itchy	
Intense	
How unpleasant	Diabetic neuropathy is associated with sharp shooting pain

the need for equal power. Holistic assessment should consider the biopsychosocial aspects of an individual's pain and identify patient's priorities. Interventions are likely to involve both pharmacological and non-pharmacological strategies. Though chronic pain sufferers cannot be seen as a uniform group with a set approach applied to all, most individuals may use a range of approaches and will most commonly be managing this at home. There are also individuals who are dependent on healthcare workers and carers, for example for clients with advanced dementia and pain, in residential nursing homes. Also, a minority may require specialist support from pain management services due to the complexity and impact that their pain has caused. The Pain in Europe report (Fricker 2003: 17) identified it as worrying that only 23% of the chronic pain patients surveyed had been referred to pain management specialists in order to explore possible interventions. In addition, the CPPC (2006: 14) indicate that improvements are required in the education of all medical school and professional training courses in order to prepare staff to support patients with chronic pain more effectively.

Biological factors and medical history will influence the treatment options, pharmacological approaches and interventions as suited to the pain type. The psychological impact and emotional responses, including the patient's beliefs and attitudes, will also be an important factor when considering appropriate interventions. As identified in the Pain Toolkit (Moore 2007), the first tool advocated for self-help is to accept the fact that the chronic pain is present. Indeed, in the toolkit, Moore (2007: 4) suggests that:

> many people go therapy or doctor shopping whilst looking for a cure for their pain and you may be wasting your time and money.

Pharmacological approaches

The appropriate use of analgesics clearly has an important role to play in the management of chronic pain. One of the major considerations when using drugs is the evidence for benefit versus risks from harmful side effects. The implication for chronic pain is that these drugs may be required over an extended period of time; therefore, the risk of adverse effects can be greater. In addition, in the older patient co-morbidities and drug interactions become an important consideration. The use of over-the-counter (OTC) medicines for self-medication in chronic pain must also be considered. Figure 2.10 illustrates the role of the nurse in the pharmacological management of chronic pain.

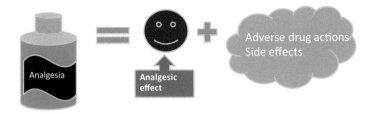

Nurses can support patients to evaluate the analgesic effects and the side effects; note all analgesics can cause side effects and acceptability of these on normal activities will impact on concordance with treatment.

For effective pain control, the correct dose of analgesic should be **taken by the clock**. Use multidimensional pain assessment to evaluate effectiveness.

As chronic pain requires long-term treatment, monitoring for side effects may be desirable. Note that OTC medications and herbal remedies may produce serious side effects, so seek advice from pharmacist.

Figure 2.10   The nurse's role in chronic pain pharmacological management.

Barber and Gibson (2009) review treatment of chronic pain in the elderly and reveal that studies consistently identify undertreatment of pain in older people, particularly those who have frailty and dementia. While the intention may be to reduce adverse effects, Barber and Gibson identify that appropriate use of simple analgesics and adjuvants can provide adequate relief without the need to escalate to risks associated with stronger opioid analgesics. Barber and Gibson (2009) explain that adverse drug reactions (ADRs) or side effects should not be considered a single entity: some are common but easily managed, for example constipation due to codeine. Other ADRs are predictable but more hazardous as they are not as easy to resolve, for example non-steroidal anti-inflammatory drugs (NSAIDs) causing gastric ulceration or renal impairment. Barber and Gibson (2009) identify that NSAIDs were reported by some studies as the leading cause of ADRs. Rarely, there are also unpredictable ADRs; for example, anaphylaxis induced by NSAIDs.

The usual self-management of acute pain, for example a headache, is to use analgesics if the pain reaches an intensity that interferes with normal activity; therefore, we take tablets to reduce the pain. However, this is not an effective approach for chronic pain management as it results in regular breakthrough pain. Effective pain management can be achieved by taking the analgesic *by the clock* to maintain effective therapeutic levels in the plasma and continuous pain control. For chronic pain management it is clearly desirable to use drugs which can maintain therapeutic levels without having to remember to take them every 4 hours, so a longer-acting drug is more practical.

Analgesics can be divided into three major categories: simple analgesics, (NSAIDs and paracetamol), opioid agents (codeine, morphine), and adjuvants (Amytriptylline, Gabapentin) which have properties to assist pain relief but are not true analgesics (McCaffery and Pasero 1999). It is helpful to consider how these drugs have an effect on the pain pathway as this helps to recognise that the type of pain will influence appropriate choice of analgesic (see Figure 2.11). For example, NSAIDs generally cause a reduction in inflammatory chemicals, particularly prostaglandins, which are associated with tissue damage; hence, NSAIDs are appropriate for inflammatory pain. If a patient is suffering from

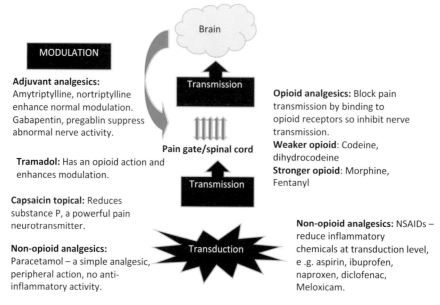

Figure 2.11   The pain gate and effect of analgesics.

post-herpetic neuralgia the pain is not inflammatory in origin and drugs which moderate the abnormal nerve firing associated with this neuropathic pain are more appropriate, for example anticonvulsants or tricyclic antidepressants (Baron 2004).

When considering appropriate analgesics the WHO analgesic ladder (WHO 2005) is also often used to guide analgesic strength ranging from mild, moderate to severe. Figure 2.12 illustrates how this applies to the management of back pain.

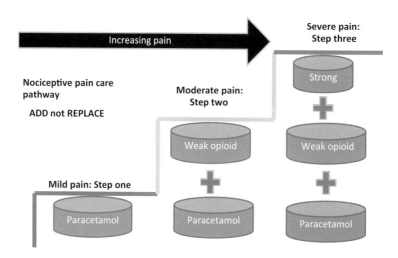

Figure 2.12   The WHO (2005) analgesic ladder applied for use with back pain drug therapy. (Adapted from Moore 2009:27.)

Mild to moderate pain: simple analgesics
Non-steroidal anti-inflammatory drugs

Mild to moderate pain will respond to simple analgesics (paracetamol, aspirin and NSAIDs), and these represent level one of the analgesic ladder. These are widely used; many NSAIDs are available without prescription. Though these drugs may be effective for the management of some chronic pain, Mann and Carr (2009: 120) state simple analgesics no longer work for many people. In addition, the risk of adverse effects increases for chronic pain sufferers. The Pain in Europe report (Breivik et al. 2006) identified NSAIDs as the most popular OTC non-prescription medications, with 55% of respondents across European countries currently taking NSAIDs, followed by paracetamol at 42%.

Gastric irritation is recognised as a common adverse effect of NSAIDs due to the prostaglandin suppression which can lead to serious gastric ulceration. There are risks of impaired renal function (nephrotoxicity) with continuing use of NSAIDs, so they are contraindicated in individuals with renal insufficiency (Field and Swarm 2008: 49, D'Arcy 2006). In the author's view, this risk is significant as many patients will self-medicate over many months or years with these drugs and the effects on renal function are not monitored. This is of particular concern in the ageing population as renal function declines naturally with ageing, so older patients are more vulnerable to these toxic effects. NSAIDs are not recommended for patients with cardiac failure, and adverse drug interactions are associated with antihypertensives, ACE inhibitors, diuretics, anticoagulants, oral hypoglycaemic agents and others (Barber and Gibson 2009). Therefore, they will not be suited to many older patients with co-morbidities. However, of importance for the elderly with co-morbidities, the use of *topical NSAIDs* has been advocated as appropriate and effective without the gastrointestinal side effects or general concerns associated with polypharmacy (Mann and Carr 2009: 88). See Figure 2.13 for a summary of NSAID side effects.

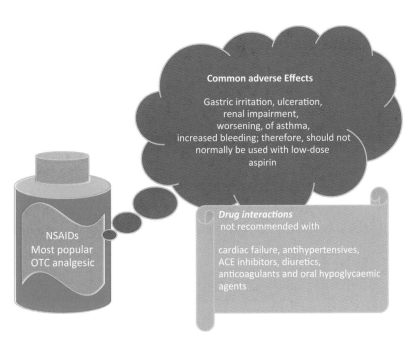

Common adverse Effects

Gastric irritation, ulceration, renal impairment, worsening, of asthma, increased bleeding; therefore, should not normally be used with low-dose aspirin

Drug interactions
not recommended with

cardiac failure, antihypertensives, ACE inhibitors, diuretics, anticoagulants and oral hypoglycaemic agents

NSAIDs Most popular OTC analgesic

Figure 2.13   Interactions and side effects of NSAIDs.

Topical analgesics

There are several preparations produced containing menthol or camphor. These are categorised as rubefacients and act by counter-irritation, causing irritation and reddening of the skin due to increased blood flow. This activates the fast non-pain sensory pathways and reduces awareness of pain, and these OTC remedies may be used to manage pain. Matthews et al. (2009) reviewed their use for chronic pain such as that from osteoarthritis, and evidence from seven studies suggested that there was a useful level of pain relief in 'one in six' individuals with rubefacients. However, this compared poorly with topical NSAIDs where substantial amounts of good quality evidence indicate that 'one in three' individuals experienced useful levels of pain relief over and above those that also responded to placebo. Some topical preparations contain a combination of rubefacients and NSAIDs. Topical application of NSAIDs appears to reduce the side-effects' risks associated with oral NSAIDs and is, therefore, useful for management of localised joint pains such as osteoarthritis of knees. Capsaicin is another topical agent, and though not a rubefacient it is a preparation which uses an extract of hot chilli peppers. It is thought to work by peripheral depletion of substance P, an important neurotransmitter for C nociceptive pain neurons (Hawksley 2006: 816). Capsaicin does cause a local intense burning sensation initially which may be an unacceptable side effect. As stated in the Chief Medical Officer's (DH 2008) report about pain, treatments such as topical preparations of capsaicin can increase flexibility and independence for chronic pain patients, and these methods may, therefore, improve effectiveness and reduce side effects.

Paracetamol

Paracetamol is simple and effective, has minimal side effects, and it is advocated as the first line of treatment for mild to moderate musculoskeletal pain in the elderly and as the primary long-term management for chronic osteoarthritic pain (Barber and Gibson 2009). However, if used in excess of the stated dose or by an individual with chronic alcohol use or liver disease, fatal hepatotoxicity can result (Field and Swarm 2008: 49). Therefore, the nurse should recognise the importance of assessing maladaptive behaviour such as excessive alcohol use as it can influence analgesic suitability. The major risk of toxicity is as a result from inadvertent overdose due to the many compound non-prescription medications available to the general public; for example, cold and flu medications.

Concordance

Banbury et al. (2008) examined experiences of analgesic use in patients with low back pain who were referred to the 'back team'. It was identified by the team that frequently patients were not taking analgesics as directed and there were common concerns shared by patients that lead to suboptimal use. The study, though small ($n = 16$), explored by semi-structured interview the views of patients about their analgesic use. It identified that patients were generally confused about the value of complying with their analgesic regimen, and insufficient explanation was provided when drugs were started. Only one patient in the study took their analgesics by the clock – they were told to do so by the pharmacist. Side effects were a major issue for patients, including fears of long-term organ damage and risks of addiction. The study identified the importance of concordance in drug administration as a partnership between doctor and patient; this, of course, relies upon effective communication. This study has important implications for the nurse's role in drug administration, and patients with chronic pain in particular should be educated appropriately so that they can optimise the chance of any prescribed regimen achieving the benefits desired and limit the chances of adverse effects. Currently, a patient information leaflet for OTC analgesics has been produced jointly by the British Pain Society and the Proprietary Association of Great Britain (PAGB). The aim of the leaflet is to tell patients how to use OTC medication most effectively. The leaflet, described by Knaggs (2010), identifies the sort of pain that may be managed with OTC analgesics, how they work and common side effects. It also promotes safety, recognising issues around physical dependence and addiction problems which can be caused by misuse of codeine (an opioid), frequently taken in combination with a simple analgesic, for example ibuprofen or paracetamol.

Moderate to severe pain

Opioids

Many patients with chronic pain require the regular use of opioids to achieve effective pain management. The Pain in Europe report (Fricker 2003) identified that 50% of UK patients with chronic pain were prescribed weak opioids (codeine, dihydrocodeine, Tramadol) and 12% required strong opioids (morphine-modified release continuous or Fentanyl patch). There is naturally general concern, both from healthcare professionals and patients, in relation to adverse effects and risks of addiction when these drugs are required over several weeks. However, as these drugs have now been used successfully without leading to escalating addiction problems for management of long-term cancer pain, it is now recognised that they can be a useful resource for some patients with severe chronic pain. Ferrell et al. (1992) argue that healthcare professionals are not educated appropriately in relation to the concepts of addiction versus tolerance and dependence, leading to an exaggerated fear of addiction which can hamper effective pain management. The British Pain Society (2010) has produced guidelines for professionals: 'Opioids for Persistent Pain: Good Practice' and 'Opioids for Persistent Pain: Information for Patients'. These guidelines should ensure that chronic pain patients who require these stronger analgesics receive appropriate information and prescriptions to achieve good pain management. NHS Quality Improvement Scotland (2006: 7) advocates that patients receiving opioids should be closely monitored, and the use and potential side effects should have been discussed and agreed between the person and health professional. Addiction risk from long-term opioids is rare; however, careful patient selection is advocated to ensure safety. Indeed, it appears that appropriate patient selection and education is essential to enable effective use of all analgesics, not just opioids.

Barber and Gibson (2009) identify that there are differences in an individual's capacity to metabolise codeine: between 7-10% of Caucasians and 1-2% of Asians cannot metabolise it, so gain no analgesic effect from its use. Therefore, an evaluation of effects is important, and if no improvement is obtained from use of the codeine-based analgesic combinations then other drugs should be considered instead.

One point of importance is that if an individual travels aboard with codeine phosphate or other combined opioids, for example co-codamol or strong opioids, they may require a doctor's letter to explain their use and protect them from criminal prosecution in countries where greater restrictions apply.

The side effects and risks associated with opioids are well known in relation to their use in acute pain management: nausea and vomiting, sedation and constipation. Of importance in chronic pain management, patients generally appear to develop tolerance to the effects of nausea and vomiting and sedation. This means that though patients may need anti-emetic medication initially, after one to two weeks this is generally no longer required. Sedation is dose-dependent but also influenced by patient factors, for example fatigue, so initially the effect of stepping up the analgesic ladder to stronger opioids may cause sedation, as the patient is catching up on sleep deprivation due to poor pain management before. This sedative effect should then reduce. A major practical concern for patients with chronic pain is the need to get on with normal activities of living, which for many individuals involves driving. For safety, when strong opioids are started patients may be advised not to drive until the effects can be reviewed. However, after this initial period the BPS Opioid for Persistent Pain: Information for Patients (2010: 8) identifies that the law in the United Kingdom allows driving whilst on opioid medication. The individual is responsible for making sure they are fit to drive, and the DVLA should be informed.

Constipation due to slowed peristalsis is not a side effect that settles with time. It is, therefore, an essential part of pain management that advice to avoid constipation is proactively provided, otherwise this can limit effective pain management as patients may choose to discontinue the analgesic. Use of both stimulant and softener aperients is usually required. There is some evidence that transdermal Fentanyl is less constipating than Morphine Sulphate (MST continuous). One study found that in an older group it was seven times less likely to cause constipation than controlled-release oxycodone, and, therefore, may have particular benefits for the elderly with chronic pain (Ackerman et al. 2004). From a practical perspective, if pain is stable it may be more convenient to use an opioid by patch, for example Fentanyl, and change this every 3 days rather than remember to take tablets twice every day.

However, it is essential, according to Barber and Gibson (2009) that slow-release opioids are not prescribed for 'opioid-naive' elderly patients before first using immediate release upload preparations to estimate the appropriate dose required and monitor sensitivity effects. For example, Tramadol is a weak synthetic opioid which also effects pain inhibition by serotonin and noradrenergic activity. The NHS Quality Improvement in Scotland (2006) identifies this as a suitable drug for neuropathic pain. However, Barber and Gibson (2009) identify that it has limited analgesic effect, and so can encourage the use of higher doses which increases the likelihood of adverse effects. On balance, there is little advantage over codeine. Overall, the elderly are likely to be more sensitive to its opioid effect, therefore, extra care is recommended through accurate pain diagnosis, evaluation, prescribing, administering and monitoring (Barber and Gibson 2009). Clearly, the nurse is in a key position to be able to support patients by monitoring and educating patients to maximise effectiveness of all analgesics; in the elderly it is recommended to follow the principle of 'start slow and go slow', with analgesic adjustments made according to an individual's responses. Barber and Gibson (2009: 469) state that:

> one consequence of this challenge is that many older people are in fact under treated and the goal of reduced pain and optimal functionality is denied.

This may also be a concern as elderly residential nursing home residents are particularly vulnerable as most direct care will be provided by unqualified staff.

When living with chronic pain an important factor is how to manage a pain flare up. Practical review and adjustment of medication may be useful. The NHS Quality Improvement for Scotland (2006: 17) identifies the importance of a patient-led action plan and effective coping mechanisms to manage alterations in pain intensity which could lead to negative thoughts and limitations on activity.

Neuropathic pain and adjuvant analgesics

Greener (2009) notes that fewer than half of people suffering from neuropathic pain respond adequately to current analgesics but several adjuvant drugs can be used to alleviate it, which act in a variety of ways. Karmarkar and Makin (2007) explain a neuropathic pain ladder based on efficacy from clinical trials and side effects. These authors identify anticonvulsants as the most useful drug in neuropathic pain, for a variety of conditions. The newer anticonvulsant drugs Gabapentin and Pregabalin are considered to have a better side-effect profile than the older drugs in this group. Wiffen et al. (2005) reviewed 14 reports on use of Gabapentin for chronic pain and identified that there is evidence that it is effective for neuropathic pain: approximately two thirds of patients who take them can expect to achieve good pain relief. The tricyclic antidepressants, for example Amytriptyline and Nortriptyline are also advocated as very important, coming second to the anticonvulsants for chronic pain; they are recognised as important for improving sleep and mood in addition to the modulating analgesic effect. Barber and Gibson (2009) identify that Nortriptyline is preferred over Amytriptyline for the elderly, and though it can achieve moderate pain relief for 'one in three' people, 'one in five' will discontinue due to side effects. Karmarkar and Makin (2007: 36) describe these drugs as relatively contraindicated in patients with cardiovascular disease and elderly patients. Neuropathic pain may also be treated with strong opioids. NICE (2010) have recently produced guidelines for the pharmacological management of neuropathic pain in adults in non-specialist settings; this supports the view that good communication with patients is essential.

From a patient support perspective, the adjuvant drugs such as anticonvulsants and antidepressants are not like conventional analgesics. When these drugs are used in a trial the aim is to achieve some degree of pain relief with minimal side effects, yet it may be that benefits cannot be evaluated until a graduated increase in dose over a period of 2 weeks has been tried! Therefore, the patient has to recognise that an immediate effect is not expected and concordance with treatment is more likely to occur if this is clearly explained. As identified in the CMO Report (DH 2008) on chronic pain, where patients understand the purpose behind different medicines it is more likely that they will take them appropriately and that they will benefit. See Case studies 2.3 and 2.4.

Case study 2.3 Mrs Smith

Rheumatoid arthritis – nociceptive pain

Pharmacological management

DMARDs and biological therapies including steroid therapy reduce the inflammation caused by the autoimmune disorder so these reduce pain. These are powerful drugs with many toxic side effects so close monitoring is required throughout treatment.

Originally when it started 14 years ago Diclofenac (NSAID) was the first analgesic as the DMARDs do not have an instant effect. Presently taking Naproxen TDS (NSAID) with Omeprazole to prevent gastric ulceration and steroids, the dose of which is adjusted with advice from the rheumatology specialist team according to the response of the condition.

Case study 2.4 Mrs Jones

Postherpetic neuralgia

Pharmacological management

Pain started as acute associated with the herpes-zoster rash; however, the pain continued after the rash had gone and allodynia was noted. Pain was spontaneous, a burning sensation and did not respond to usual simple analgesics leading to sleep deprivation and low mood. Though prompt treatment with antiviral drug Acyclovir was given, the pain persisted as PHN. Amytriptylline low dose 10–25 mg has been effective at reducing the pain and improving sleep.

Mrs Jones has also tried topical Capsaicin and though it produced an unpleasant burning feeling initially, this has lessened and she uses it most days.

(Hawksley 2006)

Points for reflection

- Identify the side effects associated with each drug used in the case studies above. Is identification of side effects of analgesics done effectively in clinical practice?
- If not, how might identification be improved?

Summary

The evaluation of benefits (analgesic effect) versus risk of adverse effects is a key issue. Patient education to maximise analgesic action such as taking correct dose by the clock is essential. Education to prevent constipation with opioids or NSAIDs by topical administration may be suitable and reduce adverse effects. Neuropathic pain requires adjuvant agents and trials to find the most effective and acceptable.

Non-pharmacological interventions for chronic pain

There are various interventions which may be recommended by healthcare professionals, and they generally focus on the recognised persistent pain cycle and promote approaches which help individuals to reduce the negative impact and control that pain has over their lifestyle. A range of possible interventions are now considered which may have a positive impact on the pain gate and be part of positive coping strategies. Particularly with neuropathic pain, where analgesics provide adequate responses in fewer than half of patients (Greener 2009), a combination of non-pharmacological approaches may be particularly valuable for managing chronic pain. Mann (2009) identifies that if nurses work with patients who have diabetic neuropathic pain using a combination of therapies, realistic achievable goals can be achieved.

Relaxation and sleeplessness
Relaxation is defined by McCaffery and Beebe (1994: 168) as:

> a state of relative freedom from both anxiety and skeletal muscle tension, a quieting or calming of the mind and muscles.

Anxiety and muscle tension are recognised as factors which can increase pain, therefore, interventions are suggested which break this pattern. Various methods, such as music and guided imagery may help the individual achieve reduced muscle tension and anxiety. Exercises may focus on breathing and encouraging a greater awareness of tension and its impact on pain perception. In the Patient Information Pain Toolkit (Moore 2007), relaxation is identified as an important skill to learn; the link between distraction and relaxation is also identified. Relaxing, reading a book, listening to music, gardening and/or meditation are all suggested as ways to relax. Persson et al. (2008) undertook a systematic review of randomised controlled studies into relaxation for chronic pain. In the 12 studies that met the inclusion criteria, various methods of relaxation were utilised, including progressive muscle relaxation, guided imagery and biofeedback. Though Persson et al. (2008) criticised the studies as medium quality, positive effects were identified such as reduced pain intensity, depression, anxiety and fatigue with reduced sleeplessness.

Snoezelen

A novel approach to promoting relaxation is Snoezelen. This is a sensory environment which supports relaxation, and is commonly used as an intervention for clients with learning difficulties and dementia. Schofield (2002) conducted a study to evaluate the impact of Snoezelen as an alternative environment for relaxation in a group of patients with chronic pain. A convenience sample of 73 patients from the pain clinic were recruited; patients were randomly assigned to relaxation taught in the pain clinic versus Snoezelen. A range of outcome measures were utilised to evaluate the effects including pain intensity, a self-efficacy questionnaire, a coping strategies questionnaire, anxiety and depression scale, and quality of life measure. Both groups received two sessions of therapy each lasting 3 hours, one in a Snoezelen environment, and the other within a traditional hospital setting. The experimental Snoezelen group demonstrated significant reduction in disability associated with recreation and over time an improved self-efficacy score. This was interesting as it had not been demonstrated in earlier studies of the benefits of relaxation. The effect was believed to be due to relaxation, distraction and leisure. When considering benefits versus risks, a consideration for any intervention, the comment of one patient from the study stands out in the authors view: 'it's the first thing that has helped without hurting'. However, Snoezelen is not an inexpensive resource and clearly many patients with chronic pain also suffer from financial constraints; all the participants in this study were non-workers. The concept, however, of developing relaxation skills in an appropriate environment, may well be suitable for many chronic pain sufferers.

Mind-body interventions

A review by Morone and Greco (2007) into mind-body interventions for chronic pain in older adults identified 20 studies involving older adults with chronic pain, with eight interventions used. These included biofeedback, progressive muscle relaxation plus guided imagery, hypnosis, tai chi, qi gong and yoga. The lack of controlled trials and small numbers recruited appeared to be weaknesses in the studies reviewed; however, they showed that such therapies were suited to this age group with a gentle approach and emphasis on self exploration. Among the studies there were no reports of adverse effects or safety issues. Morone and Greco (2007) recommend further studies in this area as there was some support for the efficacy of relaxation and guided imagery for osteoarthritic pain, and limited support for meditation and tai chi for improving function and coping in older adults with low back pain or osteoarthritis.

Heat and cold peripheral stimulation

Peripheral stimulation using heat or cold has been used through history to manage pain. It stimulates nerve transmission through fast non-pain (A-beta) neurons and can reduce pain perception due to its influence on the pain gate. The use of heat or cold may be advocated as part of coping strategies but it must be used appropriately without causing tissue damage, so suitable sources and skin protection is important to prevent burns. This is particularly important where sensitivity may be impaired due to diabetic neuropathy or stroke. Generally, heat is not advocated for acute inflammatory pain as this could aggravate the inflammation. However, for chronic low back pain heat may relieve pain. Berger (2003: 198) suggests a heated pad, microwavable seed bag or hot pack. She advises application for at least 20 minutes and states that heat is often preferred as it is more comfortable than cold. She suggests applying both of these sequentially if appropriate, and using them on a trial and error basis to see which is most helpful for the particular problem. Massage is also advocated as it uses the same theoretical basis with stimulation of peripheral non-pain neurons to reduce pain awareness at the pain gate. However, Berger (2003) identifies that it can be useful for muscle spasm pain but if it irritates, then clearly it would not be recommended.

Transcutaneous electrical nerve stimulation (TENS)

This involves passing a tiny electrical current through the skin. The current causes stimulation of the large touch fibres (A-beta). This input is known to block transmission form the smaller pain fibres (A-delta and C fibres). In addition, high frequency TENS stimulates the release of pain modulating chemicals known as the natural endorphins. Low frequency TENS stimulates the release of endorphins in various areas of the nervous system (Berger 2003: 113). Berger (2003) explains though TENS will not suit everyone, a high proportion of people can benefit from this therapy. She estimates that 20% of patients may have no pain relieving response to TENS; however, many find a beneficial effect. The correct use of TENS may be the best treatment modality that the person has ever tried. Another positive factor is that side effects are rare (though not recommended for people with pacemakers), which cannot be said for those who require long-term use of analgesics. In addition, TENS is less expensive than acupuncture and encourages patient administration and control (Wells 2009); these are important considerations for patient empowerment. Berger (2003) stresses the importance of patient control from placement of electrodes, to the set up chosen by intensity, pulse width, mode of current and duration that TENS is used for. She advocates patients should have a trial of TENS with guidance. Recent studies indicate that using higher frequencies for longer periods may provide greater effectiveness (Berger 2003: 112). Berger (2003) states that TENS should ideally be used for 8 hours a day for 3 consecutive days to detect the complete TENS responder, and used for a minimum of 40 minutes to produce effective changes in the pain. It is not recommended for use when sleeping.

Activity and exercise

Maintaining activity levels are widely advocated as beneficial in chronic pain management (Moore 2007; Wells 2009; NICE 2009). Unfortunately, one of the consequences of chronic pain is the inactivity and deconditioning that result from fear of movement which aggravates pain, which causes the person to limit their mobility. Physiologically, endorphin release through exercise aids pain modulation and has anti-depressive actions (Berger 2003, Horn and Mufano 1997). The benefits of group exercise as distraction and socialisation are also advocated as beneficial for pain management. Berger (2003) explores way of initiating exercise and reducing inactivity by exercising in warm water – either in a bath or heated pool; for example, hydrotherapy for rheumatoid arthritis. Walking and swimming are recommended as the easiest exercises to participate in. The support of a physiotherapist for guidance can reduce fears of damage to an already painful area. Berger (2003) describes the difficulties for patients who have been inactive in recognising the difference between good pain as the muscles are activated, and bad pain that is not associated with muscle movement and does not go away, suggesting a need to avoid that movement. Moore's (2007) Pain toolkit recommends talking with a physiotherapist or fitness coach about an individualised simple stretching and exercise programme

Table 2.10 Interventions for back pain compared through the UK BEAM Trial

	Intervention	Outcome
Usual best care	In general practice where practice teams were trained in active management and provide back book for patients	
Exercise programme	Best care plus exercise; involved assessment and up to 9 classes in community settings over 12 weeks	Small benefit at 3 months not at 1 year
Spinal manipulation package	Best care plus manipulation; package developed by MDT group (chiropractic, osteopathic and physiotherapy professionals) during 8 sessions over 12 weeks	Small to moderate benefit at 3 months and 1 year
Combined treatment	Best care plus manipulation and exercise; participants received 6 weeks of manipulation followed by 6 weeks of exercise	Moderate benefit at 3 months and small benefit at 1 year

Source: Manca 2006.

that can be done steadily and safely. Berger (2003) identifies the aim is to reduce fear of exercise and build confidence so that a sense of control is restored.

The NICE (2009) guidelines for early management of non-specific low back pain (focused on symptoms of 6 weeks to 12 months) advocates that patients should continue to be physically active, pursuing normal activities. Analgesics should be offered to allow patients to keep active. At this stage, one of the three treatments may be offered: participation in a group exercise programme, manual therapy (spinal manipulation, spinal mobilisation and massage performed by chiropractors osteopaths or appropriately trained doctors or physiotherapist) or acupuncture. These treatments are recommended at an early stage as they can help reduce the development of maladaptive behaviour leading to disability which is recognised as a major problem in chronic pain patients.

The UK BEAM trial (Manca 2004) was undertaken in order to compare cost and effectiveness for back pain treated by manipulation and pain exercises. This large comprehensive study compared four interventions as summarised in Table 2.10. Questionnaires were completed at baseline, 3 months and 12 months, and in addition, healthcare use was recorded.

This appears to demonstrate that both manipulation alone and manipulation followed by exercise provide cost-effective additions to care for general practice. The study showed significant improvements in function, pain, disability, physical and mental aspects of quality of life, and beliefs about back pain. The paper concludes that though manipulation appears to be desirable and effective, there is at present scarcity of trained manipulators available to meet the potential demand, so it may be some time before implementation is possible.

Combined physical and psychological programmes

Coping with persistent pain usually involves cognitive and behavioural strategies to manage and reduce the pain and its related distress and disability (Keefe et al. 2009). There appears to be general support for the application of cognitive-behavioural strategies, particularly pain-coping skills training. Cognitive-behavioural therapy involves education about chronic pain, and negative cognitions are addressed. Misconceptions, maladaptive behaviour and expectations are considered, and patients are helped to develop coping skills (Field and Swarm 2008). Mead et al. (2007) describe a pilot study of a 4-week Pain Coping Strategies (PCS) programme for chronic pain patients. This study utilised early intervention to prevent long-term negative behaviours associated with chronic pain and promote positive coping. It included all the fundamental aspects of the more traditional pain management programmes (PMP) (including exercise, relaxation, pacing, medication review, pain pathways, posture and challenging negative thoughts). This early intervention appeared to be effective at promoting self-management and teaching positive coping strategies. In another study, Ahles et al. (2006) describe using telephone-based assistance from a nurse educator for patients with pain and psychosocial problems, compared to their usual care. The group who received problem-solving strategies and basic pain management skills showed significant sustained benefit in pain and psychological problems. Keefe et al. (2009) also advocates these strategies for patients and their partners as their lives are also significantly altered by the patients' pain. Maladaptive behaviours which can aggravate pain, such as smoking or overeating and subsequent obesity, can lead to potential negative long-term pain-related consequences. Clearly, the nurse in such situations can support individuals to consider the impact on health and support them with more positive coping strategies.

NICE (2009) also acknowledges that some patients who show high levels of psychological distress and disability may require referral for combined physical and psychological (CPP) treatment programmes. These programmes should involve a cognitive-behavioural approach and physical exercises, and are high-intensity programmes. Wells (2009) criticises NICE (2009) for recommending what is considered to be a lower quality, cheaper option, rather than the previously advocated PMPs (BPS, 2006) available from some pain management teams. Wells (2009) argues that CPP treatment programmes appear to be physiotherapy-based rehabilitation programmes with a bit of psychology thrown in. A PMP which meets the criteria of the BPS (2006) would involve a multidisciplinary team approach with resources that include clinical psychologist or registered cognitive-behavioural therapist as part of the key staff; here, the patient becomes an active agent of change.

Pacing

Pacing involves learning to maintain a balance between activity and rest to optimise overall capabilities. Unfortunately, many people will fall into a cycle of overactivity when they feel stronger and try and achieve everything in one day; this is followed inevitably by underactivity caused by exhaustion, which is not good for self-esteem. By pacing activities the individual can gain a sense of control and normality, which may involve setting daily goals (Moore 2007). An occupational therapist may be involved in supporting patients to develop more achievable patterns of activity.

Empowerment

Supporting people to make their own decisions about their condition is important in all chronic conditions and is therefore appropriate for chronic pain. The CPPC identifies it as the 2nd statement in its five-point manifesto, and asks patients, professionals and parliamentarians to pledge their support. For the professionals it requires that nurses can provide accurate and accessible information and advice about managing chronic pain. Parliamentarians are required to consider services for people with chronic pain. The services may be a specific pain management programme, which is rather scarce at present, or a self-management programme. The Expert Patient Programme development in recent years is recommended by the CPPC. Becoming a member of a patient support group can

Table 2.11 House of Lords Select Committee on Science and Technology Committee, Classification of Complementary Therapies (2000)

Group 1	Those principle disciplines already regulated professionally by Acts of Parliament – 'the big five': Osteopathy, chiropractic, acupuncture, herbal medicine and homeopathy.
Group 2	Therapies that complement conventional medicine and do not embrace diagnostic skills: Aromatherapy, Alexander technique, body work therapies – including massage, counselling, stress therapy, hypnotherapy, reflexology and probably Shiatsu, meditation and healing.
Group 3	Embrace other disciplines which purport to offer diagnostic information as well as treatment. These favour philosophical approach through which various disparate frameworks of disease causation and its management are proposed. They are indifferent to scientific principles of conventional medicine. **3a** Ayurvedic medicine, traditional Chinese medicine **3b** Others which lack a credible evidence base, for example crystal therapy, iridology, radionics, dowsing and kinesiology.

be a valuable way of developing coping skills to reduce the negative impact of chronic pain – the Pain Toolkit by Moore (2007) is an example of this. The British Pain Society has compiled a list of useful organisations in the United Kingdom who can offer help; for example, Arthritis Care, Action MS and Back Care (see 'Further reading'). Nurses can act as a resource and identify appropriate support groups. Programmes are not meant to replace healthcare professionals; rather groups such as Pain Concern and Action on Pain can play a vital role in support according to the Chief Medical Officer Report (DH 2008). NHS Quality Improvement Scotland (2006) states that there should be evidence of an up-to-date directory of self-management/support groups available in each area. A revised publication for patients entitled 'Understanding and Managing Pain' has been produced by the patient liaison committee of the British Pain Society for 2010. This looks at what pain is, what can be done about it, and who can help.

Complementary therapies and pain

This general categorisation of Complementary and Alternative Medicine (CAM) is used to define approaches to diagnosis, treatment and care that are outside conventional medical treatments. The existence of chronic pain leads many individuals to explore non-conventional approaches as they seek a cure or support for managing this challenge. The Pain in Europe report (Fricker 2003) found that two-thirds of sufferers used at least one non-drug treatment for their pain, with the most popular being massage, physical therapy and acupuncture. Some of the therapies can have a positive impact on the effect of pain for individuals. For example, mind-body connections such as hypnosis, relaxation and biofeedback, and meditation can influence the pain gate and, therefore, pain perception. These therapies can, therefore, increase a sense of control and reduce anxiety. The House of Lords Science and Technology Committee (2006) have classified complementary therapies into three separate groups (see Table 2.11).

Some of these examples are practiced by registered professionally-regulated groups with recognised training (manipulation via chiropractics, osteopaths) whereas others (meditation and massage) can form part of an educational approach with information and instruction for pain sufferers. Both acupuncture and manipulation have become accepted within the framework of western medicine;

evidence supports their use in the clinical pathways for early management of persistent non-specific low back pain (NICE 2009). Clearly, therapies must only be provided by appropriately qualified and regulated practitioners. A frequent criticism of CAM is the lack of high-quality research available to support their efficacy. Studies are frequently small with poor methodology and lack randomised control comparison groups. Benefit from evidence of proven efficacy versus risk is an important consideration in relation to CAM. Therefore, at present there may be some NHS provision of 'proven' approaches such as manipulation or acupuncture, but not in less well-supported areas, for example reflexology or aromatherapy. Detail of all CAM associated with pain is beyond the remit of this book; however, nurses should only provide therapies for which they have appropriate training, in line with the NMC Code of Conduct (2008). Some nurses have undertaken courses to become registered complementary practitioners. However, these skills are only appropriate if the job description and employer agree, as in the case for pain nurse specialists who provide acupuncture or aromatherapy. Nurses should ensure that their patients are aware of advantages, disadvantages and side effects of particular therapies. However, if a therapy is safe but lacks evidence of efficacy from trials, yet provides the patient with high satisfaction levels then as a partner in care, recognition of patient satisfaction as an outcome of value is important. As identified by NHS Quality Improvement Scotland (2006), the interaction between the patient and healthcare professional may be an important mediator in treatment outcomes in relation to complementary therapies. Many of these therapies provide individual treatment with one-to-one attention from the therapist – a rare occurrence in conventional medicine and a possible reason that patient satisfaction can be high.

Acupuncture

Acupuncture originated in China and is thousands of years old. It is based on the principle from Chinese medicine that the body is controlled by a vital force or energy known as *qi*, which circulates between organs along channels known as meridians. Acupuncture points are found along the meridians and appear to correspond to physiological and anatomical features such as peripheral nerve junctions. Acupuncturists often refer to trigger points as areas of increased sensitivity within a muscle which are said to cause characteristic patterns of referred pain in a related body segment (Vickers and Zollerman 1999). It is known that acupuncture affects the pain gate as it enhances inhibition of C fibre pain impulses. It also stimulates release of endogenous opioids and serotonin, and so contributes to pain modulation. Many doctors and physiotherapists have undertaken extended training as acupuncturists and use it as an adjunct treatment.

Vickers and Zollerman (1999) describe a typical course as 6–12 sessions over a 3-month period that might be followed by top-ups. Wells (2009) states that in China, three treatments per day would be recommended because acupuncture has short-term benefits and needs to be repeated regularly. Moore (2009) indicates that evidence for the efficacy of acupuncture is still poor in quality. There appears to be no difference between sham acupuncture 'toothpick' and standardised acupuncture. From a patient's perspective it requires passive acceptance of treatment from a specialist so is not leading to independence; however, Berger (2003) notes that the overall outcome of treatment appears to cause relaxation and improved psychological state. In itself this could improve pain coping strategies by closing the pain gate, and perhaps as long as patient feels it is effective then it may be advocated. NICE (2009) guidelines for early management of non-specific low back pain have recommended acupuncture as one of the three clinical pathways for its management.

Herbal and dietary supplements

These are explored by Mann and Carr (2009: 133) as many chronic pain sufferers will try these approaches. For example, dietary restrictions may be used to identify possible links with pain associated with rheumatoid arthritis. Some supplements such as glucosamine, chondroitin or oils may be advertised for osteoarthritic conditions. It is important that patients are asked about non-prescription drugs and herbal remedies supplements, as these can have important interactions with pre-existing medication. For example, fish oil, Ginkgo, green tea, ginseng, chamomile, devil claw, saw palmeto and coenzyme Q10 can increase the activity of aspirin, warfarin and NSAIDs causing increased risk of bleeding (Gupta and Gupta 2010). This is particularly a concern for the elderly, where co-morbidities lead to higher risks of side effects when mixing drugs. Herbs like Ginkgo should be avoided in patients taking antiepileptic medication (Gupta and Gupta 2010). The pharmacist, as part of the multidisciplinary team, can be a valuable resource in this situation. Nurses as non-prescribers should, therefore, be cautious about recommending any herbal therapies as these could lead to serious interactions. The NMC (2009) identifies that the nurse:

> Must ensure that any homeopathic treatments and herbal remedies are not contra-indicated with any prescribed medications the person is taking and advise them accordingly. As with the NMC guidelines on medicines management, the same expertise is expected of a nurse or midwife as that of a pharmacist.

In addition to fears of adverse effects due to interactions, Gupta and Gupta (2010) identify serious concerns with the production and quality of some herbal medications. These have been found to contain toxic metals such as arsenic, mercury and lead, as the regulations for these preparations as dietary supplements do not meet the rigorous standards for production, uses and consumption of conventional medications.

Olsen (2009) completed a review of CAM used by people with multiple sclerosis (MS). This revealed that a high proportion of MS patients had utilised CAM. Types of CAM utilised were exercise, vitamins, herbal and mineral supplements, relaxation techniques, acupuncture, cannabis and massage. In another study, Rosenberg et al. (2008) conducted a survey ($n = 463$) in the USA with primary care patients with chronic pain, and they found 52% reported current or prior use of CAM. The most common reported therapy was vitamin and mineral supplementation, and of the people who used CAM 54% believed it helped their pain.

Case study 2.5   Mrs Smith

Rheumatoid arthritis nociceptive pain

Non-pharmacological management
Mrs Smith recognises that her pain perception is influenced by her ability to manage her lifestyle to ensure sufficient rest and sleep, and is conscious of the need to organise her time effectively and use pacing skills. She works part-time over 5 days; she has a teaching job which she values and does not allow her to be preoccupied with her condition at work (distraction). She also has a busy family life and actively participates in several hobbies. She uses warm baths with Epsom salts as a comfort measure and finds these very effective. She has adjusted her diet as she identified a connection between tomatoes and orange juice and increased joint pain, so she restricts these. She particularly values the support offered by the rheumatology specialist team who will respond quickly and review her treatment when the condition deteriorates.

Case study 2.6 Mrs White

Diabetic neuropathy

Non-pharmacological management

Mrs White suffered from burning pains it was diagnosed as diabetic neuropathy. She initially tried Amytriptylline at night and this initially helped but the pain became worse 2 years later. She then tried Gabapentin which was gradually increased to treat the pain. She found that the sedation negatively impacted her activity so Pregabapentin was substituted. This reduced the sedation but there was 30% less pain relief. Opioids were discussed but she was reluctant to use such strong medication. She was keen to try non-pharmacological interventions and she found TENS was useful at providing additional pain relief. She was also given a trial of weak opioid Tramadol for additional pain control. This provided her with good pain control when this was needed and the prolonged release preparation reduced side effects to a minimum.

  (Adapted from Mann 2009)

Points for reflection

- Do you routinely enquire about the use of complimentary or alternative medicine when assessing patients?
- What might the risks of not enquiring be in your patient group?
- How might your patients benefit from CAM?

Summary

Strategies that promote positive coping and reduced pain perception should be promoted; for example, relaxation, pacing, and appropriate activity and exercise. Support groups can help reduce isolation and help to regain a sense of control. Specific strategies like TENS and heat or cold may be useful, and specialist support from CAM has value. Evaluation of benefits versus risk is important.

Conclusion

Nurses can make a valuable contribution towards assessment and management of chronic pain. The recognition and subsequent assessment of pain is a key role. Nurses must raise awareness about the existence of pain, and as many individuals are suffering in the community, community nurses will be playing a vital role here. Once assessment has helped to identify the nature of the pain and its impact on mood and social activities, there are a range of approaches which may be utilised. The nurse can support individuals to utilise appropriate coping strategies and support groups, help the individual to feel more in control of the pain and reduce the risk of developing depression. Knowledge of prescribed and non-prescribed medication and any possible interactions and adverse effects is essential. The nurse can assist in evaluation of therapeutic effects and teach the patient how to use the drugs most effectively. Nurses should appreciate that some patients may require referral to pain specialists to find optimal treatment.

References

Abbey, J., Piller, N., De Bellis, A., Esterman, A., Parker, D., Giles, L. and Lowcay, B. (2004) The abbey pain scale: a 1-minute numerical indicator for people with end-stage dementia. *International Journal of Palliative Nursing* **10** (1), 6-13.

Ackerman, S., Knight, T. and Schein, J. (2004) Risk of constipation in patients prescribed fentanyl transdermal system or oxycodone hydrochloride controlled-release in a California medicaid population. *Consultant Pharmacist* **19** (2), 118-32.

Ahles, T., Wasson, J., Seville, J., Johnson, D., Cole, B., Hanscom-Stukel, T. and McKinstry, E. (2006) A controlled trial of methods for managing pain in primary care patients with or without co-occurring psychological problems. *Annals of Family Medicine* **4** (4), 341-350.

Alzheimer's Society (2010) Alzheimer's Society: Statistics Available at: http://www.alzheimers.org.uk/site/scripts/documents_info.php?categoryID=200120&documentID=341 (accessed 12 March /2010).

Banbury, P., Freenan, K. and Allcock, N. (2008) Experiences of analgesic use in patients with low back pain. *British Journal of Nursing* **17** (19), 1215-1218.

Bandura, A. (1990) Perceived self-efficacy in the exercise of personal agency. *Journal of Applied Sport Psychology* **2** (2), 128-163.

Barber, J. and Gibson, S. (2009) Treatment of chronic non-malignant pain in the elderly safety considerations. *Drug Safety* **32** (6), 457-474.

Baron, R. (2004) Post-herpetic neuralgia case study: optimizing pain control. *European Journal of Neurology* **11** (suppl.1), 3-11.

Berger, P. (2003) *The Journey to Pain Relief: A Useful Tool that Empowers both the Chronic Pain Sufferer and the Therapist by Providing Hands-on Information and Advice on the Treatment of Pain* South Africa Art2Print cc

Bird, J. (2005) Assessing pain in older people. *Nursing Standard* **19** (19), 45-52.

Bond, M., Simpson, K. (2006) *Pain: Its Nature and Treatment.* Edinburgh: Elsevier – Churchill Livingstone.

Breivik, H., Collett, B., Ventafridda, V., Cohen, R. and Gallacher, D. (2006) Survey of chronic pain in Europe: prevalence, impact on daily life, and treatment. *European Journal of Pain* **10** (4), 287-333.

British Pain Society (2006) Recommended Guidelines for Pain Management Programmes for Adults Available at: http://www.britishpainsociety.org (accessed 12 March 2010).

British Pain Society (2007) Concise Guidance to Good Practice No. 8: Assessment of Pain in Older Adults. Available at: http://www.britishpainsociety.org/book_pain_older_people.pdf (accessed 12 March 2010).

British Pain Society (2010) Opioids for Persistent Pain: Good Practice. Available at: http://www.britishpainsociety.org/book_opioid_main.pdf (accessed 12 March 2010).

British Pain Society (2010) Opioids for Persistent Pain: Information for Patients. Available at: http://www.britishpainsociety.org/book_opioid_patient.pdf (accessed 12 March 2010).

British Pain Society (2010) Understanding and Managing Pain: Information for Patients. Available at: http://www.britishpainsociety.org/book_understanding_pain.pdf (accessed 12 March 2010).

British Pain Society (2010) Managing your Pain Effectively Using "Over the Counter" (OTC) Medicines Available at: http://www.britishpainsociety.org/patient_pub_otc.pdf (accessed 18 May 2010).

Chamley, C. and James, G. (2007) Pain management: minimizing the pain experience. In: Brooker, C. and Waugh, A. (eds) *Foundations of Nursing Practice: Fundamentals of Holistic Care*, 653-679. Edinburgh: Mosby/Elsevier.

Chronic Pain Policy Coalition (2006) A New Pain Manifesto. Available at: http://www.paincoalition.org.uk/cppc/our-campaign (accessed 06 January 2010).

Cleeland, C. and Ryan, K. (1994) Pain assessment: global use of the brief pain inventory. *Annals of the Academy Of Medicine, Singapore* **23** (2), 129-138.

Cousins, M. (2007) Persistent pain: a disease entity. *Journal of Pain and Symptom Management* **33** (S2), S4-S10.

D'Arcy, Y. (2006) *Which analgesic is right for my patient?* Nursing **36** (7), 50-56.

Davies, E. *et al.* (2004) Pain assessment and cognitive impairment: part 1. *Nursing Standard* **19** (12), 39-42.

Davies, E. *et al.* (2004) Pain assessment and cognitive impairment: part 2. *Nursing Standard* **19** (13), 33-40.

Department of Health (DH) (2008) On the State of Public Health. Pain: Breaking Through the Barrier. Chief Medical Officer, Department of Health, Great Britain. Available at: http://www.dh.gov.uk/prod_consum_dh/groups/dh_digitalassets/documents/digitalasset/dh_096233.pdf (accessed 8 January 2010).

Elliott, A., Smith, B., Penny, K., Cairns Smith, W. and Chambers, W. (1999) The epidemiology of chronic pain in the community. *The Lancet* **354** (9186), 1248-1252.

Ferrell, B., McCaffery, M. and Rhiner, M. (1992) Pain and addiction: an urgent need for change in nursing education. *Journal of Pain and Symptom Management* **7**, 117-124.

Field, B. and Swarm, R. (2008) *Chronic Pain.* Cambridge, MA: Hogrefe & Huber.

Fricker, J. (2003) Pain in Europe: A Report Available at: http://www.paineurope.com/files/PainInEurope Survey_2.pdf (accessed 08 March 2010).

Gibson, S. (2006) Older people's pain. *Pain: Clinical Updates* Volume X1V (3), 1-4.

Godfrey, H. (2005) Understanding pain part 1: physiology of pain. *British Journal of Nursing* **14** (16), 846-852.

Greener, M. (2009) Chronic pain: nociceptive versus neuropathic. *Nurse Prescribing* **7** (12), 540-546.

Gupta, V. and Gupta, J. (2010) Complimentary and alternative medicines in pain management - being better informed. Pain News *Spring*, 34-36.

Hawksley, H. (2006) Managing pain after shingles: a nursing perspective. *British Journal of Nursing* **15** (15), 814-818.

Horn, S. and Munafo, M. (1997) *Pain Theory: Research and Intervention.* Buckingham: Open University Press.

House of Lords Select Committee on Science and Technology. Complementary and Alternative Medicine Session 1999-2000, 6th Report Available at: http://www.parliament.the-stationery-office.co.uk/pa/ld199900/ldselect/ldsctech/123/12304.htm#a15 (accessed 18 May 2010).

International Association for the Study of Pain, Taskforce on Pain Taxonomy (1994) *Classification of Chronic Pain: Descriptions of Chronic Pain Syndromes and Definitions of Pain Terms,* 2nd edn. Seattle: IASP Press.

Karmarkar, A. and Makin, R. (2007) Neuropathic pain - a drug ladder. Pain News *Spring*, 36-37.

Keefe, F., Somers, T. and Kothadia, S. (2009) Coping with pain. *Pain: Clinical Updates* **XVII** (5), 1-5i.

Knaggs, R. (2010) Managing your pain effectively using "over the counter" medicines. Pain News *Spring*, 16.

Manca, A. (2004) United Kingdom back pain exercise and manipulation (UK BEAM) randomised trial: cost effectiveness of physical treatments for back pain in primary care. *British Medical Journal* **329** (7479), 1381-1385.

Mann, E. (2009) Diabetic neuropathy part 1: pharmacology. *Practice Nursing* **20** (5), 246-250.

Mann, E. (2009) Diabetic neuropathy part 2: coping strategies. *Practice Nursing* **20** (6), 302–306.

Mann, E. (2008) Neuropathic pain: could nurses become more involved? *British Journal of Nursing* **17** (19), 1208-1213.

Mann, E. and Carr, E. (2009) *Pain: Creative Approaches to Pain Management,* 2nd edn. Basingstoke: Palgrave MacMillan.

Mann, E. and Carr, E. (2006) *Essential Clinical Skills for Nurses: Pain Management.* Oxford: Blackwell.

Matthews, P., Derry, S., Moore, R. and McQuay, H. (2009) Topical rubefacients for acute and chronic pain in adults. *Cochrane Database of Systematic Reviews* Issue 3 Art No: CD007403, DOI: 10.1002/14651858. CD007403.pub2.

McCaffery, M. (1968) *Nursing Practice Theories Related to Cognition, Bodily Pain, and Man-Environment Interactions.* Los Angeles: University of California.

McCaffery, M. and Beebe, A. (1994) *Pain: Clinical Manual for Nursing Practice,* UK edn. London: Mosby.

McCaffery, M. and Pasero, C. (1999) *Pain: Clinical Manual for Nursing Practice,* 2nd edn. St Louis: Mosby.

Section 1

McHugh, G. and Thoms, G. (2001) Living with chronic pain: the patient's perspective. *Nursing Standard* **15** (52), 33-37.

Mead, K., Theadom, A., Byron K. and Dupont, S. (2007) Pilot study of a 4-week pain coping strategies (PCS) programme for the chronic pain patient. *Disability and Rehabilitation* **29** (3), 199-203.

Melzack, R. (1999) From the gate to the neuromatrix. Pain 6 (supplement) S121-6.

Melzack, R. and Wall, P. (1996) *The Challenge of Pain*, 2nd edn. London: Penguin.

Moore, A. (2009) Back pain, NICE, and evidence. Pain News *Autumn*, 25-28.

Moore, P. (2007) The Pain Toolkit. Available at: http://www.suffolk.gov.uk/NR/rdonlyres/CEB2C11F-7C28-4595-B175-1842A28C9228/0/Paintoolkitbooklet.pdf (accessed 06 January 2010).

Morone, 3 N. and Greco, C. (2007) Mind-body interventions for chronic pain in older adults: a structured review. *Pain Medicine* **8** (4), 359-375.

Morone, N., Greco, C. and Weiner, D. (2008) Mindfulness meditation for the treatment of chronic low back pain in older adults: a randomized controlled pilot study. *Pain* **134** (3), 310-319.

National Institute for Health and Clinical Excellence (NICE) (2009) Low Back Pain: Early Management of Persistent Non-Specific Low Back Pain. Available at: http://guidance.nice.org.uk/CG88 (accessed 19 June 2009).

National Institute for Health and Clinical Excellence (NICE) (2009) Type 2 Diabetes – Newer Agents. Available at: http://guidance.nice.org.uk/CG87 (accessed 10 November 2009).

National Institute for Health and Clinical Excellence (NICE) (2010) Neuropathic Pain the Pharmacological Management of Neuropathic Pain in Adults in Non-Specialist Settings. Available at: http://guidance.nice.org.uk/CG96 (accessed 16 June 2010).

NHS Quality Improvement Scotland (2006) Management of Chronic Pain in Adults. Available at: http://www.nhshealthquality.org/nhsqis/files/BPSManage_chronic_pain%20_adults%20(Feb06).pdf (accessed 10 November 2009).

Nursing and Midwifery Council (2009) Complementary Alternative Therapies and Homeopathy. Available at: http://www.nmc-uk.org/aDisplayDocument.aspx?documentID=6430 (accessed 12 March 2010).

Nursing and Midwifery Council (NMC) (2008) Standards for Medicines Management. Available at: http://www.nmc-uk.org/aDisplayDocument.aspx?DocumentID=6978 (accessed 12 March 2010).

Nursing and Midwifery Council (NMC) (2008) The Code: Standards of Conduct, Performance and Ethics for Nurses, Midwives. Available at: http://www.nmc-uk.org/aArticle.aspx?ArticleID=3056 (accessed 13 May 2010).

Oliver, S. (2009) Understanding the needs of older people with rheumatoid arthritis: the role of the community nurse. *Nursing Older People* **21** (9), 30-37.

Olsen, S. (2009) A review of complementary and alternative medicine (CAM) by people with multiple sclerosis. *Occupational Therapy International* **16** (1), 57-70.

Persson, A., Veenhuizen, H., Zachrison, L. and Gard, G. (2008) Relaxation as treatment for chronic musculoskeletal pain – a systematic review of randomised controlled studies. *Physical Therapy Reviews* **13** (5), 355-365.

Roper, N., Logan, W. and Tierney, A. (1996) *The Elements of Nursing. A Model for Nursing Based on a Model of Living*. Edinburgh: Churchill Livingstone.

Rosenberg, E., Genao, I., Chen, I., Mechaber, A., Wood, J., Faselis, C., Kurz, J., Menon, M., O'Rorke, J., Panda, M., Pasanen, M., Staton, L., Calleson, D., Cykert, S. (2008) Complementary and alternative medicine use by primary care patients with chronic pain. *Pain Medicine* **9** (8), 1065-1072.

Sarafino, E. (2008) *Health Psychology: Biopsychosocial Interactions*, 6th edn. Hoboken: Wiley.

Scherder, E., Oosterman, J., Swaab, D., Herr, K., Ooms, M., Ribbe, M., Sergeant, J., Pickering, G. and Benedetti, F. (2005) Recent developments in pain in dementia. *British Medical Journal* **330** (7489), 461-464.

Schofield, P., O'Mahony, S., Collett, B. and Potter, J. (2008) Guidance for the assessment of pain in older adults: a literature review. *British Journal of Nursing* **17** (14), 914-918.

Schofield, P. (2002) Evaluating snoezelen for relaxation within chronic pain management. *British Journal of Nursing* **11** (12), 812-821.

Shaw, S. (2006) Nursing and supporting patients with chronic pain. *Nursing Standard* **20** (19), 60-65.

Section 1

Vickers, A. and Zollman, C. (1999) ABC of complementary medicine: acupuncture. *British Medical Journal* **319** (7215), 973–976.

Wells, C. (2009) A NICE guideline on back pain. Pain News *Autumn*, 33–35.

White, S. (2004) Assessment of chronic neuropathic pain and the use of pain tools. *British Journal of Nursing* **13** (7), 72–78.

Wiffen, P., McQuay, H., Rees, J. and Moore R. (2005) Gabapentin for acute and chronic pain. *Cochrane Database of Systematic Reviews* Issue 3 Art No. CD005452, DOI: 10.1002/14651858.CD005452.

World Health Organization (2005) Pain Ladder. Available at: http://www.who.int/cancer/palliative/painladder/en (accessed 13 May 2010).

Further reading

British Pain Society Available at: www.britishpainsociety.co.uk

Chronic Pain Policy Coalition (2006) A New Pain Manifesto. Available at: http://www.paincoalition.org.uk/cppc/our-campaign.

Crome, P., Main, C. and Lally, F. (2007) *Pain in Older People*. Oxford: Oxford University Press.

Ernst, E., Pittler, M.H. and Wider, B. (2007) *Complementary Therapies for Pain Management: An Evidence-Based Approach*. Edinburgh: Elsevier Mosby.

Field, B. and Swarm, R. (2008) *Chronic Pain*. Cambridge, MA: Hogrefe & Huber.

Mann, E. and Carr, E. (2009) *Pain: Creative Approaches to Pain Management*, 2nd edn. Basingstoke: Palgrave MacMillan.

Pain related self help group Available at: www.action-on-pain.co.uk.

Patient experience site Available at: www.dipex.org.uk

Organisations in the United Kingdom who may offer support

Arthritis Care Available at: www.arthritiscare.org.uk

Multiple Sclerosis Action MS Available at: www.actionms.co.uk

Back Care Available at: www.backcare.org.uk

Parkinson's Disease Society Available at: www.parkinsonsons.org.uk

Chapter 3

Depression and Long-term Conditions

Robert Tummey

Learning objectives

After reading this chapter, the reader will have:

- Gained an understanding of how depression is a factor in the experience of long-term conditions (LTCs)
- Developed understanding of the personal and familial acknowledgement, accurate diagnosis and recommended treatment of depression as co-morbidity with LTCs
- A greater knowledge of the psychological therapies available for successful management strategies and reduction in healthcare need

---

Introduction

This chapter addresses some of the key issues and themes around the acknowledgement, impact and subsequent treatment of depression in the person with a long-term condition (LTC). The main focus is on drawing attention to the actual prevalence of depression as a cause or consequence of an LTC and the resulting experience. It is timely that such a chapter is introduced to explore the reality of having such a debilitating, emotional difficulty that can further add to the suffering of the person and carers of those with LTCs. Indeed, the perception from an outside viewpoint may be of the person 'giving up', 'shutting down' or 'detaching'. However, this could occur as an initial coping strategy when first confronted with having an LTC and may not lead to depression itself. More entrenched difficulties occur when the emotional reaction along with a mental health diagnosis of depression is added to the actual experience of having an LTC. Fear of the unknown and a very real sense of despair may ensue.

Throughout this chapter, there are explanations of terms and definitions to help further understanding. The focus is on the experience of depression. This forms the basis through which all information has been filtered and presented.

Long-term Conditions: A Guide for Nurses and Healthcare Professionals, First Edition. Edited by S. Randall and H. Ford.
© 2011 Blackwell Publishing Ltd. Published 2011 by Blackwell Publishing Ltd.

What is depression?

Depression is fast becoming the most experienced illness in the world. It is estimated that as many as 'one in six' people in the United Kingdom have depression (NICE 2009a, NIAMH 2010, Scottish Government 2010). For people with an LTC, this increases to 'one in five'. It should be noted that there are no unique features for the person with an LTC and depression in co-morbidity. The diagnostic presentation would be the same. Within the United Kingdom, the diagnostic manual used is the *International Classification of Diseases*, 10th edition (ICD-10), which is subscribed across Europe and compiled by the World Health Organisation (WHO). The other main diagnostic manual is the *Diagnostic and Statistical Manual IV* (revised). This is the American Psychiatric Association's version, which is similar in many respects but has some variations and not generally used in the United Kingdom.

Categories

The categories of mild, moderate and severe depressive episodes should be used only for a single (first) depressive episode. Further depressive episodes should be classified under one of the subdivisions of recurrent depressive disorder:

- The disorder of recurrent depression is characterised by repeated episodes of depression as specified in depressive episode (mild, moderate or severe).
- The age of onset and the severity, duration and frequency of the episodes of depression are all highly variable.
- In general, the first episode occurs within a mean age of onset in the fifth decade.
- Individual episodes last between 3 and 12 months (median duration about 6 months) but recur less frequently.
- Recovery is usually complete between episodes, but a minority of patients may develop a persistent depression, mainly in old age.
- Individual episodes of any severity are often precipitated by stressful life events.
- In many cultures, both individual episodes and persistent depression are twice as common in women as in men.
  Source: Major Depressive Disorder 2010.

The person would fit one of three categories. These include the level of severity of the symptoms and the duration of experience within a mild, moderate or severe depressive episode.

In typical depressive episodes of all three varieties described above (mild, moderate and severe), the individual usually has depressed mood, loss of interest and enjoyment and reduced energy leading to increased fatigue and diminished activity. Marked tiredness after only slight effort is common. Other common symptoms are:

- Reduced concentration and attention
- Reduced self-esteem and self-confidence
- Ideas of guilt and unworthiness (even in a mild episode)
- Bleak and pessimistic views of the future
- Ideas or acts of self-harm or suicide
- Disturbed sleep
- Diminished appetite
  Source: Major Depressive Disorder 2010.

Section 1

It is also important to differentiate between the objective and subjective presentation of the individual. From the objective experience, the assessor may observe certain features as poor concentration, lack of eye contact, reduced motor activity, poverty of thought and loss of interest. From a subjective assessment, the presentation may include a loss of appetite, feeling of isolation, emotional numbness, low mood and poor sleep, amongst others.

Whilst the presentation can be explored through the above features, some of which are symptoms, the actual symptoms are considered more conclusive for a diagnosis in addition to the presentation. People with mild depressive episodes are common in primary care and general medical settings, whereas mental health services deal largely with patients with more severe and entrenched presentations.

There remains a debate within psychiatry and the wider mental health field as to the origins of depression and the resulting symptoms (Strickland et al. 2002). That is, whether they are biological, psychological or sociological in origin; hence the emergence of the bio-psychosocial model. However, this can be a red herring, due to its impact on all three areas of the person's life and possible origins in all three areas too.

The treatments tend to follow the bio-psychosocial model in mental health, with medication offered as a frontline treatment to bring the symptoms under some control, and then, a psychological intervention may be offered to help cement progress and explore the nature of the arising issues. Medications are prescribed on a wide scale across primary care. The main category of medication would be the anti-depressants of which there are three main types. These include the selective serotonin reuptake inhibitors (SSRIs) such as Prozac, Seroxat, Citalopram, Sertraline, which are prescribed for depression, anxiety and related mood disorders. The next are the selective noradrenaline reuptake inhibitors (SNRIs) such as Venlafaxine and Duloxetine, which are primarily indicated for depression. Older medications – tricyclic anti-depressants (TCAs) – are still in use for depression, but are being prescribed less and less and are not first-line agents. These medications are Dothiepin, Amitriptyline, Clomipramine, and so on. One of the main reasons for their decline is the additional sedating effect associated with them, which may be fatal in overdose.

Summary

The prevalence of depression in the general population has been compared with that of the population with one or more LTCs. It has been established that there are no unique features for a person with an LTC and depression as a co-morbidity. How depression is categorised has been illustrated with a discussion on the origins of depression and frontline treatments.

Recognition of depression as co-morbidity with long-term physical conditions

It is estimated that depression is associated with 50% increase in the costs of long-term medical care. These costs are associated with the adverse health risk behaviours such as smoking, diet, lack of exercise as well as a lack of compliance with self-management regimes (Katon 2003). There are many difficulties to overcome for the 17 1/2 million people estimated to have an LTC (DH 2005). The experience envelops the individual in a life of symptom management and relapse prevention. This in itself can be tiring and produce marked changes in the person's presentation, from a carefree person to a distracted and consumed person. This can also be a slow process of navigating the experience or can be an acute onset. Nonetheless, family and friends may see a sharp contrast in mood and behaviour or could indeed be so close as not to entirely notice. Also, given that the families own changes and navigating of the experience from close quarters, initially it can be rather difficult to determine any clinical features of depression as they are masked by the reality of coping and the emotional turmoil that ensues. Acknowledgement of a depressive condition should be considered for the purpose of eliminating its presence. If depression is overlooked, the feelings can worsen and the depressive symptoms become overwhelming.

Once acknowledged by the individual, their family or by a health practitioner, the need to assess the depression is necessary to establish a baseline and ascertain the full extent to which the symptoms or the distress has taken hold. Assessment of depression can take a number of forms, depending on the geographical location, referring agency and assessing practitioner. Generally, the services available that may become referring agents include general practitioner (GP), practice nurse, and any specialist clinician attending for the LTC, support groups, and so on. It could also be the relative or carer who raises concern.

Who is raising the concern will determine the route of referral. The person may have to be referred to their GP or primary care first and then referred on to mental health services or, indeed, managed within primary care. Usually, once referred to a community mental health service the person will be allocated to an appropriate team and then clinician.

Primary care liaison

If primary mental healthcare receives the referral direct, they will have a minimum waiting period and then offer assessment. Treatment may take the form of up to six sessions (Tummey and Smojkis 2005).

Mental health crisis

If it is an emergency, the mental health crisis team (also known as crisis resolution or home treatment) will pick up the referral and assess the individual within a short time period. Service availability should be over a 24-hour period. The team will provide intensive support to the person in their own home. This can occur two or three times a day during the crisis and remain until crisis is resolved (Hopkins and Niemiec 2005).

Mental health liaison

If the person is 'picked up', seen or indeed referred to the Accident and Emergency Department of their local hospital and depression is detected, the person may be visited by the Mental Health Liaison team. They provide an emergency assessment for people who show signs of mental illness, self-harm or suicide (Roberts and Whitehead 2005: 52).

If longer or more specialist treatment is necessary, the person will be referred to longer-term therapy. This process can be long and frustrating, with similarities in the assessments undertaken by various clinicians.

Further considerations

There can be many other factors that require further consideration during assessment. These are discussed in the following.

Gender

- *Masculinity/femininity*: It can be compromised, along with gender differences in personal acceptance and even service acknowledgement of an LTC diagnosis (Lockyer 2009: 120). This can take many subtle or overt forms and is a very real concern. Supportive literature or referral to self-help groups and discussion with other patients can be useful.
- *Sexuality*: The ability to perform, a person's libido and general self-consciousness/image may be reduced (Denny and Earle 2009: 23). It is also linked to masculinity and femininity.
- *Labelling/stigma*: Concern may be apparent as to the individual's perception of their situation and their role within the home. Being given a label (diagnosis) and attributed stigma can be a useful conceptualisation of the experience but could equally be damaging for self or others (Denny and Earle 2009: 10). This can result from the LTC itself or depression.
- *Provider/carer role*: People's defined role in the home may have to be re-evaluated and adjusted (Furze et al. 2008: 111). This can cause resentment and possible friction and would need consideration in adapting to an LTC.

Cultural

- *Definitions and terms*: Some ethnic groups do not recognise depression or have the language to describe it (Mallinson and Popay 2008). Each discrete ethnic group should be considered as having their own unique beliefs and ways of describing the experience of depression (Mitchell et al. 2009: 222). See Case study 3.1.
- *Expectations*: Many cultures are used to being part of a large family group, often contained and protected within. The concept of depression is what Fernando (2002) terms a 'western disease'. Therefore, the culturally defined idioms of distress might be used to express the experience of symptoms, including somatic symptoms (Ahmed and Bradby 2008). Research into ethnic experiences of mental illness identified weaknesses in the acknowledgement and management of depression amongst people of South Asian origin (Mallinson and Popay 2008).

Age

- *Child*: In point ten of standard six of DH (2007) provision for children with LTCs is apparent and it acknowledges that the aim of treatment is to manage their illness in such a way that they are able to enjoy and achieve fully in their lives. To achieve this, they should have access to services that help to develop self-confidence and self-management skills (DH 2007). Clinicians need to ensure that they are taking the wishes and feeling of the young person into account in the decision-making process. Also, all staff working with children should be able to address emotional well-being and refer to specialist services and access psychological therapies as necessary.
- *Adult*: Being a spouse or partner can be incredibly rewarding or it may become a feeling of burden due to loss of role. The LTC may have adverse effects on all aspects of life, including the perceived role of family head (paternal or maternal), protector, or provider, carer, and so on (Furze et al. 2008: 111).
- *Older adult*: It refers to increased experience of loss in life, including various aspects such as role, social network, employment, friends, mobility and bereavement. With age, physical and mental

capacity can also be impaired or restricted by any LTC and compounded by the experience of depression (Mitchell et al. 2009: 219).

- *Parents*: Being a parent with an LTC and depression can be debilitating and frustrating. The responsibility of children is a major influence on parents and this can remain so even into older age. Protecting children and continuing to provide parental stability may restrict a person in fully sharing the extent to which their difficulties are being experienced. Adaptation to the LTC may be further compromised if the person is a single parent overcoming competing concerns, a lack of resources and limited time for self.

Case study 3.1 Mrs Harpreet Kaur

Mrs Kaur is a 65-year-old Indian Sikh lady with a painful rheumatoid arthritis (RA) and increased feelings of mild depression. English is not Mrs Kaur's first language and she appears to be having difficulty in expressing her concerns. Although the family are very supportive, they are not able to understand the physical condition. The nurse needs to establish Mrs Kaur's current level of knowledge and understanding for the condition. It would then be useful to establish the frequency, duration, severity and timing of the pain and tease out the correlation between the feelings of pain and the symptoms of depression.

Mrs Kaur does not understand depression or consider the symptoms to be separate from her experience of RA. She finds it difficult to explain through her grandson (who is acting as an interpreter). The nurse will acknowledge the perspective of Mrs Kaur and provide an opportunity for her to express her fears about the illness. She can relate to the pain of RA as the total cause of her distress and so does not wish to focus on feelings of depression separately.

Points for reflection

- How could language-specific materials be used to enhance Mrs Kaur's understanding? If not available, could materials in English be given for the family to translate? If it is at all possible, an interpreter could be used to ensure the treatment is being adhered to and is effective.
- Medication for depression should still be considered to assist in the overall treatment regime for the RA, alleviation of pain and reduction of depressive symptoms that may hinder progress.
- Cultural sensitivity is necessary for this case, as Mrs Kaur is an Indian Sikh. Further research and understanding of specific cultural norms and differences would be beneficial and assist in reducing the impact on the care provided.

Summary

How depression can be recognised, why recognition is important and issues of referral have been established in this section. Factors which may affect assessment, such as gender, culture and age, have been highlighted and discussed.

Prevalence of depression as co-morbidity with long-term physical conditions

Depression is a mental health condition that is co-morbid for many people with a variety of physical health problems. People with LTCs are at increased risk of mental health problems, especially depression (Tylee and Haddad 2007). A key role for the health professional is to be alert to the possibility of depression (Haddad et al. 2009a).

The evidence suggests that coronary heart disease and diabetes have the highest prevalence (Nemeroff and Mussleman 2000; Anderson et al. 2001; Goldney et al. 2004) with stroke-related depression on the increase within an ageing population (Ormell and Von Korff 2000). Also included are some of the diseases less associated with depression but with growing evidence and attention of late. These include RA and chronic obstructive pulmonary disease (COPD). Other diseases that may impact on mental health are neurological conditions such as epilepsy, motor-neurone disease or multiple sclerosis. However, the information about their co-morbidity with depression is scant. Patients with chronic physical illness can experience life-changing effects that impact on quality of life, functioning and personal well-being. Depression as a cause or consequence may exacerbate the perceived severity of the symptoms (DH 2008: 1). Depression also decreases the adherence to medical treatment and can increase unhealthy behaviour such as smoking, substance misuse and poor diet (Prince et al. 2007; DH 2008: 1).

Stroke

The prevalence of post-stroke depression is estimated to be as high as 61% (Herrmann et al. 1998; Stenager et al. 1998). Untreated, the depressive symptoms are likely to have a negative effect on the recovery and activities of daily living. Ormell and Von Korff (2000) have shown that effective treatment for depression can enhance the person's holistic functioning. May et al. (2002) identified that middle-aged men are three times more likely to suffer a fatal stroke if they have depression.

Coronary heart disease

People with coronary heart disease are more likely to experience depression and people with depression are more likely to have coronary heart disease (Nemeroff and Mussleman 2000). Rozanski et al. (1999) reported that a state of hopelessness within an individual more than doubled the risk of developing coronary heart disease. Depression is also a predictor for 1-year cardiac mortality, but very high levels of support can mitigate the harmful effect of depression (Frasure-Smith et al. 2000) whereas low levels of emotional support will have the opposite effect and increase risk threefold (Williams et al. 1992). People who have suffered a myocardial infarction have a 30% chance of developing depression (Davies et al. 2004) and three times more likely to die if they have depression than if they do not (Frasure-Smith et al. 2000). It is estimated that 40% of admissions and half of revascularisations can be avoided by providing psychological therapy to those with angina (DH 2008: 2).

Diabetes

It is estimated that 24% of people who have diabetes will also have depression (Goldney et al. 2004) and are up to three times more likely to have depression than the general public (Boehm et al. 2004).

Poor hyperglycaemic control is also linked to severity of depression (Lustman et al. 2000). There is also evidence of poor self-care in this group (Park et al. 2004), greater loss of workdays and an increase in hospital bed use (Egede 2004). Indeed, Egede et al. (2002) highlight that diabetes and co-morbid depression have an association with increased healthcare costs.

Rheumatoid arthritis

Depression is one of the most common psychological manifestations in RA and is associated with pain intensity (Dickens et al. 2002). This results in significant societal implications because of the negative health consequences, functional limitations and higher utilisation of health services (Katz and Yelin 1993). Wright et al. (1998) found that younger individuals with RA were indeed at higher risk for developing depression than older individuals. This may be due to additional pressures such as employment and parenting. Unfortunately, depression is sometimes not recognised by clinicians as it resembles the RA disease process itself (Parker and Hart 2009). Patients with RA who have been given psychological therapy early in the course of their illness used significantly less healthcare resources for the following 5 years, with reduction in admission, injections, referrals for physiotherapy and total healthcare costs (Sharpe et al. 2008).

Chronic obstructive pulmonary disease

Depression tends to be high in COPD and is found in 50% of the patients with COPD, according to Stage et al. (2003). High levels of depression contribute to the poor quality of life for patients with COPD (Kaptein et al. 2009). This is one of the least researched areas of the LTC's co-morbidity with depression. It is estimated that up to 51% people with COPD have clinically significant symptoms of depression and up to 67% experiencing panic disorder (DH 2008: 5).

Chronic pain

Between 30% and 40% of patients attending chronic pain clinics are estimated to be clinically depressed (Banks and Kerns 1996). Consider Case study 3.2.

Case study 3.2 Mr Andrew Slater

Andy is a 46-year-old male who experiences chronic pain in his lower back following a road traffic accident 3 years ago. Because the pain has been debilitating and restricts mobility, Andy's initial low mood has deteriorated to symptoms of moderate depression. He is currently prescribed Venlafaxine 150 mg, which appears to have little impact on his symptoms. He has had to leave employment, where he worked as a long-distance lorry driver and now exists on benefits. His wife and children are a great support but Andy is withdrawn from them and isolates himself.

Points for reflection

- The experience of depression is compromising the management of his physical condition. Indeed, Andy may have more intense chronic pain, more frequently and over longer periods. The clinical presentation of depression will add to the distress of the LTC and exacerbate feelings of isolation with the pain experienced.
- Medication is currently not relieving any symptoms and needs to be reviewed with a view to increase the Venlafaxine. Discussion with the GP or care team is necessary to ensure that the correct therapeutic dose is prescribed.
- Cognitive behavioural therapy (CBT) (see Section 'Cognitive behavioural therapy') is indicated for this condition to promote improved understanding of health-related beliefs and more effective self-management (Furze et al. 2008). The approach will be similar to Case study 3.5, but applied to the experience of pain.

Summary

In this section, consideration has been given to specific LTCs and the literature reviewed on links with depression. The effect of depression on an individual's ability to engage in the decision-making process around their treatment and life course is discussed.

Diagnosis of depression

Delay in the accurate diagnosis of depression and thus the treatment can result in unnecessary suffering, investigations and health service cost (DH 2008). It is necessary to ensure accurate diagnosis. A diagnosis is considered following assessment. This will be drawn from the ICD-10 as described above in Section 'What is depression?' The depression will be mild, moderate or severe and this will determine the treatment offered. However, there should be caution for making assumptions as to the origin or reason for the depression. Severity will need to be decided. Should the symptoms and severity be mild, it may be a low mood that is transient. More moderate symptoms may impact on suicidal ideation and negative thought processing. Severe depression is concerning but usually too debilitating for any adverse action on the part of the individual.

Pre-morbid personality and mood

A baseline will need to be established as to the current mood and the effect on the individual. Thus, this can be tested against and monitored for alteration in mood. It is also necessary to find out the person's pre-morbid personality (what they were like prior to the onset of depression). This will help to realise more appropriate goals for the patient and provides knowledge to the clinician of the amount of shift in the person's functioning, presentation and mood.

Assessment methods

There are a variety of assessment methods that can help to ascertain the current mood of the patient (Barker 2004: 92). Some are more effective than others and some are preferred by some clinicians over others. The best guide is to use evidence-based methods to establish the baseline of mood. It is worth pointing out that assessment tools do not replace clinical judgement or override it. The purpose is to corroborate with the clinician and provide further evidence for the patient, as to whether the mood is worse or improved. Significant improvement can be monitored and charted.

Useful assessment tools include the following:

- Depression Inventory (Beck et al. 1961).
- Hopelessness Scale (Beck et al. 1974). Hopelessness is a factor in predicting suicide risk.
- Hospital Anxiety and Depression Scale (Zigmond and Snaith 1983). This questionnaire is designed for clinically significant levels of anxiety and depression.
- A mood diary or a negative thought diary can be a helpful assessment tool, providing further evidence of the severity of low mood.
- Localised assessment schedules ascertain the holistic picture of the individual's difficulties, including physical, psychiatric history and current perception of the problem.

Contributing factors

Grieving process

Many people may experience the grieving process as a result of loss. This may be linked to loss of role, health, employment, mobility, and so on. The process is not specific to death and can be debilitating until navigated. Depression is just one of the five stages of grief, which according to Kubler-Ross (1973) include denial, anger, bargaining, depression and acceptance. The stages do not necessarily occur in order and each stage can last for a brief moment or a prolonged period.

Change of role

The person with an LTC may also have the changing of their role to contend with and navigate. This may in turn alter their circumstances. Aspects to be effected may include home, employment, family and, indeed, their actual or perceived social standing. Their reaction could be to retreat inwards.

Adjustment

As with the change in role, adjustment to the condition can take its toll. This may be overwhelming and enforce a lifestyle that is alien to the individual. Withdrawal may be inevitable for a short period of processing events, but if prolonged, may lead to a lack of coping. Adjustment may take time and will require what Rollnick et al. (1999) term readiness to change as part of the 'motivational interviewing' model (see section 'Motivational interviewing'); a belief that individual's readiness to change is dependent on perceived importance and personal confidence to change. See Case study 3.3.

Stigma

Stigma can be a barrier to people receiving the help and treatment they may require. Concerns for what others may think or judge about the LTC and its impact and the public perception of mental illness can create a stigma that most people would not wish to experience. Avoidance of help for depression is an issue that needs to be considered for all individuals with LTCs.

Substance abuse

The use of substances to help mediate against the effects of an LTC and possibly depression is not a new phenomenon. For many people, substances used as an addition to prescribed treatment can mask the symptoms, allow a form of self-medicating in the person's control and assist in avoiding the emotional reality of having a physical condition. The substances used or abused can be identified along a wide-ranging spectrum that includes caffeine at one end, to alcohol, through to illicit drugs such as cannabis, cocaine or heroin at the other[1]. Consideration must be given for why the person is using the substance, and the duration, frequency and severity of use. Each substance will provide some benefit to the user, but will also have additional consequences physically and mentally.

Case study 3.3 Mrs Florence Makin

Mrs Makin is a 61-year-old female who suffered a stroke 4 months ago. She has a supportive husband and family who live locally and visit regularly. Prior to the stroke, Mrs Makin was a charity worker within the local community and a keen rambler on most weekends. Currently, her progress is encouraging physically, although her mood does not appear to be improving. Professional support is provided on a daily basis.

This lady is experiencing tremendous loss in her life. She can no longer engage in the activities she enjoyed, has lost her role in the family and has become withdrawn. It is more than likely that Mrs Makin has depression because of the effects of the stroke, the physical demands of recovery and the emotional strain as a result of the loss she has experienced.

Points for reflection

- The health professional needs to establish how Mrs Makin is feeling at present and her concerns for adjusting to the debilitation of the stroke.
- Treatment for the depression is necessary, as the symptoms will hinder any progress and almost certainly contribute to a marked deterioration. Medication could be used here to elevate her mood and motivational interviewing could be employed to consider her readiness to change. A referral for this may be necessary.
- It is also worth bearing in mind that the loss she is experiencing may leave her in a grieving process, feeling bereft, low in mood and withdrawn as a reaction. This could be talked through using counselling skills.

[1]With regard to illicit drug taking, the nurse is faced with the ethical dilemma of taking action against such behaviour. However, any potential action should be balanced with a duty of care to the patient, breaking confidentiality, losing their trust, and so on. Each case will be based on individual merits, as to whether to inform the police or general practitioner. Clinical supervision would play a part here and would ensure that the information is recorded appropriately.

Summary

Assessment of possible depression has been explored in the last section. Contributing factors which may be associated with LTCs have been examined.

Treatment for depression

Depression is the most common mental health problem presented in general practice (CSIP 2006). Layard (2004) estimates that one-third of people visiting their GP have mental health problems and only a one-quarter of people with mental health problems receive treatment (Layard 2004, 2005). There are many barriers to accessing referral, accurate diagnosis, treatment and therapies for depression as co-morbidity to an LTC. The following are some of the more obvious.

Medication

Anti-depressants have been used in the treatment of depression for over half a century. The principal theory of how they work focuses on their effects on neurotransmitters, noradrenaline and serotonin (Healy 2005). There are three main varieties of anti-depressants. These include TCAs, SSRIs and SNRIs.

All of the medications in Table 3.1 can be given in two doses or one single dose at bedtime. TCAs are non-addictive, and potential for abuse is minimal (Keltner and Folks 2005). The difference between a therapeutic dose and dangerous dose can be slight. This needs consideration not only in terms of impairing health but also to be avoided for patients at potential risk of suicide, as TCAs are lethal in overdose. SSRIs and SNRIs are mainly used in the United Kingdom (see Tables 3.2 and 3.3).

The SSRIs are prescribed for clinical depression, phobia, generalised anxiety disorder and related mood disorders.

The SNRIs are primarily indicated for major depression.

As with most medications, there are side effects with anti-depressants. SSRIs are less sedating and have fewer anti-muscarinic and cardiotoxic effects than TCAs; see Table 3.4.

Table 3.1 Tricyclic anti-depressants (TCAs)

Generic name	Trade name	Therapeutic dosage (mg)	Caution
Dothiepin	Prothiaden	150-225	Cardiovascular disease
Amitriptyline	Tryptizol	150-200	Epilepsy
Clomipramine	Anafranil	30-150	
Lofepramine	Gamanil	140-210	Hyperthyroidism
Imipramine	Tofranil	150-200	

Source: British National Formulary 2010a.

Table 3.2   Selective serotonin reuptake inhibitors (SSRIs)

Generic name	Trade name	Therapeutic dosage (mg)	Caution
Citalopram	Cipramil	20–60	Pregnancy
Fluoxetine	Prozac	20–60	Cardiac disease
Paroxetine	Seroxat	20–50	Diabetes
Sertraline	Lustral	50 (200 max)	
Fluvoxamine	Faverin	50–100	

Source: British National Formulary 2010b.

It is worth consulting the BNF for an understanding of the possible side effects of each specific anti-depressant medication and also the identified cautions, which may correspond with the physical condition of the person.

For further information regarding drug interaction and recommended anti-depressant, please refer to Haddad et al. (2009b: 4).

Taking more and more medications on top of those already prescribed is not preferable, but may be necessary for reducing the impact of both physical and mental conditions. Medidose packs (or similar) should be a consideration to help assist the person to take the medication at the right time and order. Monitoring of the medications taken should be necessary and a regular review by a medical practitioner is essential.

Alternative therapies

There are a range of various alternative therapies that people can use, or seek within their own localities and usually at their own cost. Although research evidence is limited, such alternatives can provide added relief from symptoms of depression and also afford the person some allocated personal time. These can be extremely valuable, but would require self-funding. Further exploration is advised (Holisticonline 2010).

Table 3.3   Serotonin and noradrenaline reuptake inhibitors (SNRIs)

Generic name	Trade name	Therapeutic dosage (mg)	Caution
Venlafaxine	Efexor	150–375 (max)	Heart disease
Duloxetine	Cymbalta	60	Pregnancy
Mirtazapine	Zisbin	30–45	Cardiac disorders and diabetes

Source: British National Formulary 2010c.

Section 1

Table 3.4   Side effects of SSRIs and SNRIs

Gastro-intestinal effects (dose-related and fairly common):
Nausea, vomiting, dyspepsia, abdominal pain, diarrhoea, constipation

Other possible effects may include:
Weight changes, hypertension, palpitation, vasodilatation, changes in serum cholesterol; chills, pyrexia, dyspnoea, yawning; dizziness, dry mouth, insomnia, nervousness, drowsiness, asthenia, headache, abnormal dreams, agitation, anxiety, confusion, hypertonia, paraesthesia, tremor; urinary frequency, sexual dysfunction, menstrual disturbances; arthralgia, myalgia; visual disturbances, tinnitus; sweating, pruritus, rash

Source: British National Formulary 2010d.

Group work

Groups can be a supportive, informative and even cathartic experience. See Case study 3.4. The NICE (2009b) clinical guidelines describe some of the group treatments offered for mild to moderate depression and an LTC combined. They include the following:

(i)   A physical activity programme that incorporates a group exercise class over a period of up to 14 weeks.
(ii) A peer support group conducted by a health professional. This would be to provide a series of weekly meetings for sharing experiences with people who have a similar condition.

Group work for more moderate depression may entail the following:

(i)   Group-based CBT, where a therapist will work with a group of six to eight people who have the same physical health problem.
(ii) Behavioural couple therapy, enabling couples to understand links between their behaviour with each other and the symptoms of depression.

Case study 3.4   Mr David Bass

David is a 58-year-old male who currently has COPD and is experiencing physical and social difficulties as a result. This has now led to a reduction in mood and a diagnosis of mild to moderate depression for the last 3 months. He has been prescribed Citalopram 40 mg and recently referred to a local peer support group to share his feelings and the experience of having COPD with other patients. David has been apprehensive and anxious about attending the group. This is not something he has ever experienced in his life as a civil servant.

The respiratory nurse consultant has been most encouraging to David and accompanies him for the first three visits to the group. David grows in confidence, due to the welcome from the group, the opportunity to relate to others' experiences and the sharing of his own isolating condition and lack of adjustment. The group engage in sharing 'tips' on their own process of adjustment and identifying ways they each overcome the physical and social difficulties

David is currently experiencing. This is invaluable to David, as the members of the group are all at various stages of their condition and offer help that he appreciates, understands and values.

Points for reflection

- Some patients will need more support than others. It can be extremely beneficial to patients if there is some consistency in their care delivery. Once a referral to a support group is made, it may be useful to ascertain the confidence of the person and support them in attending through the initial stages.
- David is in a risk category for suicide (age, isolation, adverse event, loss, depression, and so on) and so this will need consideration. If concern for risk is sufficient, a referral to mental health services should be made or requested from the GP. Any previous attempts of suicide noted will dramatically increase the real risk of suicide. Increase in mood is not an indication of reduced risk.

Psychological therapies for depression

Increased access to psychological treatment

Over the last few years, there has been an acknowledgement of the research that specifically identifies service provision that the service user populations believe should be improved and increased. The main service highlighted time and again is access to psychological treatment or therapies. In 2007 it was decided by DH (2007) and Scottish Government (2007) to instigate an initiative to be rolled out across the United Kingdom. This is the 'increased access to psychological therapies', covering the most effective, evidence-based approaches within a low-intensity (brief intervention) or high-intensity (complex) programme. The process has increased the training of clinicians to provide a wider range of therapies and widening access for people using the mental health service.

Counselling and problem solving

Some health professionals have developed counselling skills in the course of their work or through specific training to enhance their role and provide an opportunity to discuss arising issues. Often the main concern, from the practitioner's point of view, is the lack of time to be able to provide a listening ear or sounding board. This can be extremely valuable to the patient and enable time to talk through feelings of helplessness and isolation, even fear. Another opportunity that the use of counselling skills can provide is talking through concerns to help contextualise the experience and receive feedback, clarification and support. This may, in turn, help resolve some of the feelings of anger or helplessness. The success rate for this approach is unknown and rather difficult to quantify due to varying levels of counselling ability, provision of time, knowledge and understanding of the patients situation and their frustrations. Most nurses across the branches of nursing will have some degree of communication skill that can form a therapeutic rapport with a patient. The spectrum of ability is wide, with nurses and allied health professionals in a unique position to engage the patient in conversation and work towards some form of resolution.

Basic understanding of communication should include the use of skills such as paraphrasing, clarifying, summarising, through attentive listening or what Egan (1998) termed 'micro skills of attending'. The clinician should be aware of verbal content, delivery, tone, speech and meaning; also recognising that non-verbal communication conveys the majority of the message being delivered. This includes body posture, facial expression, eye contact, and so on. Mastering these basic skills and being able to use 'considered' communication is essential for gaining understanding of the patients concerns and could help alleviate fears that impact on their overall emotional well-being and affect the course of their physical illness (Heslop et al. 2009).

Engaging the patient to discuss their concerns about adjusting to life with an LTC will help and have a beneficial effect on the mood (Benison 2009). This process would be a good start and would be of particular benefit to those patients experiencing low mood as a result of their situation or illness. Mainly, it would assist those people with mild symptoms of depression, low mood and feeling down. Those with more moderate symptoms of depression would need a more established form of actual therapy, such as the following three models.

Cognitive behavioural therapy

CBT is a psychological intervention best known for its efficacy with depression. It seeks to explore the links between an individual's feelings and thinking patterns that relate to the experience of distress and relies on contracted involvement, agreement with the treatment rationale and the ability for self-help. The focus is not on concerns from the past, but on the behavioural, cognitive and physiological response to stimuli in the present. One of the major assumptions held in CBT is that anyone can experience mental health difficulties if the meanings attributed to specific events are sufficiently upsetting (Grant et al. 2004: 2).

Essentially, the practitioner would need to develop a therapeutic relationship with the individual in order to be able to work collaboratively. This would be established during the assessment process, when the practitioner is ascertaining the extent of the person's difficulties.

Assessment in CBT

This will entail the full and comprehensive exploration of the difficulty experienced. Although depression may be the diagnosis attributed, the main difficulty experienced may be avoidance of specific events or social interaction for instance. Other main concerns could be the impact of negative thoughts or constant rumination over a concern, such as an LTC. See Case study 3.5.

The assessment will need to comprise the following:

- Finding out the nature of the difficulty (problem).
- What is the frequency (how often)?
- What is the duration (how long)?
- What is the severity (how bad)?
- When does it occur (timing)?
- What does it affect (consequences)?

A useful model to help identify the relationship between all elements of difficulty created by the problem is the five aspect model developed by Greenberger and Padesky (1995). The therapist promotes understanding of the problem by identifying the interaction between the five aspects of life. These include (in no particular order) environment, thoughts, mood, behaviour and physical reaction. An example of the model in use is given in case study 3.5.

Case study 3.5 Ms Mary Smith

Mary is a 53-year-old female who lives alone. She has been suffering with COPD for the last year and requires weekly input from her local health professionals. Mary's progress seems to be limited, and through further discussion, it is discovered that she is avoiding family and any social interactions. Using the five-aspect model reveals that Mary has a number of concerns about her condition that fuel her fear and creates avoidance.

Environment
Living alone with COPD. Local family contact, but no significant friends.
Thoughts
Memory – Suffering an attack of increased symptoms at night
Thought – 'I'm not going to cope', 'I'm useless', I'm a burden'
Belief – If I cannot cope I will lose control
Moods
Depressed, angry, fearful
Behaviour
Avoiding social situations, avoiding family, overeating, avoiding sleep
Physical reaction
Tension, sleep disturbance, lethargy

Points for reflection

- This example highlights how negative experience can be exacerbated by the interaction between thoughts, beliefs and moods. The thought that she is useless leads to feeling depressed, thus leading to the experience of lethargy and avoiding family (because she thinks she is useless). Just by exploring the connections, Mary will be able to understand how each aspect influences the other and, thus, be able to take control.
- Mary will be able to take back control by providing evidence for herself. This would be achieved by keeping a thought diary, challenging the negative thoughts and managing her experience of anxiety through relaxation techniques and education around symptom reduction.

How CBT works

Following detailed assessment of the main problem (duration, frequency and severity) and agreement with the treatment rationale (process and focus of engagement), CBT is used to help construct different coping strategies and confront negative processes that maintain the problem.

In CBT, the relationship between thoughts, emotions, physiological reactions and behaviour are linked. Psychological difficulties such as depression are not caused by these, but are exacerbated. A number of factors such as stressful life events, adversity (poverty or deprivation), childhood abuse (bullying or parental abuse) and physical ill health may all contribute to the experience of distress (Furze et al. 2008; Heslop and Foley 2009). Negative thoughts and beliefs can have a powerful impact on the development and maintenance of depression (Furze et al. 2008).

Some useful questions which may help elicit negative behaviour and beliefs are:

1. What thoughts did you have when you felt low?
2. How did you feel?
3. What did that experience mean to you?
4. Did you think about what was happening around you?
5. Did you feel anything in your body at the time?
6. What did you actually do?

Depression can be an important consequence of chronic disease in its own right and has the potential to hinder any progress and undermine self-management behaviour (Newman et al. 2009; Heslop and Foley 2009). Therefore, it is important to help patients to identify and modify negative distorted thought patterns. This may include questioning how realistic the thoughts are, using positive self-talk and possibly scheduling positive, enjoyable activities to increase positive experiences (Newman et al. 2009). This may be enough, if symptoms are mild, or it may be a useful start if the symptoms are more moderate.

The initial goal of CBT is to work collaboratively to break vicious cycles that sustain or intensify the problem (Townend and Grant 2008). Using a model such as the five-aspect model explored in Case study 3.5, the problem should be identified and considered for its influence in each aspect. Once understanding has been achieved, agreement needs to be reached in partnership with the patient on how to overcome the difficulties. This would entail a treatment plan. Interventions might include the following:

- Education regarding the nature of depression, shame, role relationships, fears, and so on.
- Education regarding the five-aspect model and links between thought, behaviour, physical reaction, and so on.
- Use of a thought diary or monitoring sheet to elicit negative thoughts, measure belief, challenge the thought and measure belief again. Add a positive thought.
- Develop the patient's empathy and understanding for own distress and its consequences.
- Graded exposure to avoided situations. A list of activities that grade levels of exposure to avoided events or situations and then self-monitored for thoughts/feelings or anxiety before, during and after exposure. The specific activity is repeated until the level of anxiety is recorded as reduced to within normal range. Then the person moves to the next activity.
- Relaxation techniques and breathing exercises.
  Source: Adapted from Townend (2008: 204).

Most interventions within CBT enable the recording of a measurement on a scale of 1–10 or 0% to 100% to gauge the level of influence, provide evidence and identify progress or areas for further work. CBT therapists will have the necessary documentation. The activities will be expected to be achieved as 'homework' without the presence of the therapist.

If support is necessary, a partner, carer or family member can provide input as a co-therapist. This relationship can help keep the person on track, motivated and supported to succeed. The data that are recorded can then be evaluated and treatment adjusted to assist in maximising the potential to progress.

Motivational interviewing

Motivational interviewing evolved from the experience of treating alcoholism and drug addiction in the 1980s. Since then, motivational interviewing has gained in popularity and clinical use for a number of issues and problem behaviours. Some areas targeted include weight loss, lowering of lipid levels, increasing physical activity, diabetes, asthma and smoking cessation (Rubak et al. 2005).

The terms motivational interviewing are chosen for their distinct meanings, motivational to elicit motivation to change and interviewing, because it is quite different to therapy and implies a process of gaining information in a more egalitarian way. The model is defined as a 'client-centred, directive method for enhancing intrinsic motivation to change by exploring and resolving ambivalence' (Miller and Rollnick 2002: 25). Understanding the interviewing process is vitally important to the spirit of motivational interviewing and can be identified through the following three main areas:

1. *Collaboration*: An authoritarian one-up stance is to be avoided. The interviewer will communicate a partner-like, supportive relationship that involves exploration in an atmosphere conducive to change (Hettema, Steele and Miller 2005).
2. *Evocation*: The tone of the interviewer is one of eliciting information, not imparting it. The role is not of expert, but of an interviewer finding the intrinsic motivation of the person and evoking it, calling it forth (Rollnick, Miller and Butler 2002).
3. *Autonomy*: Responsibility for change is left with the client and must solely lie with them. The individual's autonomy must be respected. The client is free to take counsel or not. When motivational interviewing is achieved properly, it is the client who presents the argument for change (Miller and Rollnick 2002). See Case study 3.6.

Case study 3.6 Mr Muhammad Ahmed

Mr Ahmed is a 32-year-old male who has type 1 diabetes for last 6 years. He has had a trouble keeping to a healthy diet, not taking insulin on time, not reducing his alcohol intake and generally not taking care of his well-being. Currently, his blood sugar levels remain unstable. On further investigation, he admits to manipulating his diet and insulin in order to compensate for alcohol use. His mood appears low and resentful. Acceptance of his disease is limited and his health continues to be compromised.

Motivational Interviewing is indicated here to explore his commitment to adhering to treatment, changing risk behaviour and accepting his condition.

Health Professional (HP): 'So Muhammad, could you tell me your thoughts about having diabetes?'

Muhammad (MA): 'I have never really accepted it fully. I mean, none of my friends have it or have all of the inconvenience that goes with it. It makes me feel angry and trapped.'

HP: 'So none of your friends can relate to you having diabetes?'

MA: 'That's right.'

HP: 'You mention feeling angry and trapped, could you explain?'

MA: 'I never asked for diabetes and not knowing anyone else with it makes me wonder – why me? I can control it, but do feel trapped by the insulin, meals and injecting.'

HP: 'You said you can control it. To what degree do you control it?'

MA: 'Ok, I tend to eat when I should, but maybe not what I should. I have the injection when necessary, but can sometimes alter the timing to allow for my blood sugars to adjust when I drink alcohol.'

HP: 'How do you feel about that? Is it something you can sustain?'

MA: 'Well I don't think it's a problem, but I do know it has consequences. I can get away with it now, but it's not something I can sustain for a long time.'

[This statement would suggest that Muhammad is currently in contemplation in the stages of change (Prochaska and DiClemente 1982). It would be useful to 'tip the balance' with him, evoke reasons for change and strengthen his self-efficacy.]

HP: 'Tell me, what are the consequences? You are aware that you are getting away with it at the moment, so I wonder what your thoughts are on that.'

MA: 'My concentration is not great and my blood sugars can fluctuate. I probably do not have the focus with my diabetes that I should have. Sometimes it concerns me, but I do feel on top of it.'

HP: 'You feel you don't have the focus that you should have and that concerns you. What are your concerns?'

MA: 'I suppose my lack of focus concerns me, because my health is affected. I really do not want to have long-term consequences for my actions now.'

HP: 'It sounds as though you are becoming more aware of how your current actions influence your health negatively and possibly in the long term. What do you do now to protect your health?'

[This interview can continue exploring Muhammad's thoughts and behaviours and develop the discrepancy. By summarising and providing the right information for his stage of change, Muhammad can consider moving to the next stage of behaviour change - Determination.]

Points for reflection

- Motivational interviewing does not have to be provided by a psychologist or therapist. If a health professional works within the care and treatment of LTCs, it is worth exploring training options in motivational interviewing. This will add to the overall care package and help to consider working at the pace of the patient.

- Exploring his resentment of the disease will be necessary. This will be the key to progress and should be given a priority. Once accepting his situation, Muhammad should find it easier to comply with his treatment and care. General counselling skills could assist, but motivational interviewing may help move the process along.

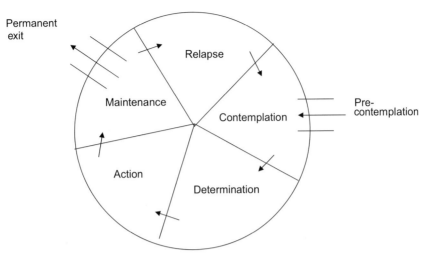

Figure 3.1   The stages of change. (Adapted from Prochaska and DiClemente, 1982).

Essentially, there are four broad guiding principles that underlie motivational interviewing. These are more specific for greater understanding in practice, compared with the general spirit described in the three areas above. The principles are:

1. *Express empathy*: Empathic communication is employed from the beginning and throughout the process. Through skilful reflective listening, the counsellor seeks to understand the client's feelings and perspectives without judging, criticizing or blaming.
2. *Develop discrepancy*: A person who presents with health-threatening behaviours can be helped to change behaviour. The interview will be intentionally directed towards the resolution of ambivalence. A discrepancy needs to be created and amplified between a present behaviour and the person's broader goal. When a behaviour is seen as conflicting with important personal goals (such as health), change is more likely to occur.
3. *Roll with resistance*: Advocating for change whilst the client argues against it is counterproductive and may press them into the opposite direction. Resistance that the person offers can be turned or reframed to create a new momentum towards change. Reluctance and ambivalence are not opposed but acknowledged as natural and understandable.
4. *Support self-efficacy*: This refers to a person's belief in their own ability. Enhance the client's confidence in their own capability to cope with obstacles and succeed in change. The person not only can but also must make the change themselves.
   Source: Adapted from Miller and Rollnick (2002).

The following explanation of the stages of change (Figure 3.1) is an appraisal of the explanation found in Miller and Rollnick (1991).

The stages of change recognise that each slip or relapse brings the client closer to recovery. Do not encourage relapse, but be realistic. Different skills are required for each stage, i.e. working in contemplation versus action. Resistance occurs when the therapist is using strategies inappropriate for a client's current stage of change.

Section 1

In *pre-contemplation*, raise doubt. Increase client's perception of risk and problems with current behaviour. Offer information and perhaps a card/telephone contact.

When the person is in *contemplation*, tip the balance, evoke reasons for change and strengthen the client's self-efficacy. They might say:

- 'I don't think I have a problem ... no more than my friends.'
- 'Sometimes I worry, but I can't stop.'
- 'I can stop or start whenever I want to.'

Help the client in *determination* to determine the best course of action to take in seeking change. They may say:

- 'I've got to do something about the problem.'
- 'This is serious! Something has to change.'
- 'What can I do?'
- 'How can I change?'

In *action* stage, help the client to take steps towards change. This is what people associate with therapy. Engage in actions to bring about change. The goal during this stage is to produce a change in problem area.

In *maintenance*, help the client to identify and use strategies to prevent relapse, sustain the change accomplished by previous action and prevent relapse where possible.

When relapse occurs, renew the process without becoming stuck and do not get disheartened. The client is to start around the wheel again. Remember that slips and relapses are normal and can happen several times before maintenance is achieved. Avoid discouragement.

Summary

In the treatment for depression section, consideration of the role of medication has been examined. As prescribing is now a key element in the role of many healthcare professionals, this provides clear guidance of what is available. Non-medical treatment options such as alternative therapies, group work and psychological therapies are considered. Case studies explore the impact of some of these interventions.

Conclusion

This chapter has considered depression and its co-morbid relationship with LTCs. A definition of depression has been identified through the ICD-10 and the basis for understanding its context to the person with an LTC has been explored. Various case examples are used to help illustrate a connection between theory and practice through the application of various therapies or treatments. The prevalence of depression with LTCs in general and specifically has been highlighted. Anti-depressants,

CBT and motivational interviewing have been explored in some detail to help health professionals understand the treatment necessary to overcome such a debilitating illness.

References

Ahmed, W. and Bradby, H. (eds) (2008) *Ethnicity, Health and Health Care: Understanding Diversity, Tackling Disadvantage*. Oxford: Blackwell Science.

Anderson, R. et al. (2001) The prevalence of comorbid depression in adults with diabetes: a meta-analysis. *Diabetes Care* **24**, 1069-1078.

Banks, S. and Kerns, R. (1996) Explaining high rates of depression in chronic pain: a diathesis-stress framework. *Psychological Bulletin* **199** (1), 95-110.

Barker, P. (2004) *Assessment in Psychiatric and Mental Health Nursing: In Search of the Whole Person*. Cheltenham: Nelson Thornes.

Beck, A., Ward, C., Mendelson, M., Mock, J. and Erbaugh, J. (1961) An inventory to measure depression. *Archives of General Psychiatry* **4**, 561-71.

Beck, A. et al. (1974) The measurement of pessimism: the hopelessness scale. *Journal of Consulting and Clinical Psychology* **42** (6), 861-865.

Benison, L. (2009) Quality of life: the key to care for long-term conditions [Meeting Report]. *Practice Nursing* **20** (8), 418-419.

Boehm, G., Racoosin, J., Laughren, T. and Kate, R. (2004) Consensus development conference on antipsychotic drugs and obesity and diabetes: response to consensus statement. *Diabetes Care* **27** (8), 2088.

British National Formulary (2010a) Available at: http://bnf.org/bnf/bnf/current/3295.htm (accessed 3 February 2010).

British National Formulary (2010b) Available at: http://bnf.org/bnf/bnf/current/3351.htm (accessed 3 February 2010).

British National Formulary (2010c) Available at: http://bnf.org/bnf/bnf/current/3358.htm (accessed 3 February 2010).

British National Formulary (2010d) Available at: http://bnf.org/bnf/bnf/current/27102.htm (accessed 3 February 2010).

Care Services Improvement Partnership (CSIP) (2006) *Long-Term Conditions and Depression: Considerations for Best Practice in Practice Based Commissioning*. London: CSIP.

Davies, S., Jackson, P., Potokar, J. and Nutt, D. (2004) Treatment of anxiety and depressive disorders in patients with cardiovascular disease. *BMJ* **328**, 939-943.

Denny, E. and Earle, S. (eds) (2009) Chronic illness, disability and the politics of health. In: *The Sociology of Long-Term Conditions and Nursing Practice*. Basingstoke: Palgrave Macmillan.

Department of Health (DH) (2005) *Supporting People with Long Term Conditions: An NHS and Social Care Model to Support Local Innovation and Integration*. London: DH.

Department of Health (DH) (2007) *National Service Framework for Children Young People and Maternity Services: Children and Young People Who Are Ill: Standard 6*. London: DH.

Department of Health (DH) (2008) *Long-Term Conditions Positive Practice Guide*. London: DH.

Dickens, C., McGowan, L., Clark-Carter, D. and Creed, F. (2002) Depression in rheumatoid arthritis: a systematic review of the literature with meta-analysis. *Psychosomatic Medicine* **64**, 52-60.

Egan, G. (1998) *The Skilled Helper: A Problem-Management Approach to Helping*. Pacific Grove, CA: Brooks/Cole.

Egede, L. (2004) Effects of depression on work loss and disability bed days in individuals with diabetes. *Diabetes Care* **27** (7), 1751-1753.

Egede, L., Zheng, D. and Simpson, K. (2002) Co-morbid depression is associated with increased health care use and expenditures in individuals with diabetes. *Diabetes Care* **25**, 464-470.

Fernando, S. (2002) *Mental Health, Race and Culture,* 2nd edn. Basingstoke: Palgrave.

Frasure-Smith, N., Lespérance, F., Gravel, G., Masson, A., Juneau, M., Taljic, M. and Bourassa, M. (2000) Social support, depression and mortality during the first year after myocardial infarction. *Circulation* **101**, 1919-1924.

Furze, G., Donnison, J. and Lewin, R. (2008) *The Clinicians Guide to Chronic Disease Management for Long-Term Conditions: A Cognitive-Behavioural Approach.* Keswick: M&K Publishing.

Goldney, R., Phillips, P., Fisher, L. and Wilson, D. (2004) Diabetes, depression, and quality of life: a population study. *Diabetes Care* **27** (5), 1066-1070.

Grant, A., Mills, J., Mulhern, R. and Short, N. (2004) An introduction to the cognitive behavioural approach and why it is needed. In: A. Grant, J. Mills, R. Mulhern and N. Short (eds) *Cognitive Behavioural Therapy in Mental Health Care,* Chapter 1. London: Sage.

Greenberger, D. and Padesky, C.A. (1995) *Mind Over Mood: A Cognitive Therapy Treatment Manual for Clients.* New York: Guilford Press.

Haddad, M., Taylor, C. and Pilling, S. (2009a) Depression in adults with long-term conditions: 1. How to identify and assess symptoms. *Nursing Times* **105** (48), 14-17.

Haddad, M., Taylor, C. and Pilling, S. (2009b) Depression in adults with long-term conditions: 2. Antidepressant and psychological treatments. *Nursing Times* **105** (49-50), 20-23.

Healy, D. (2005) *Psychiatric Drugs Explained.* London: Churchill Livingstone.

Herrmann, N., Black, S.E., Lawrence, J., Szekely, C. and Szalai, J.P. (1998) The Sunnybrook Stroke Study: a prospective study of depressive symptoms and functional outcome. *Stroke* **29**, 618-624.

Heslop, K. and Foley, T. (2009) Using cognitive-behavioural therapy to address the psychological needs of patients with COPD. *Nursing Times* **105**, 38.

Heslop, K., De Soyza, A., Baker, C., Stenton, C. and Burns, G. (2009) Using individualised cognitive-behavioural therapy as a treatment for people with COPD. *Nursing Times* **105**, 14.

Hettema, J., Steele, J. and Miller, W.R. (2005) Motivational interviewing. *Annual Review of Clinical Psychology* **1**, 91-111.

Holisticonline. Available at: http://www.holisticonline.com/remedies/Depression/dep_home.htm (accessed 17 March 2010).

Hopkins, C. and Niemiec, S. (2005) Crisis resolution/home treatment. In: R. Tummey (ed) *Planning Care in Mental Health Nursing.* Basingstoke: Palgrave Macmillan.

Kaptein, A., Scharloo, M., Fischer, M., Snoei, L. and Weinman, J. (2009) Chronic obstructive pulmonary disease. In: S. Newman, L. Steed and K. Mulligan (eds) *Chronic Physical Illness: Self-Management and Behavioural Interventions.* Maidenhead: Open University Press.

Katon, W. (2003) Clinical and health services relationships between major depression, depressive symptoms, and general medical illness. *Biological Psychiatry* **54** (3), 216-226.

Katz, P. and Yelin, E. (1993) Prevalence and correlates of depressive symptoms among persons with rheumatoid arthritis. *Journal of Rheumatology* **20** (5), 790-796.

Keltner, N. and Folks, D. (2005) *Psychotropic Drugs.* St Louis: Elsevier/Mosby.

Kubler-Ross, E. (1973) *On Death and Dying.* London: Routledge.

Layard, R. (2004) Mental health: Britain's biggest social problem. In: *Long-Term Conditions and Depression: Considerations for Best Practice in Practice Based Commissioning.* London: Care Services Improvement Partnership.

Layard, R. (2005) *Happiness – Lessons from a New Science.* London: Penguin.

Lockyer, L. (2009) Coronary heart disease: moving from acute to long-term accounts. In: E. Denny and S. Earle (ed) *The Sociology of Long Term Conditions and Nursing Practice.* Basingstoke: Palgrave Macmillan.

Lustman, P., Anderson, R., Freedland, K., De Groot, M., Carney, R. and Clouse, R. (2000) Depression and poor glycemic control: a meta-analytic review of the literature. *Diabetes Care* **23** (7), 934-942.

Major Depressive Disorder (2010) Available at: http://www.mentalhealth.com/icd/p22-md01.html (accessed 24 August 2010).

Mallinson, S. and Popay, J. (2008) Describing depression: ethnicity and the use of somatic imagery in accounts of mental distress. In: W.I.U. Ahmad and H. Bradby (eds) *Ethnicity, Health and Healthcare: Understanding Diversity, Tackling Disadvantage.* Oxford: Blackwell Science.

May, M., McCarron, P., Stansfield, S., Ben-Schlomo, Y., Gallacher, J., Yarnell, J., Smith, G., Elwood, P. and Ebrahim, S. (2002) Does psychological distress predict the risk of ischaemic stroke and transient ischaemic attack? The Caerphilly Study. *Stroke* **33**, 7-12.

Miller, W. and Rollnick, S. (2002) *Motivational Interviewing: Preparing People for Change*, 2nd edn. New York: Guilford Press.

Miller, W. and Rollnick, S. (1991) *Motivational Interviewing: Preparing People to Change Addictive Behaviour*. New York: Guilford Press.

Mitchell, A., Denny, E. and Earle, S. (2009) Social perspectives of depression. In: E. Denny and S. Earle (eds) *The Sociology of Long-Term Conditions and Nursing Practice*. Basingstoke: Palgrave Macmillan.

Nemeroff, C. and Mussleman, D. (2000) Are platelets the link between depression and ischaemic heart disease. *American Heart Journal* **104** (4 suppl.), 57-62.

Newman, S., Steed, L. and Mulligan, K. (2009) *Chronic Physical Illness: Self-Management and Behavioural Interventions*. Maidenhead: Open University Press.

NIAMH (2010) Available at: http://beacon-ni.org/dispfactsheet.php?parent=Informationandsubmenu= Mental%20Health%20statisticsandid=30 (accessed 30 April 2010).

NICE (2009a) *Treating Depression in Adults*. London: National Institute for Health and Clinical Excellence.

NICE (2009b) *Treating Depression in Adults with a Long-Term Physical Health Problem*. London: National Institute for Health and Clinical Excellence.

Ormell, J. and Von Korff, M. (2000) Synchrony of change in depression and disability. *Archives of General Psychiatry* **57**, 381-382.

Park, H., Hong, Y., Lee, H., Ha, E. and Sung, Y. (2004) Individuals with type 2 diabetes and depressive symptoms exhibited lower adherence with self-care. *Journal of Clinical Epidemiology* **57** (9), 978-984.

Parker, J. and Hart, E. (2009) Rheumatoid arthritis. In: S. Newman, L. Steed and K. Mulligan (eds) *Chronic Physical Illness: Self-Management and Behavioural Interventions*. Maidenhead: Open University Press.

Prince, M. et al. (2007) No health without mental health. *Lancet* **370**, 859-877.

Prochaska, J. and DiClemente, C. (1982) Transtheoretical therapy: toward a more integrative model of change. *Psychotherapy: Theory, Research, and Practice* **19**, 276-288.

Roberts, D. and Whitehead, L. (2005) Mental health liaison. In: R. Tummey (ed) *Planning Care in Mental Health Nursing*. Basingstoke: Palgrave Macmillan.

Rollnick, S., Mason, P. and Butler, C. (1999) *Health Behaviour Change: A Guide for Practitioners*. London: Churchill Livingstone.

Rollnick, S., Miller, W.R. and Butler, C. (2008) *Motivational Interviewing in Health Care: Helping Patients Change Behaviour*. New York: Guilford Press.

Rozanski, A., Blumenthal, J. and Kaplan, J. (1999) Impact of psychological factors on the pathogenesis of cardiovascular disease and implications for therapy. *Circulation* **99**, 2192-2217.

Rubak, S., Sandbek, A., Lauritzen, T. and Christensen B. (2005) Motivational interviewing: a systematic review and meta-analysis. *British Journal of General Practice* **55**(April), 305-312.

Scottish Government (2007) Increasing the availability of evidence-based psychological therapies in Scotland: Phase 1. Plan. Scotland: Scottish Government.

Scottish Government (2010) Available at: http://www.scotland.gov.uk/Topics/Statistics/Browse/Health/TrendMentalHealth (accessed 30 April 2010).

Sharpe, L., Allard, S. and Sensky, T. (2008) Five year follow up of a cognitive-behavioural intervention for patients with recently diagnosed rheumatoid arthritis: effects on health care utilization. *Arthritis Care and Research* **59** (3), 311-316.

Stage, K., Middleboe, T. and Pisinger, C. (2003) Measurement of depression in patients with chronic obstructive pulmonary disease (COPD). *Nordic Journal of Psychiatry* **57**, 297-301.

Stenager, E., Madsen, C., Stenager, E. and Boldsen, J. (1998) Suicide in patients with stroke: an epidemiological study. *British Medical Journal* **316**, 1206.

Strickland, P., Deakin, J., Pervical, C., Dixon, J., Gater, R.A. and Goldberg, D.P. (2002) Bio-social origins of depression in the community: interactions between social adversity, cortisol and serotonin neurotransmission. *British Journal of Psychiatry* **180**, 168-173.

Section 1

Townend, M. (2008) A case study and formulation of chronic depression in a client with high self-criticism. In: A. Grant, M. Townend, J. Mills and A. Cockx (eds) *Assessment and Case Formulation in Cognitive Behavioural Therapy*, p. 204. London: Sage.

Townend, M. and Grant, A. (2008) Assessment in CBT: the ideographic approach. In: A. Grant, M. Townend, J. Mills and A. Cockx (eds) *Assessment and Case Formulation in Cognitive Behavioural Therapy*, p. 8. London: Sage.

Tummey, R. and Smojkis, M. (2005) Primary mental health care. In: R. Tummey (ed.) Planning Care in Mental Health Nursing. Basingstoke: Palgrave Macmillan.

Tylee, A. and Haddad, M. (2007) Managing complex problems: treatment for common mental disorders in the UK. *Epideliologaie e Psychiatra Sociale* **16** 302-308. In: Haddad, M., Taylor, C., Pilling, S. (2009) Depression in adults with long-term conditions: 1. How to identify and assess symptoms. *Nursing Times* **105**(48), 14-17.

Williams, R., Barefoot, J., Califf, R., Haney, T., Saunders, W., Pryor, D., Hlatky, M., Siegler, I. and Mark, D. (1992) Prognostic importance of social and economical resources among medically treated patients with angiographically documented coronary artery disease. *Journal of the American Medical Association* **267**, 520-524.

Wright, G., Parker, J., Smarr, K., Johnson, J., Hewett, J. and Walker, S.E. (1998) Age, depressive symptoms, and rheumatoid arthritis. *Arthritis and Rheumatism* **41** (2), 298-305.

Zigmond, A. and Snaith, R. (1983) The Hospital Anxiety and Depression Scale. *Acta Psychiatrica Scandinavica* **67**, 361-370.

Further reading

Denny, E. and Earle, S. (eds) (2009) *The Sociology of Long-Term Conditions and Nursing Practice*. Basingstoke: Palgrave Macmillan.

Section 2

Empowerment

Chapter 4

Adaptation in Long-term Conditions: The Role of Stigma Particularly in Conditions that Affect Appearance

Andrew R Thompson

Learning objectives

By the end of this chapter, the reader will be able to:

- Understand the psychological impacts associated with living with a long-term condition (LTC) affecting appearance
- Understand the social threat of oppression faced by those living with an LTC affecting appearance and have an understanding of the process of stigmatisation
- Understand the high level of individual variability in adjustment and the limited relationship between adjustment and biomedical factors
- Have an awareness of some of the key psychological, social, and cultural factors that have been found to account for adjustment
- Feel more confident in assessing for the presence of such factors and be aware of interventions available to both facilitate psychological adjustment and empower people in managing their own lives

---

Introduction

This chapter explores the concept of adaptation in relation to LTCs. Clearly, the occurrence of a chronic condition as outlined in Section 1 of this book can have a significant impact across all areas of a person's life not only affecting the physical, but the relational and emotional aspects as well. Put simply, a new type of life might need to be built, and the process by which this occurs is called

---

adaptation. Adaptation is often confused with adjustment. Adjustment refers to the outcome of the process and has been used to describe a successful end point (see Miller Smedema et al. 2009 for a fuller discussion). What actually constitutes successful adjustment has been widely discussed and debated, and many doubt that adaptation is a simple linear process (Thompson and Kent 2001 Thompson and Broom 2009). Indeed, LTCs by their very nature tend to involve continued changes in health and functioning, and in any event almost always require ongoing engagement with both internal psychological processes and external factors in order to maintain well-being.

This chapter primarily focuses upon conditions that have a disfiguring or appearance-altering effect although most of the issues discussed will also be applicable to other types of LTCs. It begins by briefly revisiting the range of psychosocial impacts that can be experienced by those living with an LTC. It goes on to describe the high degree of individual variation found in relation to both the presence and severity of such impacts. It discusses the role played by psychological, social, and cultural variables in accounting for individual variation in adjustment. The relevance of theoretical perspectives on stigma and related concepts of shame are discussed. The chapter demonstrates how interventions can facilitate adaptation and reduce stigmatisation, and the overall emphasis is upon empowerment. Finally, the chapter makes practical suggestions for clinical practice.

LTC, Visible difference, disfigurement and body-image

Body image

Body image has been utilised as a term to capture a variety of constructs, most of which have relevance to many living with LTCs. Pruzinsky and Cash (2002) in their overview of the historical development of the concept describe how early research in this area focused almost entirely at a neurological level, and was concerned with how body movement and posture were controlled. They detail how a bio-psychosocial view of body image emerged within the work of Schilder who described body image as 'the picture of our own body which we form in our own mind' (Schilder 1935, p. 11, as cited by Pruzinsky and Cash 2002, p. 7). Yet Pruzinsky and Cash point out that this simple definition does not capture the modern multidimensionality of the concept which has been used to explore rarefied concepts as diverse as size perception accuracy and body satisfaction, to name but a few.

Given the array of complex conceptual areas that have been considered under the heading of body image, it is not surprising that it has been suggested that the term 'body image' is unhelpful without specification as to the nature of the actual area or concept being discussed (Fisher 1990, Thompson and Kent 2001, p. 667). This chapter focuses on 'disfigurement', which can be thought of as part of the perception of appearance aspect of body image. The perception of the person living with a disfigurement and the perception of others are equally important in the adaptation process, as we shall see as we progress through the chapter.

Disfigurement and visible difference

Disfigurement itself is not easily defined and some people do not like the term as it may be equated with negativity. Further, the term may be particularly unhelpfully applied when it is not perceived as a relevant concern for the actual person himself or herself, regardless of whether their condition affects their appearance (*note disfigurement is in the eye of the beholder*). An alternative term, 'visible difference' has been used by some (see Harcourt and Rumsey 2008) although this term is also problematic as it can be used to refer to almost anything. The UK charity Changing Faces (www.changingfaces.org.uk), which is concerned with improving quality of life and empowering people living with a disfigurement, recommends, where possible, using the correct medical name for the causative underlying condition as this promotes understanding. However, it does also recommend the use of the term disfigurement for its succinct and generic qualities. The term is also used in British law in the Disability Discrimination Act (DDA: 1995, now superseded by the Equality Act 2010) and, therefore, has the potential to be used to seek redress when discrimination has occurred. Changing Faces point out that the word is better used as a noun and best avoided as an adjective (*i.e. a 'person who has a disfigurement' rather than 'a disfigured person'*).

The prevalence of conditions affecting appearance

A significant number of LTCs have either a direct or indirect effect upon appearance; for example, skin conditions such as psoriasis and neurofibromatosis, and vitiligo noticeably affect the appearance of the skin, rheumatoid arthritis can alter the shape as well as the functioning of limbs, and neurological conditions such as stroke and Parkinson's disease can alter appearance through palsy and loss of functioning. Surgical treatment for diseases such as cancer can cause significant alterations in appearance (for example mastectomy and treatment for head and neck cancer). Many types of traumatically acquired injuries (for example burns, limb loss, spinal and head injuries) can also be arguably viewed as LTCs and such injuries often lead to sudden alterations in appearance.

In 2007, Changing Faces conducted an epidemiological study reported in their 'Face Equality Campaign' (Changing Faces 2010) that indicates that 542,000 (or 'one in 111') people in the United Kingdom have a facial disfigurement; the number rises to 1,345,000 (or 'one in 44') if significant disfigurements affecting the body are also included. Whilst a significant number of people will either be living with a disfigurement resulting from a congenital condition (such as a cleft lip/palate), Changing Faces estimate that a significant number will result from LTCs or from an accident (see Table 4.1).

> ### Summary
>
> In summary, many LTCs lead to alterations in appearance. The term body image has been applied to many different areas and it is preferable to use a less generic term to reflect the precise concerns of an individual. Whilst disfigurement is a useful term, succinctly describing an objective change in appearance, applicable to many living with an LTC, it is also not a very positive word, and it is important in practice to use the specific medical term or preferably to find a term that the individual is comfortable with themselves. It also follows that a good assessment of an individual's needs should sensitively explore the impact of the condition on the perception of appearance, and it is to this area we shall now turn.

Psychosocial, social and cultural impact of living with an LTC affecting appearance

Social impacts

Individuals living with visible LTCs often report encountering intrusive and sometimes discriminatory reactions from others (Thompson and Kent 2001, Rumsey and Harcourt 2004). Many experimental and observational studies have demonstrated that there is a reality to these reactions with people

Table 4.1   The Changing Faces estimated prevalence and incidence of disfigurement as related to cancer treatment and paralysis.

	Number of face and body disfigurement	Number of facial disfigurements	Annual cases of facial disfigurements
Cancer treatments			
Skin	75,000	15,000	37,500
Head and neck	16,000	16,000	8,000
Eye conditions			
Loss of eye, squints	25,000	25,000	10,000
Paralysis			
Bell's palsy	40,000	40,000	12,000
Stroke	60,000	60,000	140,000
Accidental causes			
Burns	60,000	12,000	2,000
Scarring and fractures	360,000	54,000	18,000
Skin conditions			
Acne and eczema	125,000	104,000	125,000
Epidermolysis bullosa and neurofibromatosis	28,000	14,000	2,000
Psoriasis	262,500	78,750	30,000
Vitiligo	75,000	22,500	20,000
Total (includes congenital conditions not shown)	1,345,000	542,250	415,550

Source: Adapted from information available on www.changingfaces.co.uk.

offering less help to actors made up to look as if they had a disfiguring condition (for example Bull and Stevens 1981; for a full account of studies in this area see Rumsey and Harcourt 2005). The reactions experienced by people can be extremely abusive and it is not uncommon for children living with LTCs to report being bullied (Frances 2004) as described below in Case study 4.1.

Case study 4.1   Child with severe eczema (From Thompson and Worthington 2007)

Talking about school experiences, she said:
   "They'd call me names because of it, 'scabby fish cake', what they called me because my skin's quite scaly."

Points for reflection

- What would your reactions be if you experienced such 'bullying'?
- What would your reaction be if your child experienced such bullying?

It is not surprising that being subjected to such reactions can cause severe acute distress and may also impact upon long-term psychological and family functioning. We will return to this shortly when the psychological impact is discussed (Thompson and Kent 2001).

Cultural impacts

It is somewhat artificial to separate out cultural impacts from wider social impacts; however, it is important to be aware that beliefs about illness are linked to psychosocial adjustment and there is some evidence that such beliefs vary according to culture and ethnicity. For example, even the well-known appearance stereotype of Dion, Berscheid and Walster (1972: the phenomenon of attributing positive characteristics to those viewed as attractive) has been shown to be influenced by cultural values in relation to both what aspects of appearance are valued and what constitutes positive characteristics (Eagly et al. 1991).

There has generally been a dearth of studies that have explored cultural issues in relation to disfigurement but as Case study 4.2 below shows there is clearly a need to sensitively explore these issues with people.

Case study 4.2 Young British Asian Woman with Vitiligo (from Thompson et al. 2010)

A young British Asian woman discusses one of the impacts of living with vitiligo:
"... once we had this huge argument ... when my mum just said, well who's going to marry you with your skin like that, because a lot of arranged marriages are pretty much based on looks and like status."

Point for reflection

- What might the psychosocial impact be of this perception of the value of appearance?

Thompson et al. (2010) conducted a qualitative study to explore the ways in which British Asian women adapt to vitiligo. Their participants described feeling visibly different and reported experiencing stigmatisation to some extent and avoidance and concealment were commonly used as methods of coping, as has been reported by other groups (Thompson et al. 2002). However, for some the experience of stigmatisation was often perceived to be associated with subtle cultural values related to appearance, status, and myths linked to the cause of the condition. The condition was perceived as impacting upon social acceptability and influencing the prospect of marriage. Cultural nuances as to how stigmatisation operates have recently been reported by studies exploring community views on disfigurement (Hughes et al. 2009). This is an important area, not least because of its influence upon social support, which has been reported time and again to play a crucial role in adaptation to almost all LTCs (for a useful summary see Chronister 2009).

Section 2

Psychological impacts

Thompson and Kent (2001) have written that: 'given the reality of negative reactions directed at people with disfigurements, it is not surprising that many individuals experience higher than average levels of psychological distress' (p. 666). However, they also point out that what is crucial is the way these reactions are perceived, internalised, and managed (which will be further considered below). The predominant difficulties reported by people include higher levels of depression, anxiety (particularly social anxiety), and shame and lower levels of self-esteem. For example, Rumsey et al. (2002) found high levels of anxiety, depression and lower quality of life in up to half of their sample of 650 people attending outpatient appointments for treatment of a range of disfiguring conditions. Often people will have multiple concerns (as one might expect with the issues associated with living with an LTC) and a thorough individual assessment is always required as is suggested by the fictitious examples based on clinical referral to the author shown below in Case study 4.3.

> **Case study 4.3** Typical problems associated with referral for psychological therapy (all names reported are pseudonyms)
>
> Example 1
> David has acne and also a stoma following surgery to treat Crohn's disease; he is depressed and rarely leaves the house. He was bullied at school in relation to both his gastric condition and later his acne. He sees himself as 'disgusting' and is unable to see how is life could be different without resolution of his medical conditions. He feels suicidal and is desperate, and the referral indicates urgent support is required although he is ambivalent about discussing his feelings and coping strategies.
>
> Example 2
> Shirley has had a stroke. She is making a good recovery and is very engaged in rehabilitation yet berates her own progress. She has lost muscle tone since the stroke and has some palsy. She is finding emotional and physical intimacy difficult, and complains that she's now 'old and ugly'. The rehabilitation team are concerned that she may become depressed once their input is complete and would like additional support in managing this situation.
>
> Example 3
> Bill is in his early 50s and is recovering from an upper gastrointestinal cancer and has lost a significant amount of weight. He states that he no longer feels like a 'proper bloke' and avoids meeting his old friends. He has also lost his libido, anticipating that his wife sees him as unattractive. He's not sure how things could change but recognises he needs to do something differently as he is tempted to start drinking. He has discussed this with his consultant who has referred him for help in 'improving his coping strategies'.
>
> Example 4
> Joel suffered an industrial accident that left him with severe crush injuries to his leg that was eventually amputated. The rehabilitation team report that he is 'demotivated' and hostile. He has stopped socialising and ended the relationship he had. He says he is furious towards his employer as he believes the accident could have been prevented. He has flashbacks to the accident itself which trigger rumination as to how his appearance has 'changed for the worse'. He's happy to be seen as part of his compensation claim but sceptical as to how psychological intervention might help.

Example 5

Shauna has had cancer of the mouth and had extensive reconstructive surgery. She does have some facial scarring and palsy, and she now feels less attractive to her partner and feels unable to continue to associate with her friends who 'always talk about appearance'. She says her mood fluctuates between rage and sadness. She is really keen to talk about how she feels having had a prior experience of counselling and has asked for a referral.

Points for reflection

- What factors might present barriers to people seeking assistance with psychological issues?
- How might we facilitate people to engage with psychological interventions?

As can be seen from the examples above, many of the psychological issues people present with share similarities that go well beyond disease-specific issues and over-focus on the specific disease may lead to some of these issues being missed. Also evident from the examples discussed in Case study 4.3 is that a large number of people living with LTCs will be reluctant to discuss their psychological needs. This can result from a variety of reasons:

- There can be stigma associated with being seen to be 'not coping'.
- There can be a lack of awareness as to what forms of psychological support and intervention are available and how these might help.
- There can be an expectation that only physical/medical intervention can resolve the issues.
- The psychological issues themselves may present a barrier (for example depression-related hopelessness, anxiety-related fears of being judged, self-esteem-related sense of the issues not being important enough to trouble professionals with).
- Service-related issues including an environment that socialises patients into discussing only medical issues.

The above list is not exhaustive but covers many of the main concerns of people. It is important that nurses and healthcare professionals, in general, inquire into psychological well-being, as doing this raises the acceptability of disclosing such issues and such disclosure may be a sufficient intervention in its own right for some patients. There is no substitute for directly asking about mood and the concerns of the patient, and this of course should be part of routine nursing and allied healthcare professional practice. In addition, there are now lots of condition specific and general questionnaires that can provide a quick and standardised picture of mood and quality of life. The Derriford Appearance Scale is one such scale, and whilst not commonly used, provides an excellent short measure of appearance concern (Carr et al. 2005, see Carr 2002, for discussion of other measures relevant to assessing appearance concerns).

Routine provision of information about typical psychological issues can be easily incorporated into patient information packs and be available in clinics – this can serve to normalise psychological reactions. Many charities produce excellent disease specific and more general information and

Section 2

signposting patients towards such information can be useful (see the 'Further information' section at the end of this chapter). Having access to psychological consultation can assist nurses and other healthcare professionals in establishing and maintaining psychosocial assessment and intervention skills. Clear care pathways for referral on for further psychological assessment and intervention are also essential, and access to such additional support should ideally be presented as being part of the multi-disciplinary approach, so as to reduce the risk of stigmatisation often associated with referral to 'mental health services' (Thompson, 2009).

Positive adjustment and individual variation

One of the problems with much of the literature on adjustment to LTCs and disfigurement is that there has been a focus on exploring negative functioning and in doing so this has inadvertently highlighted the difficulties people can experience, and this may serve to unwittingly contribute to marginalisation and disempowerment. Whilst it is of course essential to acknowledge the sorts of difficulties described above, it is also important to recognise that the majority of people adapt (Taylor and Aspinwall 1996). Providing people with this information can in itself be empowering (if it is done in a manner that avoids conveying the message that *they should be coping*). The account contained in Case study 4.4 below is not an untypical description of adaptation (Ms Romanay provides a fuller account of her experience on the webpages of The Vitiligo Society www.vitiligosociety.org.uk).

> **Case study 4.4** Gurdeep Romanay successfully living with the skin condition vitiligo (excerpt reproduced with the permission of Ms Gurdeep and The Vitiligo Society www.vitiligosociety.org.uk)
>
> 'Vitiligo affects people in so many different ways – be it mentally, emotionally or cosmetically. One thing which it has taught me though is to love the person you are. I have tried many different treatments, some have worked, others have made it worse. It is very easy to try and hide the patches and cover it up with make up. This is what I did for a while and it made me feel so much worse as I felt as if I was leading a double life. I shut out people closest to me for a while and kept the pain to myself. I turned it around though by talking to my friends and family. They reminded me that they did not even see the patches on me as they knew me for me – not someone who has white patches on their skin. Suffering on your own is not the answer. It is very easy to hide away from the condition and to try and cover it up but that just makes it worse'.
>
> ### Points for reflection
> - What factors are described that may have helped adaptation?
> - What factors are described that may have hindered adjustment?

Only recently has research started to actively explore positive and protective factors. Meyerson (2001), for example, interviewed people with moebius syndrome (a condition associated with facial paresis) and identified several psychosocial factors including, humour and faith, as being linked to positive adjustment. Similarly, Lobeck et al. (2005) interviewed men who had had a stroke and reported that although they initially felt different about their appearance they developed a variety of strategies including humour to manage this. Saradjian et al. (2008) found in their study with men who had lost an arm as a result of trauma or disease, that the men were coping well and employing a range of strategies to minimise distress. Thompson et al. (2002) interviewed women living with vitiligo and found that they had spontaneously developed coping skills akin to the sorts of strategies taught in psychological therapy such as tackling avoidance as described above in Case study 4.3. They also commented on how their participants reported that maintaining stability required effort and recently, Thompson and Broom (2009) have found similar findings with participants living with a range of disfigurements. However, what is clear is that a large number of people adapt and ascertaining how they do so is a crucial issue for research in order to inform future interventions.

Summary

In summary, the impact of living with an LTC can be wide ranging influencing psychological, social, and cultural life. The presence of high levels of psychological distress is reported in some studies, yet many if not the majority of people achieve a good degree of satisfactory adjustment. Clearly, the presence of the psychosocial and cultural issues described above need to be routinely assessed for and clear care-pathways need to be in place. As Pruzinsky (1992) has stated people with a disfiguring condition face two challenges: dealing with their own emotional responses to the condition, and dealing with the response of others. One connecting theoretical concept joining the psychological, social and cultural is the concept of stigmatisation, and it is to this we shall now turn.

Stigmatisation and LTCs

Erving Goffman (1963) described stigma as mark that designates the affected person as 'spoiled' and, therefore, less valued than others. Stigmatisation as a process for Goffman was essentially a relational one and put very simply is socially constructed. Goffman's work is still important today and all modern accounts of stigmatisation are built on his theory (see Scambler 2009). In their seminal research on epilepsy, Scambler and Hopkins (1986) proposed the distinction between 'enacted' and 'felt' stigma. They describe enacted stigma as *actual* rejection of a person as a result of their condition, and compared this to felt stigma, stated as an individual's expectation that they *might* be subject to stigmatisation. This can lead to the person concealing to avoid enacted stigma, which can be useful in the short term but maintain distress in the long term (Scambler and Hopkins 1986, Jacoby 1994). This theory goes a long way to accounting for the high levels of avoidance coping reported by people living with LTCs and has now been supported by a huge number of studies (Falkner 2006).

Kent (2002, 2005) and Kent and Thompson (2002) present models of disfigurement, in which it is suggested that stigmatisation is a central aspect of the disfigurement experience, and is a consequence of the interaction between the objective 'medical condition' and 'social norms' (i.e. the judgements that individuals and groups may make about disfigurement in the light of social rules about normality and deviance: Falkner 2006, p. 3).

Section 2

Shame

The concept of stigma is closely related to the concept of shame. Goffman (1963) acknowledged that shame was the main effect implicated in stigma. Gilbert (1997) has argued that humans have an innate need to be perceived as attractive by others, and that shame and humiliation are associated with attacks on, and losses of, social attractiveness; this seems central to the process of stigmatisation (Kent and Thompson 2002). Indeed, Gilbert (2002) has coined the terms internal and external shame which bear many similarities to enacted and felt stigma. Thompson and Kent have posited that shame is likely to play a crucial role in disfigurement and have developed a model that describes how this might operate (Thompson 1998, Thompson and Kent 2001, Kent and Thompson 2002, Thompson 2003, Thompson 2005). They suggest that repeated experiences of being excluded, in the absence of social support, can lead to the development of beliefs of low worth in relation to appearance, which in turn are then associated with increased anxiety about social encounters, sensitivity to further rejections, and avoidance and concealment.

Summary

Stigmatisation theory can assist in making sense of why people living with LTCs might become distressed and engage in behaviours such as avoidance which may hinder adaptation. More recent theories of shame consider how cognitive processes may operate to further hinder adaptation; however, further research is required to test these models. These models also suggest that there is a need for interventions that target not just the individual but consider the wider social context.

Psychosocial interventions

There are now many psychological interventions directly geared up to facilitate adaptation in LTCs (for excellent texts see Kennedy and Llewelyn 2006, and White 2001). However, as this chapter has primarily discussed disfigurement, we will now focus on the psychosocial interventions that have been developed to manage distress in this area. Interventions for people living with a disfigurement can be grouped into those, which focus on the individual (including social skills training, psychotherapy, and non-invasive physical interventions, such as cosmetic camouflage), and interventions that focus on the community. A variety of delivery methods or therapeutic formats have also been used including individual therapy, group therapy, and self-help.

Individual

Social skills training

Social skills training facilitates the development of competencies in managing social interactions, with the aim of increasing confidence and reducing anxiety. For the person living with a disfigurement, the acquisition of a set of skills that help them deal with intrusive reactions is likely to be highly empowering.

Rumsey et al. (1986) have experimentally tested whether people might be able to influence the impact of their disfigurement on others by the use of effective social skills. Participants rated people acting in four conditions: severely disfigured versus non-disfigured and competent versus incompetent social skills. Importantly, they found that participants' ratings were significantly more favourable towards the competent social skills condition, over and above the presence or absence of the disfigurement. Thus, indicating that effective social skills may indeed be able to counteract the effects of any immediate impact of disfigurement.

The earliest reported evaluation of social skills training was conducted by Fiegenbaum (1981) who assessed a ten-week group programme provided for head and neck cancer patients. The programme was reported as successful and focused on the development of specific skills such as initiating contact with other people. The charity Changing Faces has, for a number of years, been pioneering the development and use of social skills training and an evaluation of their social skills workshops suggested a significant decrease in self-reported social interaction problems, increased social confidence, and significant decreases in anxiety and social avoidance at six-weeks and at six-months follow-up (Robinson et al. 1996).

While social skills training might be effective, the existing studies have a number of methodological weaknesses, which prevent firm conclusions being drawn. In addition, it is difficult to know which part(s) of the approach(es) (which have included instruction, modelling, role-play, feedback and discussion) is(are) important, and the degree to which other elements, such as sharing experiences or feeling supported by professionals play a role.

Cognitive behavioural therapy (CBT)

CBT has been adapted by some with the specific aim of helping people change their beliefs about their appearance and their associated coping behaviours, particularly the use of avoidance (see Cash and Grant 1996). There are relatively few studies that have directly examined its applicability to disfiguring LTCs, but those that exist have supported its utility to some extent (Bessell and Moss 2007).

Papadopoulos et al. (1999) evaluated an individually delivered eight-session course of cognitive behavioural approach designed to assist people living with vitiligo. The intervention centred upon using positive self-talk following negative comments, and reframing staring as curiosity rather than rejection – both designed to manage the effects of stigmatisation. A significant improvement was reported in quality of life, self-esteem, body image distress and body image related negative automatic thoughts, compared to minimal changes in a waiting list control group, and this was maintained at five-months follow-up. The study had a small sample size, which limits confidence in the findings, and it failed to compare CBT with other treatments.

Kleve et al. (2002) evaluated the effectiveness of the three to six sessions of individual cognitive-behavioural intervention offered by the only NHS specialist clinic providing interventions for people with a disfigurement (Outlook: Frenchay Hospital, Bristol). The results suggested that CBT led to significant improvements in social anxiety, appearance-related distress, general anxiety and depression, which were maintained at follow-up. Participants also reported finding the intervention acceptable. Whilst the study lacked a control group, the findings are clearly promising.

Papadopoulos et al. (2004) conducted a further investigation into the effects of group CBT compared to another therapeutic approach (person-centred therapy), also delivered in a group format, as compared to a control group who did not receive an intervention. Both group therapies were reported as leading to improvements for patients Fortune et al. (2002, 2004) have also reported that group CBT can be useful for psoriasis patients. Whilst both Papadopoulos et al. (2004) and Fortune et al. (2002, 2004) studies indicated improvement with the interventions delivered, these studies that have looked at the efficacy of group interventions have a number of limitations (Bessell and Moss 2007).

Newell and Clarke (2000) conducted a randomised control trial of a CBT self-help leaflet targeting avoidance using simple techniques for managing anxiety. The results indicated that participants who received the leaflet benefited from it although the findings did not suggest that there had been large changes.

Camouflage

The potential to experience stigma may be reduced by the use of camouflage and this is available in a number of NHS clinics. Kent (2002) examined the effects of camouflage (provided by The British Red Cross, see www.redcross.org.uk) upon well-being and anxiety, in people with a range of dermatological conditions. The results suggested that the use of camouflage was associated with an increase in confidence and a reduction in avoidance; however, participants still reporting high levels of fear of negative evaluation and consequently camouflage may not address underlying fears of stigmatisation. Ongenae et al. (2005) have also examined the psychosocial benefit of camouflage in relation to supporting people in managing vitiligo. They reported significant improvement on a well-known dermatology measure of quality of life but they did not have any measure of underlying fear of negative evaluation.

Clearly, camouflage can be helpful in empowering people to overcome avoidance. However, little is known about its long-term effect, and several qualitative studies indicate that it may foster dependence and serve to maintain fear of negative evaluation (Thompson et al. 2002, 2010).

Systemic interventions

The interventions described above place emphasis on changing the appearance or the skills of the affected individual, and do not address the wider issues of stigmatisation in society. This is important, given that issues arising from disfigurements are as much a product of others' reactions and culturally defined expectations, as they are personal responses (Winchell and Watts 1988, cited in Falkner 2006).

Rachman (2001) has proposed a six-level anti-stigmatisation campaign. The six levels relate to the origins of stigma and are each associated with a specific type of intervention and include the following:

- *Cognitive:* Educational intervention
- *Affective:* Psychological intervention
- *Discrimination:* Legislative intervention
- *Denial:* Linguistic intervention
- *Economic:* Political intervention
- *Evolutionary*: Intellectual and cultural intervention

Rachman suggested that destigmatisation needs to address fundamental human tendencies and so anti-stigmatisation campaigns must be continuous, open-ended projects (Rachman 2001, as cited in Falkner 2006).

There are few studies that have attempted to address negative attitudes towards disfigurement. Cline (1998) attempted to change school children's attitudes towards children with visible differences, and Frances (2004) attempted to make schools more inclusive of children with visible differences. Recently, Changing Faces have run a web-based campaign based on the work of Grandfield et al.

(2005) whereby people can participate in a survey that reveals how one perceives disfigurement. The survey uses a test of implicit attitudes and relies on reaction speed and is likely to reveal that we have an automatic reaction to disfigurement. However, the results of this survey and the impact of it upon peoples' attitudes are yet to be revealed.

Summary

Bessell and Moss (2007) conducted a systematic review of the interventions available for individuals living with a disfigurement and reported that there was relatively little published research in the area, with them finding only twelve papers that met their inclusion criteria. Further, they found that the existing studies had a number of limitations, but nevertheless as we have seen above those studies that do exist show promise. Clearly, further work is needed to develop specific interventions and existing treatment approaches developed to assist in social anxiety are highly likely to be useful (Thompson and Kent 2001).

Conclusion

This chapter has reviewed adaptation to LTCs paying particular attention to conditions that affect appearance. Many of the issues discussed are directly transferable to other LTCs and indeed the concept of stigmatisation that has been discussed in detail here has been applied to many other conditions.

 The need to assess and intervene at both a psychological and social level has been outlined, and there are some simple techniques that can be applied to empower people to discuss their psychological needs. Further research is needed to elaborate the precise mechanisms by which adaptation becomes stuck and to evaluate new psychological therapies. Nonetheless, there is emerging evidence that many people living with an LTC, can benefit from psychological intervention.

Acknowledgements

I would like to thank Dr Lucy Broom *nee* Falkner, Clinical Psychologist, for her assistance in reviewing the literature on stigmatisation. I would also like to thank the anonymous and named individuals who gave permission for sensitive areas of their lives to be shared with others in the case studies that have been presented.

References

Bessell, A. and Moss, T. (2007) Evaluating the effectiveness of psychosocial interventions for individuals with visible differences: a systematic review of the empirical literature. *Body Image* **4**, 227-238.

Bull, R. and Stevens, J. (1981) The effects of facial disfigurement on helping behaviour. *Italian Journal of Psychology* **8**, 25-32.

Carr, A. (2002) Body shame issues of assessment and measurement. In: P. Gilbert and J. Miles (eds) *Understanding Body Shame*, pp. 90-102 Hove, UK: Brunner-Routledge.

Section 2

Carr, T., Moss, T. and Harris, D. (2005) The DAS24: a short form of the Derriford appearance scale DA59 to measure individual responses to living with problems of appearance. *British Journal of Health Psychology* **10**, 285-298.

Cash, T. and Grant, J. (1996) Cognitive-behavioural treatment of body image disturbances. In: V. Vanen and M. Hersen (eds) *Sourcebook of Psychological Treatment Manuals for Adult Disorders*, pp. 567-614. New York: Plenum Press.

Changing Faces (2010) The Face Equality Campaign - The Evidence Available at: www.Changingfaces.org.uk (accessed 03 April 2010).

Chronister, J. (2009) Social support and rehabilitation: theory, research and measurement. In: F. Chang, E. DaSilva Cardoso and J. A. Chronister (eds) *Understanding Psychosocial Adjustment to Chronic Illness and Disability: A Handbook for Evidence Based Practitioners in Rehabilitation*, pp. 149-184. New York: Springer.

Cline, T., Proto, A., Raval, P. and Di Paolo, T. (1998) The effects of brief exposure and of classroom teaching on attitudes children express towards facial disfigurement in peers. *Educational Research* **40**, 55-68.

Dion, K.K., Berscheid, E. and Walster, E. (1972) What is beautiful is good. *Journal of Personality and Social Psychology* **24**, 285-290.

Eagly, A., Ashmore, R., Makhijani, M. and Longo, L. (1991) What is beautiful is good but... A meta-analytic review of research on the physical attractiveness stereotype. *Psychological Bulletin* **110**, 109-128.

Falkner, L. (2006) What does the current literature tell us about the impact of stigma on people living with a visible difference? Unpublished literature review: University of Sheffield.

Fiegenbaum, W. (1981) A social training program for clients with facial disfigurations: a contribution to the rehabilitation of cancer patients. *International Journal of Rehabilitation Research* **4**, 501-509.

Fisher, S. (1990) The evolution of psychological concepts and the body. In: T.F. Cash and T. Pruzinsky (eds) *Body Images: Development, Deviance and Change*, pp. 3-20. New York: Guildford Press.

Fortune, D.G, Richards, H., Kirby, B., Bowcock, S., Main, C. and Griffiths, C. (2002) A cognitive-behavioural symptom management programme as an adjunct in psoriasis therapy. *British Journal of Dermatology* **146** (3), 458-465.

Fortune, D.G, Richards, H., Griffiths, C. and Main, C. (2004) Targeting cognitive-behavioural therapy to patient's implicit model of psoriasis: results from a patient preference controlled trial. *British Journal of Clinical Psychology* **43**, 65-82, part 1.

Frances, J. (2004) *Educating Children with Facial Disfigurement: Creating Inclusive School Communities*. London: Routledge Falmer.

Gilbert, P. (1997) The evolution of social attractiveness and its role in shame, humiliation, guilt and therapy. *British Journal of Medical Psychology* **70**, 113-147.

Gilbert P. (2002) Body shame a biopsychosocial conceptualisation and overview with treatment implications. In: P. Gilbert and J. Miles (eds) *Understanding Body Shame*, pp. 3-54. Hove, UK: Brunner-Routledge.

Goffman, E. (1963) *Stigma: Notes on the Management of a Spoiled Identity*. Englewood Cliffs, NJ: Prentice-Hall.

Grandfield, T., Thompson, A. R. and Turpin, G. (2005) An attitudinal study of responses to a range of dermatological conditions using the implicit attitudes association test. *Journal of Health Psychology* **10**, 821-829.

Great Britain Parliament (1995) *Disability Discrimination Act (Act of Parliament)*. London: HMSO.

Great Britain Parliament (2010) *The Equality Act (Act of Parliament)*. London: HMSO.

Harcourt, D. and Rumsey, N. (2008) Psychology and visible difference. *The Psychologist* **21**, 486-489.

Hughes, J., Naqvi, H., Saul, K., Williamson, H., Johnson, M.R.D., Rumsey, N., Charlton, R. and The Appearance Research Consortium (2009). South Asian community views about individuals with a disfigurement. *Diversity in Health and Care* **6**, 241-253.

Jacoby, A. (1994) Felt versus enacted stigma: a concept revisited. *Social Science and Medicine* **38** (2), 296-274.

Kent, G. (2002) Testing a model of disfigurement: effects of a skin camouflage service on well-being and appearance anxiety. *Psychology and Health* **17** (3), 377-386.

Kennedy, P. and Llewelyn, S. (2006) *The Essentials of Clinical Health Psychology*. Chichester, UK: Wiley.

Section 2

Kent, G. and Thompson, A. R. (2002) Models of disfigurement: implications for treatment. In: P. Gilbert and J. Miles (eds) *Understanding body shame*, 106–116. Hove, UK: Brunner-Routledge.

Kent, G. (2005) Stigmatisation and skin conditions. In: L. Papadopoulos and C. Walker (eds) *Psychodermatology: The Impact of Skin Disorders.* Cambridge, UK: Cambridge University Press.

Kleve, L., Rumsey, N., Wyn-Williams, M. and White, P. (2002) The effectiveness of cognitive-behavioural interventions provided at outlook: a disfigurement support unit. *Journal of Evaluation in Clinical Practice* **8** (4), 387–395.

Lobeck, M., Thompson, A. R. and Shankland, M. C. (2005) The importance of social context in adjustment: an exploration of the experience of stroke for men in retirement transition. *Qualitative Health Research* **15**, 1022–1036.

Meyerson, M.D. (2001). Resiliency and success in adults with moebius syndrome. *Cleft Palate Craniofacial Journal* **38**, 231–235.

Miller Smedema, S., Bakken Gillen, S. K. and Dalton, J. (2009). Psychosocial adaptation to chronic illness and disability: models and measurement. In: F. Chang, E. DaSilva Cardoso and J. A. Chronister (eds) *Understanding Psychosocial Adjustment to Chronic Illness and Disability: A Handbook for Evidence Based Practitioners in Rehabilitation*, 51–74. New York: Springer.

Newell, R. and Clarke, A. (2000) Evaluation of a self-help leaflet in treatment of social difficulties following facial disfigurement. *International Journal of Nursing Studies* **37**, 381–388.

Ongenae, K., Dierckxsens, L., Brochez, L., Van Geel., N. and Naeyaert, J.M. (2005) Quality of life and stigmatisation profile in a cohort of vitiligo patients and effects of the use of camouflage. *Dermatology* **210**, 279–285.

Papadopoulos, L., Bor, R. and Legg, C. (1999) Coping with the disfiguring effects of vitiligo: a preliminary investigation into the effects of cognitive-behavioural therapy. *British Journal of Medical Psychology* **72**, 385–396.

Papadopoulos, L., Walker, C. and Anthis (2004) Living with vitiligo: a controlled investigation into the effects of group cognitive-behavioural and person-centred therapies. *Dermatology and Psychosomatics* **5** (4), 172–177.

Pruzinsky, T. (1992) Social and psychological effects of major craniofacial deformity. *Cleft-Palate Craniofacial Journal* **29**, 578–584.

Pruzinsky, T. and Cash, T. (2002) Understanding body images: historical and contemporary perspectives. In: T. Cash and T. Pruzinsky (eds) *Body Image: A Handbook of Theory, Research, and Clinical Practice*, 3–12. New York: Guildford Press.

Rachman, H. (2001) A unitary theory of stigmatisation: pursuit of self-interest and routes to destigmatisation. *The British Journal of Psychiatry* **178**, 207–215.

Robinson, E., Rumsey, N. and Partridge, J. (1996) An evaluation of the impact of social interaction skills training for facially disfigured people. *British Journal of Plastic Surgery* **49**, 281–289.

Rumsey, N., Bull, R. and Gahagen, D. (1986) A preliminary study of the potential of social skills for improving the quality of social intervention for the facially disfigured. *Social Behaviour* **1**, 143–145.

Rumsey, N, Clarke, A. and Musa, M. (2002) Altered body image: the psychosocial needs of patients. *British Journal of Community Nursing* **7**, 563–566.

Rumsey, N. and Harcourt, D. (2004) Body image and disfigurement: issues and interventions. *Body Image* **1**, 93–97.

Rumsey, N. and Harcourt, D. (2005). *The Psychology of Appearance.* Buckingham: Open University Press.

Saradjian, A., Thompson, A.R. and Datta, D., (2008) The experience of men using an upper limb prosthesis following amputation: positive coping and minimizing feeling different. *Disability and Rehabilitation* **30**, 871–883.

Scambler, G. (2009) Health-related stigma. *Sociology of Health and Illness* **31**, 441–455.

Scambler, G. and Hopkins, A. (1986) Being epileptic: coming to terms with stigma. *Sociology of Health and Illness* **8**, 26–43.

Schilder, P. (1935) *The Image and Appearance of the Human Body.* London: Kegan Paul, Trench, Trubner.

Section 2

Taylor, S.E. and Aspinwall, L.G. (1996) Mediating and moderating processes in psychosocial stress: appraisal, coping, resistance and vulnerability. In: H.B. Kaplan (ed.) *Psychosocial Stress: Perspectives on Structure, Theory, Life-course, and Methods*, 71-110. San Diego: Academic Press.

Thompson, A. and Kent, G. (2001) Adjusting to disfigurement processes involved in dealing with being visibly different. *Clinical Psychology Review* **21** (5), 663-682.

Thompson, A. R. (2005). Coping with chronic skin conditions: factors important in explaining individual variation in adjustment. In: L. Papadopoulos and C. Walker (eds) *Psychodermatology: The Impact of Skin Disorders*. Cambridge, UK: Cambridge University Press.

Thompson, A. R. (2009) Managing the psychosocial impact of skin conditions: theory and the nursing role. *Dermatological Nursing* **8**, 43-48.

Thompson, A. R. (2003) The development and maintenance of shame in disfigurement: individual and societal factors. *Invited Presentation at The Centre for Appearance Research, University of the West of England*. Bristol.

Thompson, A., Kent, G. and Smith, A. (2002) Living with vitiligo: dealing with difference. *British Journal of Health Psychology* **7** (2), 213-225.

Thompson, A. R. and Broom, L. (2009) Positively managing intrusive reactions to disfigurement: an interpretative phenomenological analysis of naturalistic coping. *Diversity in Health and Care* **6**, 171-180.

Thompson, A. R., Clarke, S. A., Newell, R., Gawkrodger, G. and The Appearance Research Collaboration (2010) Vitiligo linked to stigmatisation in British South Asian women: a qualitative study of the experiences of Living with vitiligo. *The British Journal of Dermatology* **163**, 481-486.

White, C. (2001) *Cognitive Behavioural Therapy for Chronic Medical Problems*. Chichester: Wiley.

Winchell, S.A. and Watts, R.A. (1988) Relaxation therapies in the treatment of psoriasis and possible pathophysiologic mechanisms. *Journal of the American Academy of Dermatology* **18** (1), 101-104.

Resources

Changing Faces Available at: www.changingfaces.org.uk
Comment: UK charity championing the rights of people living with a disfigurement. Provides practical support/information to healthcare professionals and individuals. Maintains list of condition specific webpages.

Disability Alliance Available at: www.disabilityalliance.org.uk
Comment: UK charity campaigning to relieve poverty and improve quality of life for people living with a disability. Publishes the Disability Rights Handbook and provides advice on benefits.

Equality and Human Rights Commission Available at: www.equalityhumanrights.com
Comment: Promotes equality through the provision of advice and guidance on rights.

Expert Patients Programme Available at: www.expertpatients.co.uk
Comment: Self-management courses for chronic conditions largely facilitated by tutors with personal experience of living with a long-term health condition.

Macmillan Cancer Support Available at: www.macmillan.org.uk
Comment: Wide range of support and information, both emotional and practical in relation to cancer. Support group locations, benefits advice, and information provision. Information on other groups/organisations also cited on the website.

Further reading

Rumsey, N. and Harcourt, D. (2005) *The Psychology of Appearance*. Buckingham: Open University Press.
Comment: Thorough text covering research on appearance.

Thompson, A. and Kent, G. (2001) Adjusting to disfigurement. Processes involved in dealing with being visibly different. *Clinical Psychology Review* **21**, 663-682.

Section 2

Comment: This short literature review provides a useful summary of the literature on disfigurement and summarises the interventions available.

Veale, D., Wilson, R. and Clarke, A. (2009) *Overcoming Body Image Problems Including Body Dysmorphic Disorder: A Self-Help Guide Using Cognitive-Behavioural Techniques*. London: Constable and Robinson.

Comment: A good self-help book that has lots of practical techniques for tackling 'body image' distress.

White, C. (2001) *Cognitive behavioural therapy for chronic medical problems*. Chichester: Wiley.

Comment: This clinician-focused textbook provides a useful guide to using cognitive-behavioural techniques with a range of LTCs and also briefly discusses the adaptation issues.

Section 2

Chapter 5

Self-management in Long-term Conditions

Sue Randall and Andy Turner

Learning objectives

By the end of this chapter, the reader will be able to:

- Define self-care and self-management
- Consider the importance of self-management as a fundamental part of the patient/healthcare professional partnership
- Have an understanding of the theories which underpin self-management
- Identify relevant resources for readers to explore in self-directed study

---

Introduction

This chapter considers the move in relationships between healthcare professionals and patients. It considers a definition of self-care and self-management and explores the context of self-management for those individuals living with a long-term condition (LTC). It considers underpinning theories on which models to empower individuals in self-management are based. Through the use of case studies, examples of the effectiveness of self-management as a cornerstone of the management of LTCs will be explored. As this is a topic on which a whole book could be written, it will point the reader to further reading.

Context

As other chapters have already highlighted, demographic changes in the makeup of society, especially the growth in the ageing population, have meant that consideration is urgently required around effectively managing individuals with LTC. Lord Darzi (DH 2008) reports that by 2031, the population

---

Long-term Conditions: A Guide for Nurses and Healthcare Professionals, First Edition. Edited by S. Randall and H. Ford.
© 2011 Blackwell Publishing Ltd. Published 2011 by Blackwell Publishing Ltd.

over the age of 75 will be 8.2 million. Without context it is hard to make sense of such figures, so consider the current situation where the population of over-75s is 4.7 million. There are important differences between what is considered to be an acute health condition and what is a chronic or an LTC (Epping-Jordan et al. 2004, Hall and Roter 2007, Wilson 2001). The former tends to be episodic and generally treatable. LTCs, however, are ongoing, incurable and need to be managed for life. This generally implies that the quality of life and the patient's work and family may be affected further than in an episodic event of ill health (Boyle, Clarke and Burns 2006a, Wagner et al. 2001).

LTCs currently affect more than 17 million people in the United Kingdom and they fill 80% of consultations in primary care (Department of Health (DH) 2005a). It is recognised that healthcare professionals and the system of healthcare they operate within are not supporting people with an LTC adequately. The DH has signalled clear support for self-care over recent years. The NHS Plan (DH 2000) highlighted the importance of self-care, and this was expanded in the White Paper 'Our Health, Our Care, Our Say' (DH 2006). This emphasised the importance of helping people with LTCs take control of their conditions and care through self-care and self-management, and stipulated that commissioners and service providers should consider self-care as a high priority. Aspirations included providing all those with LTCs and their carers with information about their condition and access to self-care support, and to influence professional education in order to develop a culture and skills to support empowerment and self-care. A subsequent DH paper provided guidance on supporting local strategies and developing practice to support self-care (DH 2005b).

The 2006 Community Health White Paper 'Our Health, Our Care, Our Say: A New Direction for Community Services' promised an increase in self-management training for people living with an LTC from 12,000 to > 100,000 course places by 2012. This is reiterated in the 2010 White Paper (DH 2010). It sets out the agenda for user involvement in a whole range of social and health services, especially for those with long-term needs, and encourages greater links between services. Recent NHS quality improvement programmes have positioned patient centredness and patient involvement, as well as self-management interventions for people with long-term health conditions, at the heart of government initiatives (Cayton 2004). The self-care pyramid (see Figure 5.1) shows that the vast majority of healthcare is actually self-care, and that input and support from healthcare professionals is reserved for patient with complex and co-morbid conditions.

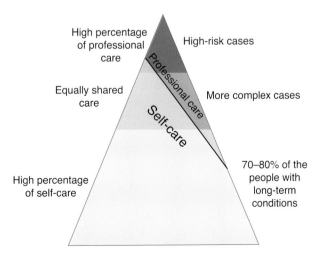

Figure 5.1 Self-care among people with long-term health conditions. (DH 2006a.)

Point for reflection

Think about the clinical placements to which you have been allocated.

- How will a growth in this older age group of population affect the service provided?
- Is change required to enable effective care to continue?
- Who and what needs to change – service provision, staffing, ways of working, or new technologies?

Summary

The changes in population mean that working with and supporting patients to enable them to self-manage to the best of their ability is one way of meeting the needs of individuals with LTCs.

Historical perspective

Up until the 1990s the medical model of health was dominant, despite attempts to weaken the power balance through consideration of the psychosocial model of health. In its simplest terms, the medical model explains illness in terms of biological malfunction or pathophysiology and as such is entirely independent of psychological and social factors. Engel (1977) was one of the first people to challenge the medical model with a fundamental assumption that health and illness are consequences of the interrelationship between biological, psychological and social problems. The International Council of Nurses has stated its concern that traditional training in healthcare has largely focused on diagnosis and treatment of acute illness (the biomedical model) at the expense of the growing number of individuals with LTC (ICN 2005). Over the last 10 years, there has been a significant shift towards partnership working which truly puts the individual at the heart of healthcare.

In so doing, the concept of paternalism in health is also less dominant. Paternalism can be defined as: 'one individual assuming the right to make decisions for another' (Marquis and Huston 2009: 74). Patients have been used to being told what to do and healthcare professionals have been used to telling patients what to do and expecting them to comply with instructions (White and Clegg 2009). Those who did not comply were often blamed by the professionals, and Redman (2004) considers the issue of compliance to be a way of maintaining control for the doctor. That healthcare professionals value information-giving issues above quality of life, which may be far more important to the individual with an LTC, and may ignore patients' views and coping skills can undermine the concept of self-management (Thorne et al. 2000). Compliance with treatment has been superseded by the concept of concordance. Concordance was originally used in the context of patients becoming effective in understanding about and taking their prescribed medication correctly through negotiation with a healthcare professional (Royal Pharmaceutical Society of Great Britain 1997). The chair of the group, Professor Marinker (2000), stresses that concordance is not a synonym for compliance, but is, in effect, a means of respecting the beliefs and wishes of the patient, who is empowered to make their own informed decision. In so doing, however, this process may clash with best-known evidence. Wilson (2001) concurs, suggesting that if an individual's decision to refuse treatment is an informed one, then this should not be viewed negatively by healthcare professionals. The Mental Capacity Act (Great Britain Parliament 2005) enshrines this point in law by stating that individuals must retain the right to make what might be seen as eccentric or unwise decisions.

Building on the idea of concordance, Bodenheimer et al. (2002) consider a true partnership approach to be a new paradigm in the care of individuals with LTCs. In this work, the authors state the importance of asking patients to identify their problems. For example, they quote the case of Ricky, who has long-term health problems and despite regular attendance at health appointments, and the doctor carrying out all the correct tests and prescribing appropriately the outcomes are disappointing. It becomes apparent that Ricky's main problem is not his health but the daily struggle he faces to look after his developmentally disabled son. In order to improve the self-management of his own health, Ricky needs help to care for his son. The complexities of life, health related or otherwise, can be major factors in an individual's ability to self-manage. Therefore, making appropriate referrals, and working with patients to develop their problem solving skills are all elements that healthcare professionals require when working with those with LTCs. For Bodenheimer et al. (2002), in cases such as Ricky, simply seeing his problems as non-compliance is missing the point.

Summary

This section has considered the changes which have occurred in the healthcare professional–patient relationship over time. Paternalism, where the healthcare professional knows best and the patient does as they are instructed has largely been replaced with a partnership approach. The partnership approach allows healthcare professionals to offer expert guidance to work with specific problems which the patient has in dealing with their disease, and which may be affecting both quantity and quality of life.

Self-care and self-management

These terms are often used synonymously due to conceptual overlap. Earlier in the chapter, the use of the terms 'compliance' and 'concordance' was examined. In the same way that compliance and concordance have very different meanings, so do the terms self-care and self-management.

Self-care

In attempting to find a clear definition for self-care, there is noted to be confusion (Wilson et al. 2006, Wilkinson and Whitehead 2009). Makinen et al. (2000) suggests that self-care comprises the ability to evaluate one's own health and to adjust behaviour accordingly. The DH (2009: 5) give the following definition:

Self-care is an integral part of daily life and is all about individuals taking responsibility for their own health and well-being with support from the people involved in their care. Self-care includes the actions people take for themselves every day in order to stay fit and maintain good physical and mental health, meet their social and psychological needs, prevent illness or accidents, and care more effectively for minor ailments and long-term conditions.

Section 2

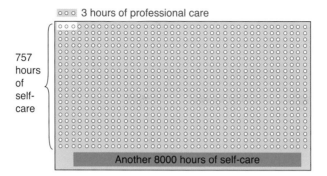

Figure 5.2 Professional care versus self-care in a year. (DH 2005b.)

In examining the term 'self-care' across several different disciplines, Gantz (1990) found agreement on four aspects. Self-care was seen as follows:

- Situation and culture specific.
- Requires the ability to make choices and to act on them.
- Is affected by knowledge, skills, values, motivations and efficacy.
- Focuses on healthcare over which individuals have control.

Analysis of the literature by Wilkinson and Whitehead (2009) found that literature around self-care revealed opposing ideologies of paternalism associated with compliance versus empowerment of individuals through self-care. When considering individuals with a diagnosis of an LTC, it is likely that they have developed self-care and expertise through living with their condition day by day (Boddenheimer et al. 2002a, Wilson 2001, Wilson and Kendall 2007). This is not least because the DH (2005) consider that individuals with LTC can receive as little as 3 hours of professional care in a year, resulting in the patient self-managing for the rest (see Figure 5.2). According to Coulter and Elwyn (2002), the real epiphany is the realisation that patients self-manage all the time (see Figure 5.2).

Some of the original ideas around self-care developed from the work of Orem. You may be familiar with Orem's Nursing Model of self-care. Orem (2001) considers the purpose of self-care is to maintain life, by keeping physical and mental functions active, and maintaining the integrity of functions and development of the individual within a framework of conditions that are essential for life. As a seminal work, Orem's theories have been examined in great detail and other writers have developed some of her ideas. One such writer is Chambers (2006) who suggests that self-care is on a continuum flowing from individual choice to care entirely dependent on healthcare professionals. This can be seen pictorially below in Figure 5.3.

Wilkinson and Whitehead (2009) report Clark's argument that self-care does not involve professional input and so is in direct opposition to the idea of a continuum. For individuals with LTCs there is some degree of professional involvement and as a result, the idea of self-care does not fit, in Clarke's opinion.

Self-management

In the context of LTCs, 'self-management' has become a widely used term especially since the spread of formal self-management programmes initially in the United Kingdom through the voluntary sector (for example Arthritis Care, Multiple Sclerosis Society, Long-term Medical Conditions Alliance) and

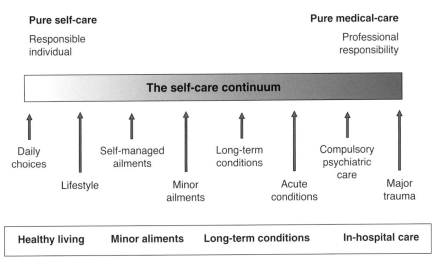

Figure 5.3 Self-care continuum. (Colin-Thome 2006.)

more recently through the Expert Patients Programme Community Interest Company (EPPCiC). For Wilkinson and Whitehead (2009: 1145), self-management is seen as a 'subset of self-care', which is linked to an individual's ability to adapt their lifestyle in order to live with an LTC. To be successful, receiving support from family, the community and healthcare professionals is important to manage aspects of life such as:

- Symptoms
- Treatments
- Physical
- Psychosocial
- Cultural
- Spiritual

There are several definitions of self-management. Clark et al. (1991) suggest that successful self-management requires sufficient knowledge of the condition and its treatment, performance of condition management activities and application of the necessary skills to maintain adequate psychosocial functioning.

Thus, self-management has been defined by Barlow (2001) as follows:

Self-management refers to the individual's ability to manage the symptoms, treatment, physical and psychosocial consequences and life style changes inherent in living with a chronic condition. Efficacious self-management encompasses ability to monitor one's condition and to effect the cognitive, behavioural and emotional responses necessary to maintain a satisfactory quality of life.

Thus, a dynamic and continuous process of self-regulation is established. The term 'supported self-management' recognises that the person living with an LTC may require support from a varied range of agencies and interventions, which include formalised training programmes such as the Expert Patient Programme, DAFNE (Dose Adjusted For Normal Eating Study Group 2002), DESMOND (Diabetes Education and Self Management for Ongoing and Newly Diagnosed Diabetics) (Davies et al. 2008), and of course health and social care services and personnel. The Co-Creating Health

Project (2008) defined supported self-management as 'what health services do in order to aid and encourage people living with a long-term condition to make daily decisions that improve health-related behaviours and clinical and other outcomes.' (www.health.org.uk/). This may be particularly pertinent when thinking about younger people living with an LTC.

How self-management differs from patient education

Concepts such as patient education, health education and health literacy reinforce a health 'expert' and an uninformed public (Cayton and Blomfield 2008). Traditional patient education, the content of which is determined by health providers, teaches patients' disease-specific information and technical skills (for example blood glucose monitoring in diabetes and management of inhalers in asthma). The most effective interventions utilise cognitive and behavioural modification, in addition to providing information (Lorig 1995). Information provision alone is unlikely to result in initiation of and mainte-nance of behaviour change and self-management of LTCs (Coulter and Ellins 2006). A meta-analysis of interventions to increase HIV preventative behaviours found that teaching self-management tech-niques and behaviour change strategies which accompanied and reinforced information provision led to changes in behaviour (Albarracin et al. 2005). Bodenheimer et al. (2002) maintain that self-management complements traditional patient education. The provision of information is an impor-tant part of self-management; however, self-management differs because of its focus on the patient's own agenda, improving problem solving skills, and improving confidence (self-efficacy) to use those skills in coping with a broad range of consequences of living with an LTC. In some group-based self-management, the course leader acts as guide or model sharing similar characteristics with par-ticipants (for example having an LTC). This approach is in contrast with patient education typically delivered by a health professional (see Figure 5.4). Bodenheimer et al. (2002) believe that only 'true' self-management interventions include patient focused goals (goal setting). In their review of arthritis and LTC self-management interventions, they found that interventions which included goal setting tended to demonstrate more improvements than those without a goal setting component.

Self-management may be one means of bridging the gap between patients' needs and the ca-pacity of health and social care services to meet those needs. A diverse range of approaches have been employed in attempts to improve physical and psychosocial well-being among people with an LTC. Self-management interventions can be group-based, individualised, or a combination of both (Barlow et al. 2002) and include computer-assisted programmes (for example Horan et al. 1990), mail-delivered programmes (for example Fries et al. 1997), telephone contacts (for example Weinberger et al. 1993) and individual and group education programmes (for example Simeoni et al. 1995).

A review by Barlow et al. (2002) found broad similarities in the type of self-management approaches developed for people with LTCs, particularly in terms of course content. However, there will always be disease-specific management tasks. A diverse range of self-management components was identified. These were broadly classified as providing information, drug management, symptom management, dealing with psychosocial consequences, lifestyle (including exercise), social support, communication and other self-management strategies such as problem-solving, goal-setting, action-planning and accessing support services.

Self-management courses

An example of self-management interventions encompassing these techniques and which have an established evidence base in the UK (Kennedy et al. 2007, Foster et al. 2007) is the Expert Patients Programme (EPP). The EPP is based on the Chronic Disease Self-Management Course (CDSMC), developed at Stanford University in the Unites States by Professor Kate Lorig. The EPP has evolved as an example of collaboration between 'motivated patients, enlightened professionals

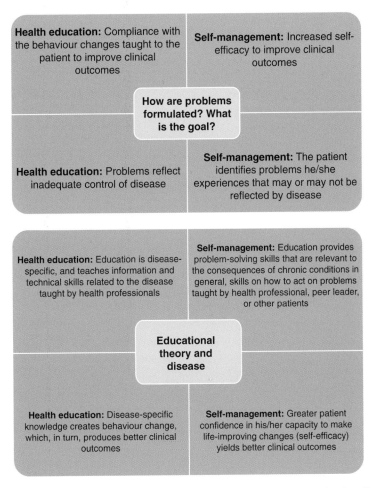

Figure 5.4   Comparison of traditional patient education and self-management education. (Adapted from Bodenheimer et al. 2002, p. 2471.)

and progressive government' (Cayton and Blomfield 2008). These concepts can be seen in the NHS and Social Care Model (see Chapter 8). Few interventions have dealt with more than one disease or with the problems of co-morbidity (Lorig et al. 1999a). The EPP recognises the common issues faced by many people with an LTC. It has been estimated that people aged 60 years and older have, on average, 2.2 LTCs (Hoffman et al. 1996) and, therefore, have to manage these diseases and their consequences simultaneously. Equally, there are many generic skills that are needed. Analyses of self-management tasks faced by people with three of the most common LTCs presenting in primary care (i.e. arthritis, asthma and diabetes) show that there are many commonalties (Barlow et al. 2002). Tasks include making lifestyle changes (for example exercise, diet, giving up smoking), dealing with the psychological distress, and communicating effectively with health professionals. The format and content of the EPP are shown in Table 5.1

The EPP comprises six weekly sessions, each lasting approximately two and half hours, delivered by pairs of lay leaders, most of whom have an LTC themselves (although this is not the delivery model adopted in some parts of the world where courses are delivered using a mixed model of lay and health professional tutors). Co-creating Health has similarly adopted a mixed model approach.

Table 5.1 Format and content of expert patient programme

Format	Content
• Lay-led • 6 weekly 2.5 hour sessions • Group • Interactive • Goal setting • Problem solving • Role modelling	• Guided imagery • Exercise • Nutrition • Dealing with depression and anger • Communicating with health professionals • Relaxation • Breathing exercises

The model of shared delivery between a health professional and a peer facilitator is potentially more effective on participant outcomes, than either a lay tutor alone (as in the EPP) or with a professional tutor alone (Griffiths et al. 2007, Foster et al. 2009). For the EPP, course format and content is guided by a manual to ensure programme fidelity. The use of a structured manual has methodological and outcome advantages. It helps to ensure consistent standard of content delivery by lay tutors who often do not come from an education or training/counselling background. The course is multi-component and topics include: disease information, an overview of self-management principles, exercise, cognitive symptom management (for example distraction, visualisation and guided imagery), dealing with depression, nutrition, communication with family and health professionals, and goal setting and action planning. The last of these involves the setting of realistic goals to be achieved during the forthcoming week. Goals should be personally relevant, be achievable, but at the same time challenging, have proximal outcomes and depend largely upon a person's own efforts. The importance of participants selecting personally relevant goals is underscored by the following quote from Duncan et al. (2007), which describes the importance of client-directed goals in cognitive-behavioural therapy, but which apply equally well to self-management programmes and of course to consultations between patients and clinicians:

> When we ask clients what they want, what they want to be different, we give credibility to their beliefs and values regarding the problem and its solution. We are saying to them that their opinion is important and we are there to serve them. As simple an act as it is, it invites clients to see themselves as a collaborator in making their lives better. Regardless of how they sound, we accept client's goals at face value because those are the desires that will excite and motivate the client to initiate action in their own behalf. If we are serving the alliance master, we know that agreement with the client about goals is essential to positive outcome. It begins the process of change, wherever the client may ultimately travel. (Duncan et al. 2007)

Case study 5.1 captures the benefits of attending a self-management programme in which the participant described the value of many of the techniques he learnt including goal setting and action planning.

Case study 5.1 Before the arthritis self-management course

Mr X's problems started while he was on holiday about ten years ago when he heard a loud 'bang' in his right knee. A diagnosis of osteoarthritis (OA) was not a shock to him given his age but it did make him feel a bit depressed because it signified old age. His primary symptoms are pain and stiffness arising from performing weight-bearing activities. He feels that the stiffness is a bigger problem than pain. Mr X uses ibuprofen prior to some activities such as gardening and prolonged walking. He has been told that he might eventually need a new knee joint but he is not keen on this option in case it further decreases his limited flexibility. Mr X knows people who are unable to bend their artificial knee joint and he is keen not to experience a similar fate. Mr X feels that his OA was probably caused by normal wear and tear and playing sport when he was younger, particularly because he has a heavy frame. Mr X has recently developed pain in his right thigh but after being given exercise recommendations from his local GP practice nurse this has improved. Mr X also has pain in his left knee and spine.

Mr X is extremely active and busy with his involvement in domestic (for example gardening), community and church activities. Mr X feels that his activities distract him from thinking and focusing on his OA. Having OA, however, means that he is restricted in some of his activities, which he finds very depressing at times. Holidays involving extensive walking are particularly problematic. Singing in the church choir entails prolonged periods of standing and he is finding this an increasingly more difficult and less pleasurable activity, and as a result is considering withdrawing from overseas choir singing. It is upon initial activity that Mr X experiences the worst discomfort and stiffness. Mr X has purchased a vibrating massage chair which he uses occasionally. Mr X would be satisfied if the pain does not worsen and he can maintain the lifestyle and activities he currently enjoys. He would like to lose weight because he is aware that being overweight is likely to contribute to worsening pain and disability. However, he finds this extremely difficult to do and would welcome advice and help from either his GP or from the course. Mr X occasionally carries out some of the exercises he was advised to do when he had the problem with his right thigh and occasionally rides his exercise bike. Mr X used to swim regularly but now struggles to find the time or inclination.

Four months after the course

Mr X thought the course was extremely comprehensive, informative, practical, relevant and very beneficial. Mr X thought that the tutors were very professional, helpful and interested both in what they were delivering and the participants. The message that the tutors put across was the importance of not giving in to arthritis, staying active and doing things which distract from focusing on arthritis. Mr X thought that it was very helpful that the tutors had arthritis as this meant they identified with the participants' problems. He was motivated to join a swimming club after hearing that one of the tutors with rheumatoid arthritis (RA) swam to exercise her hands and fingers. He now swims at least once a week benefiting from the exercise and the social contact involved, which he feels along with his other social activities has maintained his emotional well-being.

Mr X enjoyed the relaxed social atmosphere of the course and the fact that everyone was encouraged to actively participate. After the second week everyone was on first name basis and Mr X valued the friendly atmosphere. He thought the action planning was extremely useful for involving everyone and also beneficial for motivating people to set and achieve small goals. Mr X drinks more water now and he understood the benefits of doing so are in increasing the potency of medications and assisting the kidneys in removing any potential side effects. Mr X felt grateful that he wasn't as severely affected as some of the other participants, particularly the participants with RA. He was not concerned that his OA would worsen and Mr X remained positive and felt comforted that if it did he would be able to approach the tutors for advice and information.

Mr X has bought the course manual and has found it useful for illustrative advice about exercise. He considers that the exercises help strengthen his muscles, which in turn reduce stiffness. The course provided the motivation, techniques and the positive mental attitude to carry out additional exercises to those he was doing before then course. Mr X also bought the course relaxation tape and he initially found it useful in helping him sleep at night. Mr X has not used it recently. He would recommend the course to other people with arthritis.

Points for reflection

- Attending a group is not popular with everyone. How could you encourage attendance, without putting undue pressure on a patient to attend?
- What are the key benefits which Mr X reports?
- How do these fit in with wider issues of caring for someone with an LTC?

A key concept of caring for individuals with LTCs is that of partnership, as the chapter has discussed. Although the individuals with whom healthcare professionals work may be active self-managers, this does not mean that they will never need professional support in the future. A continuing link to healthcare professionals is important to refocus patients on potentially changing needs which may or may not require a different plan to maintain effective self-management. Case study 5.2 can be seen as a cautionary tale, but should not be seen as a reason to limit the promotion of self-management for individuals living with LTCs.

Case study 5.2 Peter

Peter is in his mid-50s and lives with a T6 spinal injury sustained 8 years ago. With the support of his wife, Peter is an active self-manager following an intensive rehabilitation and education programme in 2002. The GP practice had received a request from Peter's wife for the District Nursing team to assess what was described as a small discoloured area on his sacrum.

On assessment, the District Nurse found Peter had developed a large necrotic grade 4 pressure sore which appeared infected. As a result, Peter was at risk of developing autonomic dysreflexia.

Spinal injury patients are extremely knowledgeable with regard to self-management and are often considered the ultimate expert patient. Despite this expert knowledge, Peter and his wife failed to recognise the initial development of the pressure sore and its importance. Peter considered himself to have adjusted well to life changes, was married and considered his risk of pressure sore development reduced having read some research which confirmed this. Despite yearly appointments at the Specialist Spinal Injury Unit, Peter and his wife had no clear understanding of who to refer to in the community if he experienced a problem.

Points for reflection

- This example highlights the need for healthcare professionals to work in partnership with patients, even when they appear to be effective and competent self-managers.
- Reconsider the point: 'Health-care professionals are experts on diseases, but patients are experts in living and coping with their disease' (Bodenheimer et al 2002).
- What safety measures could be put in place so that Peter's care remains proactive and does not become reactive?
- How can healthcare professionals work with Peter, so as to continue his great work as a self-manager?

Self-management programmes in minority ethnic groups

In the United Kingdom, people from black and ethnic minority (BME) communities tend to have poorer health, a shorter life expectancy and have greater difficulty accessing healthcare than the majority of the population (NIMH 2003). In an ethnicity-specific randomised controlled study with 300 Sylheti-speaking Bangladeshis in Tower Hamlets, Griffiths et al. (2005) aimed to establish the effectiveness of EPP among Bangladeshis living in Tower Hamlets and to understand the structural and cultural barriers to success of EPP. The EPP course was adapted into the Sylheti dialect and Islamic culture. Courses were lay-led by trained and accredited Bangladeshi tutors with an LTC, with men and women attending separate courses. Participants attending three or more sessions showed greater improvements than the control group in self-efficacy, cognitive symptom management and had improved depression scores at four months, but no change in health service usage. The EPP is now available in nine languages and is delivered by bilingual trainers.

International research also confirms the effectiveness of Stanford University developed or inspired self-management programmes for use in minority ethnic groups. It has so far been translated into several languages and delivered in 30 countries. For example, Lorig et al. (1999b) evaluated a Spanish-language course for use with US Hispanics, Dongbo et al. (2006) examined a Chinese version of the CDSMC and Swerissen et al. (2006) examined the effectiveness of the CDSMC among Vietnamese, Greek, Chinese and Italian communities in Australia. These studies confirmed the effectiveness of the Course with these divergent populations. Recently, Australian research has investigated the extent to which the CDSMC required modification so that concepts around self-management could be made more relevant to Vietnamese, Greek, Chinese and Italian communities with various LTCs (Walker et al. 2005). Conceptual aspects of the course required little modification, with myths around the importance of fatalism, that is believing that health and well-being are beyond personal control and instead are determined by external factors such as luck, God, Allah and so on were largely dispelled. However, high levels of illiteracy in participants' own language and in English require the course materials to be made accessible and equitable for non-English speakers (Walker et al. 2005).

Self-management research has mainly been conducted among patients with physical LTCs (e.g. arthritis, diabetes) although there are a few exceptions (Lawn et al. 2007). However, mental health is a clear priority in the government's definition of self-care: 'the care taken by individuals to-wards their own health and wellbeing' and includes the actions taken to 'maintain good physical and mental health' and 'meet social, emotional and psychological needs' (DH 2005a). Recent developments in mental healthcare have begun a move towards an environment more conducive to self-care and self-management. Turner and Barlow (2007) have described the potential of self-management programmes including the EPP and Coventry University's HOPE programme (Turner 2010) for supporting LTC patients with co-morbid mild to moderate anxiety and/or depression and patients with anxiety and/or depression as a primary condition. Principles of the recovery approach (hope, personal responsibility, self-advocacy, education, support) (www.mentalhealthrecovery.com), which underpin mental health services are consistent with self-management approaches. Several mental health organisations have developed mental health self-management programmes including a self-management approach for people living with a diagnosis of schizophrenia (Rethink 2003), a self-management programme (http://www.mdf.org.uk/?o=1622) developed by the Manic Depression Fellowship, the TIDAL model (http://www.tidal-model.co.uk) and Wellness Recovery Action Plan (WRAP) (www.mentalhealthrecovery.com).

For those writers who make a distinction between self-care and self-management, it is this: 'that in self management, work which was once performed by health care professionals is now undertaken by those with long-term conditions, themselves' (Redman 2007). Wilson et al. (2006) concur with this view by highlighting prescribing drug dosages as an example of change in role from the professional arena to the patient. Examples are included in Table 5.2.

However, the change in role associated with self-management may work best in a community setting rather than a hospital setting. Although, as nurses and healthcare professionals we talk in terms of holistic care of patients, and tailoring care to the needs of the individual, it may be argued that the gulf in care provided in the community to that provided in hospital is great. For example, when individuals with LTCs are admitted to hospital, perhaps due to an exacerbation of their condition, or even something unrelated, they are stripped of their medication and given it at times to suit the ward routine and not that of the individual. Even if the ward ethos is one of encouraging self-care, risk and health and safety are often quoted as reasons for what is arguably disempowering to individuals. This concept is further discussed in Chapter 7.

With this in mind, the need to work with patients to build their capabilities in self-management is a key skill for healthcare professionals in the 21st century. Such skills are required to negate the

Table 5.2   Patient responsibility with medications and self-care regimes

Individuals with asthma	• Adjusting inhaler dosages • Starting oral steroids
Individuals with Chronic Obstructive Pulmonary Disease (COPD)	• Adjusting inhaler dosages • Commencing 'rescue' packs, which contain oral steroids and oral antibiotics, in line with a personal care plan
Individuals with diabetes	• Altering insulin doses • DAFNE (Dose Adjustment for Normal Eating) (DAFNE Study Group 2002) • DESMOND (Diabetes Education and Self Management for Ongoing and Newly Diagnosed Diabetics) (Davies et al. 2008)

findings by Glasgow and Anderson (1999), who state that patients are in control and irrespective of what healthcare professionals do or say, when left alone patients can choose to ignore any recommendations. Although true in some cases, maintaining professional accountability through, for example, the Nursing and Midwifery Code (2008) is key. Extracts from The Code that are applicable include the following:

- You must listen to the people in your care and respond to their concerns and preferences.
- You must support people in caring for themselves to improve and maintain health.
- You must respect and support people's rights to accept or decline treatment or care.

Most individuals with LTCs are amenable to being self-managed with the support and encouragement from the patient's healthcare team and most patients welcome the opportunity to become more involved in their healthcare and improve their lifestyles. An example is seen in Case study 5.3.

Case study 5.3 The Expert Patient Programme gave me my life back

I had been living with a variety of LTCs for several years and managing to keep them under control with an assortment of medications, but when I was diagnosed with Chronic Obstructive Pulmonary Disease (COPD) in 2002, I was devastated, both physically and mentally, not least because my father had died with the same condition and I had cared for him and watched him deteriorate until he died.

I allowed the disease to take control of my life and lost my coping skills, I became disabled because of my inactivity and my health rapidly worsened, I had to give up work and my social life was non- existent, I was scheduled to have major lung surgery in 2005/2006.

Then in April 2005, I heard about an Expert Patients course in my area, I signed up for the course and it changed my life! I learned new skills, action planning, problem solving, better breathing, exercise and many many more. I began to get my life back.

When I saw the surgeon late in 2005 he deferred my operation for a year as my breathing was showing signs of improvement and when he saw me in 2006 he took me off his list saying "I no longer needed surgery as my lung function and breathing had improved so much."

I am now a volunteer tutor with the EPP and also the Looking After Me carers course. I help at a parent toddler group once a week and corun a social group for lonely and elderly people. I even joined an amateur drama group in 2006 and discovered hitherto unknown acting skills. In our latest production I even sing two songs (the better breathing technique really helps there!).

So as you can see The Expert Patients Programme has really given me my life back.

Malcolm Benny

Points for reflection

- How did receiving a diagnosis of COPD affect Malcolm?
- Consider his reaction and those reported in Chapter 4 on adaptation to illness.
- What effect has the Expert Patient Programme had on Malcolm?
- List the benefits to the wider community, which are apparent from Malcolm's personal account.

Section 2

Coulter and Ellins (2006) maintain that if healthcare professionals undermine patients' coping skills, they can expect to see patients utilising their services more often. There is growing call for healthcare professionals to receive training in supporting their patients' self-management attempts and given the limited contact that healthcare professionals have with patients (see Figure 5.1). It is important that the interaction is as productive as possible with both parties maximising the opportunity for successful self-management outcomes. Newman and Cooke (2008) have argued that health professionals tend to use verbal persuasion and information giving, both of which are poor at building patients' self-efficacy for self-management. One of the recommendations by a King's Fund working paper was that health professionals should attend training programmes to learn how to develop and foster self-management skills among their patients (Corben and Rosen 2005). The General Medical Council (2001) also recommends communication and self-management skills training for clinicians.

Summary

This section has considered issues of terminology and has considered the differences between self-care and self-management, and has considered the role of programmes such as the Expert Patient Programme in assisting individuals with LTCs to gain a greater understanding of their conditions and their own needs within this.

Co-creating health initiative (CCH)

Co-creating health (CCH) is a national programme commissioned by The Health Foundation (http://www.health.org.uk/), which aims to embed self-management support within mainstream health services in order to achieve measurable improvements in the quality of life of patients with an LTC. CCH recognised that one of the limitations of self-management policy and research in the United Kingdom has been the over-emphasis on providing training to patients without either providing training to clinicians to support patients self-management behaviours or making service improvements to embed self-management within service provision. This has led to limited outcomes for patients of self-management programmes who can quickly lose the confidence and motivation to self-manage when faced with unresponsive and unsupportive clinicians and services.

> We believe that to take a more active role in their health, people need self-management skills and easier access to information about their conditions. They also need skilled support and motivation from their clinicians and healthcare systems that operate very differently from those we have today.
>
> *-http://www.health.org.uk/*

CCH is working with eight sites, in four LTCs (pain, diabetes, COPD, depression) integrating three programmes:

- *A Self-Management Programme (SMP) for patients with LTCs*: The SMP is designed to develop the knowledge and skills patients require in order to manage their LTC and work in effective partnership with their clinicians.

- *An Advanced Development Programme (ADP) for clinicians*: The ADP aims to help clinicians to develop the skills required to support and motivate their patients to achieve behaviour change and to take an active role in their own health and healthcare.
- *Service Improvement Programme (SIP):* This is an organisational development programme including quality improvement methods. The SIP aims to support patients and healthcare professionals, working together, to identify and implement new approaches to health service delivery that enable patients to take a more active role in their own health and healthcare.

Patients and heathcare professionals are being trained to develop shared agendas for clinical consultations, and to set collaborative goals, which are regularly and routinely monitored. Case study 5.5 gives an example. One of the challenges for CCH is to train clinicians to engage in co-production with their patients. Co-production of health in consultations is a crucial part of a system to support self-management (Bodenheimer et al. 2002). The ADP consists of three half-day workshops cofacilitated by a health professional and a patient living with an LTC. It teaches communication and motivational interviewing skills and techniques to assist the patient in initiating and maintaining self-management activities. Training clinicians in motivational interviewing skills has been recommended as part of a strategy to improve self-management support (Glasgow et al. 2008).

CCH is set with the Wagner chronic care model (1998), which has been adopted by the NHS as the generic model for LTCs (Epping-Jordan et al. 2004). According to the model (see Figure 5.5), one of the main tasks for health services should be to support self-management. This is an important task and needs to be embedded in a system which includes activated patients, prepared clinicians, and a responsive and flexible administrative structure (Wagner 1998). There is strong evidence that suggests that self-management support is more likely to work if transformation in every part of the system takes place instead of the implementation of isolated strategies which have no long-lasting impact (Wagner et al. 2001). The system should integrate the expertise and skills of the health providers, ensure the provision of health education and support to patients, guarantee the provision of planned and team-based care delivery and enforce the use of clinical registers (Coleman et al. 2009).

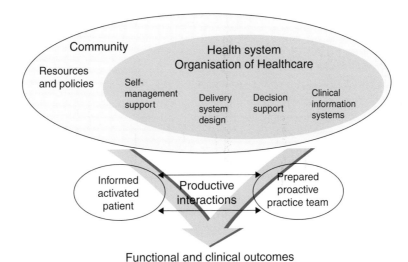

Functional and clinical outcomes

Figure 5.5 The chronic care model: Wagner 1998. (Reproduced with kind permission of American College of Physicians: Effective Clinical Practice.)

Section 2

Case study 5.4 Co-creating Health

Patient's experience of attending the self-management programme

"When I started on the self-management programme I was really sceptical about it, but by the end of the seven weeks I'd changed, and I think both clinicians and other patients feel the same. I think for the clinicians, they see the change with their patients who've been through the programme because it does change your life dramatically from what you had before. In the group, the first week, it's kind of strained. The second week, it gets a bit better. By the third week, everybody's pals and how can we help each other – someone may say 'I had trouble with such and such', and someone else will say 'oh, have you tried such and such' – so we're all helping each other in that way. They've sown the seed here and I think it will grow to a great maturity."

Consultant's experience of attending the Advanced Development Programme

"The Advanced Development Programme (ADP) was a real eye-opener to me and it showed me a completely new way how to deal with an encounter with the patients and how to interact with the patient in a much more meaningful, effective and satisfying way. Because the old way, there was always that feeling in the back of your mind you weren't quite satisfied with this consultation, as a clinician, and you got a feel the patient wasn't quite satisfied as well. We hadn't achieved what could have been achieved in that consultation. And I think the ADP has really showed me the way how this could be done. It's sort of stepping back, letting the patient take the lead, listen to what the patient really wants to talk about, what the patient is ready to talk about. Tune into the patient's journey really; where are they and what are they ready to talk about and embrace, you know. That's fantastic, you know, it really is, it makes you feel almost happy after a consultation, you know."

Points for reflection

- In the descriptions above, how have the patient and the consultant changed their views of the patient/healthcare professional relationship?
- Consider areas in which you have worked. How often do you see an interaction between patient and healthcare professional which shows a partnership approach to planning care?
- What are your personal views about a changed way of working, with an alteration in the power balance between professionals and patients?

Summary

This section has considered another programme, the Co-Creating Health initiative, to enable patients and healthcare professionals to better understand the importance of self-management. This programme is considered in the context of the chronic care model (Wagner 1998), which underpins much theory surrounding the care and effective management of individuals with LTCs in the wider context.

Underpinning theories

Understanding behaviour and factors which affect individuals ability to change their behaviour are central to understanding self-management of chronic disease (Serlachius and Sutton 2009). This chapter examines three theories which consider interventions which need to be developed in order to increase self-management behaviour in individuals with LTCs. The theories examined are Socio-Cognitive Theory, Health Belief Model and Stages of Change Model.

Social cognitive theory

This theory was developed by Alfred Bandura in the United States of America (1986–1997). It under-pins a lot of self-management practice including the Expert Patient Programme. This theory helps to understand and predict behaviour, and as a result of this an individual's behaviour can be modified and changed. An individual's expectations, beliefs, self-perceptions, goals and intentions give shape and direction to behaviours. Biological and personal factors also have an impact. These include sex, ethnicity, temperament and genetic makeup. Of specific importance from this theory is the notion of self-efficacy, which is defined as an individual's belief in their own ability to achieve an action, which in turn, produces a specific expected outcome (Wilson and Mayor 2006). The concept of self-efficacy is important because it is often referred to as the patients' confidence in their own ability to manage (Lau-Walker and Thompson 2009). The majority of people will avoid self-managing their disease if they believe it is beyond their capabilities or if the expected outcome does not provide sufficient reward for the amount of effort put into the activity (Wilson and Mayor 2006).

> **Points for reflection**
>
> - You may or may not have experience of living with an LTC.
> - If you do not, consider self-efficacy in an area that you do have experience in. For example, undertaking your training may present many challenges. You may feel that you do not have the ability to complete an assignment for university which allows you to reach the pass mark. That may stop you from trying to manage the difficulty.
> - Equally, if you put a lot of effort into your assignment and are then disappointed with the mark, then this may also affect your self-efficacy.

For Bandura, there is a distinction in the way individuals use information (Bandura 1997). Bandura considers these to be two types:

1. Information gained through an experience
2. Information that is given, and then has to be processed by the individual

As a consequence, Bandura developed a hierarchy of information as follows (see Figure 5.6):

This may seem complicated and the reader may wonder what this has to do with self-management, but one of the key elements from social cognitive theory is that therapeutic interventions, such as those developed in partnership between healthcare professionals and patients should allow

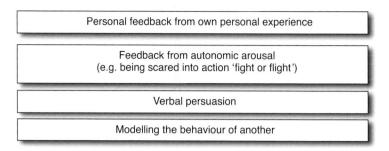

Figure 5.6 **Hierarchy of information.**

patients to gain mastery in looking after their LTCs. In order to attain mastery, specific skills need to be acquired to meet the needs of the patient as an individual. Contracting around specific goals is commonly used in cognitive-behavioural therapy. Without specific goals, an individual with coronary heart disease may understand that undertaking regular exercise is likely to help them remain healthy, but because they have low efficacy expectancy, because they have never enjoyed exercise or participated in it much, they can't see themselves starting now or if they do start, have the ability to keep the action going. These individuals would need specific goals to address confidence to manage the exercise in order to self-manage. The argument here is for specific rather than generic materials, as one size does not fit all (Lau-Walker and Thompson 2009).

The use of SMART goals is an example (Brooker and Nicol 2003).

S: specific
M: measurable
A: achievable
R: realistic
T: timely

Case study 5.5 Mr Jones

Mr Jones has suffered a right cerebral vascular accident (CVA) and has been left with a right hemiplegia. As you care for him, he tells you that he wants to be able to walk to his allotment where he meets up with his friends, but he feels that this will never happen again.

Mr Jones goal is not SMART at this time. In discussion with his physiotherapist and Mr Jones, a SMART goal is set around moving from bed to chair independently, using any necessary aids, in the first instance. Mr Jones can see that this is a specific goal, which is an incremental in his journey to his ultimate goal. Moving from bed to chair independently is measurable, achievable, realistic and timely in his rehabilitation. There is clear outcome expectancy for Mr Jones, which will aid his self-esteem and assist in his ability to self-manage by gaining mastery, following a CVA.

Coping skills are a vital part of building self-efficacy. As such, Mr Jones' ability to adapt to his stroke will be key. These aspects are explored further in Chapter 4.

Section 2

> ### Points for reflection
> - Consider how important it is to involve Mr Jones's family in understanding the reasons behind goal setting.
> - Which other members of the multidisciplinary team should be involved?
> - Ensure plans are communicated to everyone, so that the goals are understood and there is no room for 'crossed wires'.
> - Continue to assess Mr Jones and refer to psychology team if slower progress affects his mental well-being.

How social/cognitive theory is operationalised through the Expert Patient Programme
The EPP enhances perceived ability to control various aspects of living with an LTC through four major efficacy-enhancing strategies: skills mastery, modelling, persuasive communication and reinterpretation of symptoms.

Skills mastery is considered to be the most potent efficacy enhancing strategy. This involves learning and practising appropriate behaviours. New behaviours should be broken into smaller, manageable ones to ensure that each is successfully executed. It is important that course participants set their own written goals in the form of a contract. Personal goals serve to provide greater incentive for task accomplishment. Making a contract and receiving feedback provide an opportunity for participants to monitor progress.

Modelling is a technique whereby a realistic, positive, role model who is successfully managing aspects of their life serves as a source of inspiration to course participants. In the context of the an EPP, this role model is represented by the course leaders who themselves have an LTC. Course participants also act as models when encouraged to share their knowledge and strategies for overcoming disease-related problems.

Persuasive communication is most effective when it involves encouraging participants to attempt a little more than they are currently doing. Evidence suggests that group members can influence a member who is reluctant to initiate a course of action. Persuasion is most effective when used in combination with other techniques.

Reinterpretation of physiological symptoms is the final type of efficacy-enhancing strategy. Participants are taught to distinguish between physiological disease-related symptoms such as pain, fatigue, muscle soreness and similar symptoms that can arise from therapeutic exercise for example.

Social cognitive theory places considerable emphasis on self-efficacy, but it is important to remember that self-efficacy relates to a specific behaviour and not a personality trait (Nieuwehuijsen et al. 2006). The same authors also stress that individuals can have strong self-efficacy in one behaviour, such as exercise, but not in another such as eating healthily.

The health belief model

Developed in the 1950s by Hochbaum and colleagues, this theory is based on individuals believing that an issue associated with an LTC poses a threat and as a result, they are motivated to take

Section 2

Table 5.3   Constructs and concepts of the health belief model

Constructs:	Examples
1. Perceived susceptibility	Jane Evans, who is 55, has Type 2 diabetes and is concerned that she may have a heart attack (Myocardial infarction).
2. Perceived severity of a condition	Jane's mother had Type 2 diabetes and died following a fatal myocardial infarction at the age of 60.
3. Perceived benefits of treatment	Jane has been offered the chance to attend an Expert Patient Programme, which will help her manage her diabetes more effectively.
4. Perceived barriers to treatment	Jane is not keen on groups of people. She is anxious that she may not fit in.

Concepts:	Examples
• Self-efficacy	Jane needs to have the belief in herself to overcome this barrier.
• Cues for action	These encourage people to engage in activities which may benefit their health. They can be internal or external. Jane's own desire to try and manage her condition better may win through (internal).
	The practice nurse who works with Jane and who suggested the course, asks if she would like to speak with someone who has already attended to try and allay Jane's anxieties (external).

action, provided that barriers can be overcome (Nieuwehuijsen et al. 2006). The model comprises four constructs and two additional concepts, as illustrated in Table 5.3.

To recap, the health belief model considers how preventative health behaviours can be explained by health actions which arise out of an individual feeling threatened by a health problem. The individual's appraisal of the problem and the strategies for preventing or managing the problem influence this theory.

Stages of change model

This model was originally conceived by Prochaska in the late 1970s and then further developed by Prochaska and DiClemente (1984, 1986). It considers change as a process, which can be cyclical if individuals are unable to maintain the change. A number of attempts at change may be required before it is successful, but all attempts provide experience which the individual can use in future attempts. A diagrammatic representation of the model can be seen in Figure 5.7.

Although this model is commonly used for individuals who have addictive behaviours, it can usefully be used to underpin change in individuals who have an LTC. The first stage is *precontemplation*, which is when an individual has not really considered a need for change. This may be as a result of the shock of diagnosis, but as they become aware of potential problems they may move to the next stage.

The second stage is *contemplation*. Here an individual is aware of the benefits of making a change in their behaviour. This may be as a result of discussions and information exchange with healthcare professionals or through their peers at a support group, but they are not quite ready to implement the change.

Preparation for change is the third stage. At this point, the perceived benefits appear to outweigh other considerations. The change appears worthwhile and expert support may be sought and required at this point.

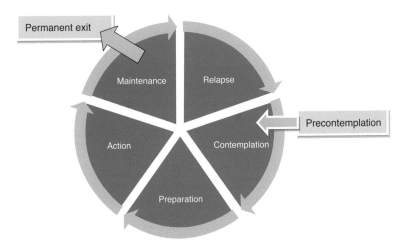

Figure 5.7   Stages of change model. (Adapted from Prochaska and DiClemente, 1984.)

The fourth stage is *action*, and at this point a clear goal and a realistic plan are required (may be SMART goals as discussed earlier). A discussion with the Practice Nurse on quitting smoking may form a catalyst on this occasion for action (Randall 2006). The foundations of this action may have been built over many years through the patient's own experience of worsening breathing as a result of COPD, as well as discussion about the harmful effects of smoking by other healthcare professionals.

Maintenance, as the fifth stage, can prove the most challenging. With support from family and friends and healthcare professionals, as well as motivation from the individual themselves it possible for the change to become permanent. This links with Social Cognitive Theory and outcome expectancy where the change has to feel worth the effort and with perceived benefits from the Health Belief Model. Without these the result may be *relapse*.

Relapse is very different from failure, however. For some individuals they may need to go around the cycle several times before the change is effective. Indeed, Prochaska et al. (1992) suggest that stages may not be followed in order and that all stages are valuable. On each occasion the individual is gaining more experience around issues which went well or not so well, which will then strengthen future attempts at behaviour change.

Summary

As highlighted in the text, this section has considered various models and the similarities which can be seen in the models discussed. Having some understanding of human behaviour is important for nurses and other healthcare professionals in order that they have an evidence base on which to build partnerships with patients who live with LTCs. In so doing, improving patients ability to self-manage should result.

Conclusion

Developing an LTC can occur at any age, but changes in an ageing population mean that increasing numbers of people will live with LTCs and it is important that they are supported by healthcare professionals and the health service to self-manage. Most Patients with an LTC want to be actively involved with their care. This chapter has described the benefits of attending of group self-management programmes, such as the EPP, although it is important to remember that not everyone needs or welcomes this type of support. There is no single approach to self-management, and it is important to ascertain patients' preferences for the type and level of support they require. Whole systems approaches such as CCH leading to self-management, which involve services, healthcare professionals and patients are needed to achieve optimal patient outcomes. Early findings from CCH show that collaborative interactions between patients and healthcare professionals are more satisfying and more productive for both parties. Changes in the way healthcare professionals work with patients and changes whereby patients are active partners in their care is a cornerstone of practice required to effectively manage individuals with LTCs, so as to enable them to have fulfilling lives with an LTC whenever possible.

References

Albarracin, D., Gillette, J., Earl, A., Glasman, L. R., Durantini, M. R. and Ho., M. H. (2005) A test of major assumptions about behavior change: a comprehensive look at the effects of passive and active HIV-prevention interventions since the beginning of the epidemic. *Psychological Bulletin* **131**, 856-897.

Bandura, A. (1997) *Self Efficacy, The Exercise of Control*. New York: WH Freeman.

Barlow, J.H. (2001) How to use education as an intervention in osteoarthritis. In: M. Doherty, and M. Dougados (eds) *Osteoarthritis. Balliere's Best Practice Research Clinical Rheumatology* **15**, 545-58.

Barlow, J.H., Sturt, J. and Hearnshaw, H. (2002) Self-management interventions for people with chronic conditions in primary care. Examples from arthritis, asthma and diabetes. *Health Education Journal* **61** (4), 365-378.

Bodenheimer, T., Lorig, K., Holman, H. and Grumbach, K. (2002) Patient self-management of chronic disease in primary care. *Journal of American Medical Association (JAMA)* **288** (19), 2469-2475.

Brooker, C. and Nicol, M. (eds) (2003) *Nursing Adults: The Practice of Caring*. Philadelphia: Mosby.

Cayton, H. (2004) *Patient-engagement and Patient Decision-making in England*. Paper presented at the Improving Quality of Health Care in the United States and the United Kingdom: Strategies for Change and Action.

Cayton, H. and Blomfield, M. (2008) Health citizenship - leaving behind the policies of sickness. In: Christopher Exeter (ed) *Advancing Opportunity: Health and Healthy Living*, Chapter 1. The Smith Institute.

Chambers, R. (2006) The role of the health care professional in supporting self care. *Quality in Primary Care* **14** (3), 129-131.

Clark, N.M., Becker, M.H., Janz N.K., Lorig, K. et al. (1991) Self-management of chronic disease by older adults: a review and questions for research. Journal of Aging Health **3**, 3-27.

Coleman, K., Austin, B., Brach, C. and Wagner, E.H. (2009) Evidence on the chronic care model in the new millennium. *Health Affairs* **28**, 75-85.

Colin-Thome, D. (2006) Key Note Speech in Self Care: Turning Rhetoric into Reality. Available at: http://www.selfcareconnect.co.uk/135 (accessed 31 October 2009).

Corben, S. and Rosen, R. (2005) Self-Management for Long-term Conditions: Patients' Perspectives on the Way Ahead. London: King's Fund. Available at: www.kingsfund.org.uk (accessed 31 October 2009).

Coulter, A. and Elwyn, G. (2002) What do patients want from high quality general practice and how do we involve them in improvement? *The British Journal of General Practice* **Oct 52**, S22- S56.

Coulter, A. and Ellins, J. (2006) Patient-Focused Interventions: A Review of Evidence. London: The Health Foundation. Available at: www.health.org.uk/publications (accessed 31 October 2009).

Davies, M., Heller, S., Khunti, K. and Skinner, T. (2008) The DESMOND educational intervention. *Chronic Illness* **4**, 38-40.

Department of Health (DH) (2000) *The NHS Plan*. London: The Stationery Office.

Department of Health (DH) (2005a) *Self Care – A Real Choice: Self Care Support – A Practical Option.* London: The Stationery Office.

Department of Health (DH) (2005b) *Supporting People with Long-term Conditions: An NHS and Social Care Model to Support Local Innovation and Integration.* London: The Stationery Office.

Department of Health (2006) *Our Health, Our Care, Our Say: A New Direction for Community Services.* London: The Stationery Office.

Department of Health (2008) *High Quality Care for All: The Darzi Report.* London: The Stationery Office.

Department of Health (2010) *Equity and Excellence: Liberating the NHS.* London: The Stationery Office.

DAFNE Study Group (2002) Training in flexible, intensive management to enable dietary freedom in people with Type 1 diabetes: dose adjustment for normal eating (DAFNE) randomised controlled trial. *British Medical Journal* **325** (7367), 746.

Davies, M., Heller, S., Skinner, T., Campbell, M., Carey, M., Cradock, S., Dallosso, H., Daly, H., Doherty, Y., Eaton, S., Fox, C., Oliver, L., Rantell, K., Rayman, G., and Khunti, K. (2008) Effectiveness of the diabetes education and self management for ongoing and newly diagnosed (DESMOND) programme for people with newly diagnosed Type 2 diabetes: cluster randomised controlled trial. *BMJ* **336**, 491-495.

Dongbo, F., Ding, Y., McGowan, P. and Fu, H. (2006) Qualitative evaluation of chronic disease self management program (CDSMP) in Shanghai. *Patient Education and Counseling* **61** (3), 389-96.

Duncan, B.L., Miller, S.D. and Spark, J. (2007) Common factors and the uncommon heroism of youth. *Psychotherapy in Australia* **13** (2), 34-43.

Engel, G. (1977) The need for a new medical model: a challenge for bio-medicine. *Science* **196**, 129-136.

Epping-Jordan, J.E., Pruitt, S.D., Bengoa, R. and Wagner, E.H. (2004) Improving the quality of health care for chronic conditions. *Quality and Safety in Health Care* **13** (4), 299-305.

Foster, G., Taylor, S., Eldridge, S., Ramsay, J. and Griffiths, G. (2007) Self-management education programmes by lay leaders for people with chronic conditions (systematic review). *Cochrane Database of Systematic Reviews* **4**.

Fries, C., Carey, C. and McShane, D.J. (1997) Patient education in arthritis: randomized controlled trial of a mail-delivered program. *Journal of Rheumatology* **24** (7), 1378-1383.

Gantz, S. (1990) Self-care: perspectives from six disciplines. *Holistic Nursing Practice* **4** (2), 1-12.

General Medical Council (2001) Good Medical Practice. Available at: http://www.gmc-uk.org/static/documents/content/GMC_GMP_0911.pdf. (accessed 12 February 2010).

Glasgow, R. and Anderson, R. (1999) In diabetes care, moving from compliance to adherence is not enough. *Diabetes Care* **22**, 2090-2092.

Glasgow, N.J., Jeon, Y.H., Krauss, S.G. and Pearce-Brown, C.L. (2008) Chronic disease self-management support: the way forward for Australia. *Medical Journal of Australia* **189** (10 suppl.), S14–S16.

Great Britain Parliament (2005) Mental Capacity Act (Act of Parliament) London: HMSO.

Griffiths, C., Foster, G., Ramsay, J., Eldridge, S. and Taylor, S. (2007) How effective are expert patient (lay led) education programmes for chronic disease? *British Medical Journal* **334** 1254-1256.

Griffiths, C., Motlib, J., Azad, A., Ramsay, J., Eldridge, S., Feder, G., Khanam, R., Munni, R., Garett, M., Turner, A. and Barlow, J. (2005) Randomised controlled trial of a lay-led self-management programme for Bangaldeshi patients with chronic disease. *British Journal of General Practice* **55** 831-837.

Hall, J.A. and Roter, D. (2007) Physician-patient communication. In: H. Friedman and R. Silver (eds) *Foundations of Health Psychology* New York: Oxford University Press.

Health Foundation's Co-Creating Health Project (2008) Available at: http://www.health.org.uk/ (accessed 12 April 2010).

Hoffman, C., Rice, D. and Sung, H.Y. (1996) Persons with chronic conditions. Their prevalence and costs. *Journal of the American Medical Association* **276**, 1473-1479.

Horan, M.C., Yarborough, G., Besigel and Carlson, D.R. (1990) Computer-assisted self-control of diabetes by adolescents. *Diabetes Education* **16**, 205-211.

International Council of Nurses (2005) *Supporting Statement. Preparing a Health Care Workforce for the 21st century.* Switzerland: World Health Organisation.

Kennedy, A., Reeves, D., Bower, P., Lee, V., Middleton, E., Richardson, G., Gardner, C., Gately, C., and Rogers, A. (2007) The effectiveness and cost effectiveness of a national lay-led self-care support programme for patients with long-term conditions: a pragmatic randomised controlled trial. *Journal of Epidemiology and Community Health*, **61** (3), 254-261.

Lawn, S., M. Battersby, R. G. Pols, J. Lawrence, T. Parry and M. Urukalo (2007) The mental health expert patient: findings from a pilot study of a generic chronic condition self-management programme for people with mental illness. *International Journal of Social Psychiatry* **53** (1), 63-74.

Lau-Walker, M. and Thompson, D. (2009) Self-management in long-term health conditions: a complex concept poorly understood and applied? *Patient Education and Counselling* **75**, 290-292.

Lorig, K. (1995) Patient education: treatment or nice extra? *British Journal of Rheumatology* **34**, 703-706.

Lorig, K.R., Sobel, D.S., Stewart, A.L., Brown Jr, B.W., Ritter, P.L., González, V.M., Laurent, D.D. and Holman, H.R. (1999a) Evidence suggesting that a chronic disease self-management program can improve health status while reducing utilization and costs: a randomized trial. *Medical Care* **37** (1), 5-14.

Lorig, K., Gonzalez, V.M. and Ritter, P. (1999b) Community-based Spanish language arthritis education program: a randomized trial. *Medical Care* **37** (9), 957-63.

Makinen, S., Suominen, T. and Lauri, S. (2000) Self care in adults with asthma: how they cope. *Journal of Clinical Nursing* **9**, 557-565.

Marinker, M. (2000) *Viewpoint.* Primary Care Pharmacy **4**, 93-95.

Marquis, B. and Huston, C. (2009) *Leadership Roles and Management Functions in Nursing*, 6th edn. Philadelphia: Walters Kluwer/Lippincott, Williams and Wilkins.

Newman, S. and Cooke, D. (2008) Conclusions. In: S. Newman, E. Steed and K. Mulligan (eds) *Chronic Physical Illness: Self-Management and Behavioural Interventions*. Maidenhead, UK: McGraw Hill Open University Press.

Nieuwehuijsen, E., Zemper, E., Miner, K. and Epstein, M. (2006) Health behaviour change models: contributions to rehabilitation. *Disability and Rehabilitation* **28** (5), 245-256.

Nursing and Midwifery Council (2008) *The Code*. London: NMC.

Orem, D. (2001) *Nursing: Concepts of Practice*, 6th edn. St Louis: Mosby.

Prochaska, J. and DiClemente, C. (1984) *The Transtheoretical Approach: Crossing Traditional Foundations of Change*. Harnewood, Illinois: Don Jones/Irwin.

Prochaska, J. and DiClemente, C. (1986) Towards a comprehensive model of change. In: Miller, W. and Heather, N. (eds) *Treating Addictive Behaviours: Process of Change*. New York: Plenum.

Prochaska, J., DiClemente, C. and Norcross, J. (1992) In search of how people change. *American Psychologist* **47**, 1102-1114.

Randall, S. (2006) Secondhand smoke: not just a community issue. *Paediatric Nursing* **18** (2), 28-31.

Redman, B. (2004) *Patient Self-Management of Chronic Disease*. Sudbury: Jones and Bartlett.

Redman, B. (2007) Responsibility for control: ethics of patient preparation for self-management of chronic disease. *Bioethics* **21** (5), 243-250.

Rethink (2003) Self-Management: The Experiences and Views of Self-Management of People with a Diagnosis of Schizophrenia. Available at: www.rethink.org/document.rm?id=130 (accessed 12 April 2010).

Royal Pharmaceutical Society of Great Britain (1997) *From Compliance to Concordance: Achieving Shared Goals in Medicine Taking*. London: RPSGB.

Serlachius, A. and Sutton, S. (2009) Self-management and behaviour change: theoretical models. In: S. Newman, L. Steed and K. Mulligan (eds) *Chronic Physical Illness: Self-Management and Behavioural Interventions*. New York: McGraw Hill, Open University Press.

Simeoni, E., Bauman, A., Stenmark, J. and O'Brien, J. (1995) Evaluation of a community arthritis program in Australia: dissemination of a developed program. *Arthritis Care Res.* **8**, 102-107.

Swerissen, H., Belfrage, J., Weeks, A., Jordan, L., Walker, C., Furler, J., McAvoy, B., Carter, M. and Peterson, C. (2006) Randomised control trial of a self-management program for people with a chronic illness from Vietnamese, Chinese, Italian and Greek backgrounds. *Patient Education and Counseling* **64** (1-3), 360-368.

Thorne, S., Nhylin, K. and Paterson, P. (2000) Attitudes towards patient expertise in chronic illness. *International Journal of Nursing Studies* **37**, 301-311.

Turner, A. (2010) The HOPE Course. In: F.R. Jones (ed) *Perspectives on Lay Led Self-Management Courses for People with Long-term Conditions* p 26-33, Oxford: Oxford University Press.

Section 2

Turner, A.P. and Barlow, J.H. (2007) The expert patients programme: a resource for GPs treating chronic disease and co-existing common mental health problems? *Mental Health Review Journal* **12** (2), 4-6.

Wagner, E.H., Austin, B.T., Davis, C., Hindmarsh, M., Schaefer, J. and Bonomi, A. (2001) Improving chronic illness care: translating evidence into action: interventions that encourage people to acquire self-management skills are essential in chronic illness care. *Health Affairs* **20**, 64-78.

Wagner, E.H. (1998) Chronic disease management: what will it take to improve care for chronic illness? *Effective Clinical Practice* **1**, 2-4. Available at: www.acponline.org/clinical_information/journals_publications/ecp/augsep98/cdm.pdf (accessed on 22 April 2010)

Walker, C., Weeks, A., McAvoy, B. and Demetriou, E. (2005) Exploring the role of self-management programmes in caring for people from culturally and linguistically diverse backgrounds in Melbourne, Australia. *Health Expectations*, **8** (4), 315-323.

Weinberger, M., Tierney, W.M., Cowper, P.A., Katz, B.P. and Booher, P.A. (1993) Cost-effectiveness of increased telephone contact for patients with osteoarthritis. A randomized controlled trial. *Arthritis and Rheumatism* **36** (2), 243-6.

White, L. and Clegg, A. (2009) Encouraging and supporting patients living with long-term conditions to self-care. *Nursing Times* **105**, 31.

Wilkinson, A. and Whitehead, L. (2009) Evolution of the concept of self care and implications for nurses: a literature review. *International Journal of Nursing Studies* **46**, 1143-1147.

Wilson, P. (2001) A policy analysis of the expert patient in the United Kingdom: self care as an expression of pastoral power? *Health and Social Care in the Community* **9** (3), 134-142.

Wilson, P. and Mayor, V. (2006) Long-term conditions 2: supporting and enabling self care. *British Journal of Community Nursing* **11** (1), 6-10.

Wilson, P., Kendall, S. and Brooks, F. (2006) Nurses' responses to expert patients: the rhetoric and reality of self management in long-term conditions: a grounded theory study. *International Journal of Nursing Studies* **43**, 803-818.

Wilson, P. and Kendall, S., (2007) The expert patient programme: a paradox of patient empowerment and medical dominance. *Health and Social Care in the Community* **15** (5), 1-13.

Resources

- Self Care Connect Available at: www.selfcareconnect.co.uk/
- Health Foundation Available at: www.health.org.uk/
- Expert Patient Programme Available at: www.expertpatients.co.uk/

Further reading

Jones, F.R. (ed) (2010) *Working with Self-management participants, planners and policy-makers*. Oxford: Oxford University Press.

Mayor, V. (2005) Long-term conditions 3: Being an expert patient. *British Journal of Community Nursing*, **11** (2), 59-63.

Salter, B. (2004) *The New Politics of Medicine*. Basingstoke: Palgrave Macmillan.

Section 2

Chapter 6

Assistive Technology – A Means of Empowerment

Darren Awang and Gillian Ward

Learning objectives

By the end of this chapter, the reader will be able to:

- Establish the policy context of assistive technology (AT)
- Review key terms and define and explain the potential of AT with reference to LTCs
- Provide examples of how AT might be used
- Use reflective exercises around the use of AT
- Identify relevant resources for readers to explore in self-directed study

Introduction

This chapter highlights the important role that AT can play in enabling, maintaining and supporting the lifestyles of individuals with LTCs. Advances in AT have and continue to develop at pace within western societies. In this first section the policy background that supports the AT agenda is explored to give readers a clear sense that the government's commitment to the effective use of technology is a common policy theme in different parts of the United Kingdom.

Given that potential resource restrictions affecting many sectors (including health and social care provision) will become much more apparent in the coming years it is likely that the emphasis on the utilisation of AT will grow rather than diminish.

It is argued by the Foundation for Assistive Technology (FAST 2006) that the role of AT should be seen to complement a range of interventions to support both individuals and their families. With the emphasis on the need for health and social care professionals to select and justify the right kinds of interventions that fully take into account the needs, wishes, capacities and circumstances of the individuals concerned and the available evidence and resources, AT is no different to any other intervention that professionals may consider.

Long-term Conditions: A Guide for Nurses and Healthcare Professionals, First Edition. Edited by S. Randall and H. Ford.
© 2011 Blackwell Publishing Ltd. Published 2011 by Blackwell Publishing Ltd.

Subsequent sections of this chapter explore what AT is, how it works, and what evidence there is to underpin its use to support individuals with a variety of LTCs.

Policy background

Since the late 1980s successive governments in the United Kingdom have identified the increasing preference for people that use health and social care services to retain their independence and remain in their own homes or homely environments rather than move into costly residential or nursing care (Griffiths 1988). This sentiment was enshrined within the NHS and Community Care Act (Great Britain Parliament 1990). Since then there has been a series of policies to support these goals. Consultation received on the Green Paper 'Independence, Wellbeing and Choice' has reaffirmed this position (Department of Health (DH) 2005a).

Recognition of the potential of AT to complement health and social care provision in the United Kingdom has been steadily growing. For example, the report by the Royal Commission for Long-term Care *With Respect to Old Age* (DH 1999: 2, 159) identified that new technology and information technology would become increasingly important to enhance future quality of life. This document was important as it recognised that the modernisation of financial resource systems was required to adapt to the changing demographics of the growing older population and the subsequent need to plan effectively to meet living, housing and personal care costs.

In 2000, The NHS Plan (DH 2000) set out a commitment to modernise and reform the NHS. It was underpinned by ten NHS core principles. At the centre of reform was the vision to redesign the NHS around the patient. Although the vision placed emphasis on the development of information technology infrastructures, other technological advances within intermediate care and promoting independence highlighted the need to make use of community equipment services and 'more sophisticated equipment such as fall alarms and remote sensor devices' (DH 2000 126).

The NHS Plan was complemented by a series of National Service Frameworks (NSFs) (NHS 2010) that attempted to establish a range of healthcare standards for identified areas. These NSFs identified clear quality requirements and strategies that organisations could use to achieve these. To date NSFs have been introduced covering the following:

- Cancer
- Children
- Coronary heart disease
- Diabetes
- LTCs
- Mental health
- Older people
- Renal services

A national strategy for stroke was developed and a strategy for Chronic Obstructive Pulmonary Disease (COPD) is in development.

Within the NSF for Older People (DH 2001) specific mention is given to the wider application of 'new technologies' to support the safety and security of older and disabled people using, for example, fall alarms and sensors (p. 37) extending the use of Telecare or environmental control technologies (including passive alarms) to provide 'added safety for those who are particularly vulnerable.'

Section 2

(p. 85). Those with community-based mental health needs should receive service that includes out-reach facilities, including Telecare and environmental technologies (p. 105).

Of particular interest is the emerging role of AT particularly in the Long-term Conditions NSF (DH 2005b) where the need to provide 'appropriate assistive technology/equipment and adaptations to accommodation to support them to live independently, help them with their care, maintain their health and improve their quality of life.' (p. 4) is recognised for example with people with rapidly deteriorating conditions, long-term neurological conditions and brain injury conditions.

Examples are given of the application of AT. These include the use of a falls detector as part of Telecare package to provide an alert to a call centre for someone with epilepsy; the provision of communication aids to support social participation and prevent the potential development of depression; and the use of an electric standing frame to reduce the number of carers needed to transfer and position a person.

The Long-term Conditions NSF (DH 2005b) also identifies the need for a holistic assessment that considers the home environment, lifestyle and the need for practical advice on how to use AT/equipment not only for patients but also for staff training. In addition, specialist assessments to meet complex needs with coordinated approaches are highlighted.

In terms of obtaining equipment, the Long-term Conditions NSF refers to good models of practice linking in Integrated Community Equipment Services (ICES) and advisory/information services to encourage choice to enable people to assess their own needs and advise them on using direct payments to buy basic items of equipment.

The momentum for the development of AT was further enhanced by the introduction of Building Telecare in England (DH 2005c). This confirmed the investment of £80 million to local authorities during 2006-2008 to develop Telecare-related services to support people to remain independent.

The White Paper 'Our Health, Our Care, Our Say' (DH 2006) set out the government's vision in bringing health and social care much closer to the person's home rather than being provided in acute hospital care settings. Drawing upon two reports (Wanless 2002, 2004) the White Paper outlined a 10-15 year strategy to transform social care to enable service users to have more control, choice and help to decide how to meet their needs and to give them the best quality of support and protection to those with the highest needs. The *intensive* use of assistive and home monitoring technologies was highlighted as having a clear role in this vision. For example, people with LTCs could use in-home touch screen units to feedback data to health professionals remotely so the detection of episodes of illness could be identified earlier thereby minimising or eliminating acute admissions. Putting People First Concordat (DH 2007a) reiterated how adult users of social care services should be able to take a greater role in their own personal care to maximise choice, control and power over their services. Included at the heart of this personalisation drive (see also the Darzi Report, DH 2008a) was the increased emphasis on personal (or individual) budgets (to be extended to NHS resources in the form of personal health budgets), targets to be increased for service users to take up direct payments and the transformation of community equipment services to adopt a retail market model.

Summary

AT has been identified as an important aspect in the transformation of health and social care over the next decade. It will play an increasingly vital role in enabling people to remain at home, offering innovative choices on how care is provided. Current and future health and social care workers need to understand what AT is available and how it can be used to empower the individuals and families they work with to support their health and social care needs.

Defining key terms

An important aspect to consider with regard to AT is deciding upon an overarching definition. There has been an ongoing debate as how to define AT and the different aspects or subcategories that have developed. The rapid development of new technologies, whilst providing new opportunities in terms of the scope of its applications, has also meant that consensual agreement on what we understand by various AT-related terminologies is constantly shifting.

Several definitions have emerged over the last decade. For example, the US *'Tech Act'* definition has been cited widely as:

Any item, piece of equipment, product or system, whether acquired commercially, off the shelf, modified or customized, that is used to increase, maintain or improve the functional capabilities of individuals with cognitive, physical or communication disabilities. (The Technology-Related Assistance for Individuals with Disabilities Act, 1988)

This definition clearly identifies that AT has a remit specifically for disabled people to enhance functional abilities.

Perhaps a more straightforward definition was adopted by Royal Commission on Long-term Care (1999b: 325) as:

An umbrella term for any device or system that allows an individual to perform a task they would otherwise be unable to do or increases the ease and safety with which the task can be performed.

Here, the emphasis appears more inclusive indicating that AT can have benefits to the wider population. The focus is on the enabling nature of AT rather than it being designed for a particular group of people.

According to Blackhurst and Lahm (2000: 7) assistive technologies (ATs) include:

mechanical, electronic, and microprocessor-based equipment, non-mechanical and non-electronic aids, specialized instructional materials, services, and strategies that people with disabilities can use either to (a) assist them in learning, (b) make the environment more accessible, (c) enable them to compete in the workplace, (d) enhance their independence, or (e) otherwise improve their quality of life. These may include commercially available or 'home made' devices that are specially designed to meet the idiosyncratic needs of a particular individual.

This definition demonstrates the wide scope of what can be considered as AT, the context in which it can be used and the concept that it can be both mainstream *and* person specific. Here AT could span what is commonly called 'community equipment', environmental adaptations and/or control systems, information and communication technologies and monitoring technologies.

Doughty et al. (2007) have reviewed how terminology around AT, Telehealth and Telecare is used. They suggest a model that incorporates three major categories. These are AT, Telecare and Telemedicine. These categories exist across a continuum where the focus may shift from the home or institution (in terms of where care is being provided) and the increasing or decreasing use of telecommunication technology.

Within this model AT refers to fixed or portable adaptations or community equipment that may be mechanical or non-mechanical and may have electronic components. Telecare covers a multitude of equipment and systems that includes alarms or alerting equipment and systems, intelligent monitoring (ambient) systems, and Telehealth systems. Telemedicine focuses on the remote consultation between medics with other medics or directly, and with patients (Doughty et al. 2007).

These examples indicate the potential ambiguity around the use of the term 'assistive technology' and how it can mean different things to different people. According to Doughty et al. (2007), there is a real need to adopt a range of standard definitions to simplify the process of delivering service improvements, establishing best practice and the integration of technologies. As this debate continues the following sections of this chapter adopt a broad approach to what can be considered as AT and specific definitions for each subcategory addressed are provided for the reader.

Telecare

Telecare has become an umbrella term for all assistive and medical technologies that depend on electronic devices and/or telecommunication systems to enable people to maximise their independence within their environment (Doughty et al. 2007). This is mainly within the person's own home but it can be used within a ward or residential/care setting. Telecare has advanced and developed through three generations and continues to develop with the integration of environmental controls and Telehealth monitoring.

Common Telecare sensors include the following:

- Pull cords
- Fall detectors
- Smoke detectors
- Flood detectors
- Gas and CO_2 detectors
- Door exit sensors
- Bogus caller alarms

First generation telecare

Community alarms were the first generation of Telecare devices; these simple devices have no embedded intelligent system and are reliant on the user raising an alarm in an emergency situation, to detect a fall, for example, through pulling a cord or pressing a button on a pendant alarm worn around the neck (Advanced Care Technologies Programme 2010). Community alarms are the most common assistive technology device, even in light of the technological advances in AT over the last fifteen years. Yet, the simplicity of the community alarm system is also its major limitation – the lack of an intelligent mechanism embedded within the device relies on the user to raise the alarm, which is impossible if the person is unconscious or out of reach of the alarm when they fall (Porteus and Brownsell 2000). Community alarms are usually linked to a call centre and afford the benefit of providing 24-hour care while being potentially cost-effective for health and social care services. In a survey of 2,596 community alarm users in Birmingham, 80% of the participants thought that 24-hour care from the control centre was a very important feature of the community alarm service (Birmingham City Council Housing Department 1997, cited in Brownsell et al. 2000). Within the sample, 86% thought the community alarm system worked well. Though Brownsell and colleagues acknowledged that this positive attitude towards community alarms might be due to participants having no alternative to community alarms to aid comparison.

Second generation telecare

The second-generation Telecare systems are based on the first generation but have an embedded level of intelligence (Porteus and Brownsell 2000). Depending on the device, some can either be placed on the user or placed within the user's environment, which reduces the need for the user's participation in raising an alarm (Porteus and Brownsell 2000). The second generation includes some fall detection devices and life-style monitoring systems.

Worn automatic fall detectors are second generation devices. The device is based on the simple mechanism of first generation but in addition will provide an immediate response to a fall without a trigger being pressed by the user (Doughty et al. 2000).

Third generation telecare

The third generation of Telecare systems are based on the automatic detection functions of the second generation systems (Porteus and Brownsell 2000), but with added support identified through activity or life-style monitoring devices and devices to include medical/vital signs monitoring (Telehealth), virtual consultations (Telemedicine) and neighbourhood communication and networks (Brownsell and Bradley 2003).

Brownsell et al. (2000) investigated whether a sample of 179 older people who lived within sheltered housing in Birmingham would prefer Telecare instead of a traditional community alarm service. Mixed opinions were given on the usefulness of four types of Telecare defined within this study as: Telemedicine, automatic fall detection, lifestyle monitoring and video conferencing. Focusing on prevention and detection of falls in older people, 77% of the participants said they were fearful of falling and were interested in the fall detector. Lifestyle monitoring equipment was also viewed highly, with 68% of residents interested in the system, and interestingly they were not deterred by the suggestion of a monitoring unit in the bathroom and suggested this would have potential benefits. Overall just over half (57%) of the residents were interested in AT to support them, indicating that there is a need for healthcare professionals to be aware of the benefits of AT and be able to offer this within the service that they provide, or at least provide information about where the service user can access this technology.

Ward-based use of telecare to monitor falls

Falls by inpatients on hospital wards are common, with the National Patient Safety Agency (NPSA 2007) reporting that, on average, an 800-bed acute trust can expect to have at least 1260 inpatient falls every year and these are only the ones that are reported to the NPSA. There has been an increasing focus on risk management to prevent falls in the hospital environment (Oliver 2004). A controlled clinical trial over 8 weeks by Spetz et al. (2007) that incorporated vital signs monitoring and a bed exit sensor into the existing bedside call system demonstrated the overall effectiveness of the system in reducing the rate of inpatient falls. However, the cost-effectiveness analysis found that use of the system was associated with higher measured costs, although they concluded that it was likely that the system was saving overall due to unmeasured costs (i.e. the treatment of injury sustained through a fall).

Who benefits from telecare?

The absence of published information about cost and clinical effectiveness has been given as a major reason why Telecare has not become embedded as a routine service (Brownsell et al. 2008). Although evidence is emerging on a small scale as reported here, the potential impact of AT on a larger scale will be better understood when the Whole System Demonstrator (WSD) sites in England are evaluated in 2011 (see section 'Whole system demonstrators').

In Scotland, the National Telecare Development Programme (TDP) has estimated savings to be over £11 million. In the evaluation report compiled by the York Health Economics Consortium at York University, it is estimated that over 81,000 bed days have been saved in Scotland in only 1 year as a result of the Telecare services installed. This is broken down into 5,668 hospital bed days saved by facilitating quicker hospital discharge, 13,870 reduced unplanned hospital admissions, and 61,990 care home bed days saved by avoiding the need for people to move into care homes (York Health Economics Consortium/Scottish Government 2009).

However, as Gatward (2004) states 'Telecare cuts across three funding streams; there is a mismatch of budget and benefit': the NHS benefits considerably because of reduced admissions and faster discharge after a fall; Social Services will bear most of the costs; however, over time a reduction in residential care costs will accumulate if Telecare is used to its full potential. Also, the Supporting People agenda benefits as the technology enables people to stay in their own homes at a more affordable cost.

Summary

Telecare uses technology to support people to live independently, primarily within their own home but can be used within other environments. Community alarms connected to a 24-hour call centre are the most common type of AT but it is continuing to develop with a range of sensors that are more intelligent in the way that they detect a potential risk and with the integration of environmental controls and Telehealth monitoring.

Telehealth

In the United Kingdom, Telehealth can be described as the reliable and accurate remote monitoring of patients' vital signs. It is used in the management of LTCs such as diabetes, chronic heart failure and COPD (Barlow et al. 2007).

Typically, Telehealth systems are customisable so that specific parameters can be set for individual patients which provide an alert through a variety of media to the healthcare professional when parameters are exceeded. Patients would be trained in the use of the peripheral equipment (such as a blood pressure cuff) and be responsible for taking their own measurements which are then transmitted electronically to a healthcare professional or delegate responsible for reviewing their care.

The range of peripheral devices is evolving and physiological measurements that can be taken include the following:

- Blood pressure
- Blood glucose levels
- Pulse rates
- Oxygen saturation
- Temperature
- Weight

In addition, systems can also incorporate care plans that can be updated by healthcare professionals. This can include individual questionnaires or access to specific information or guidance (smoking cessation, exercise programmes, alcohol advice). Data are kept securely and can be sent to relevant parties including patients if they manage their own records.

Portable Telehealth equipment is being developed and there are medical applications that can, for example, turn the Apple iPhone into a personal medical assistant through its capability for direct connectivity to hardware, in particular medical monitoring devices. Combined with an accelerometer (an instrument that measures acceleration in mobility) built into the iPhone these new advancements offer unprecedented opportunities for falls prevention (Richardson 2009).

In their systematic review of the benefits of home Telecare, Barlow et al. (2007) concluded that the most effective intervention appeared to be automated vital signs monitoring (to reduce health service use) and telephone follow-up by nurses, though the cost-effectiveness of these interventions was less clear. Nearly two-thirds of these studies related to the management of diabetes and heart failure. A number of Telehealth projects have been instigated throughout the United Kingdom; some, for example, funding through the Preventative Technology Grant and others through the more recent Regional Innovation Fund. This £220 million fund is based on the vision to create an innovative NHS as set out in 'High Quality Care for All' (DH 2008) that has enabled Strategic Health Authorities to pilot Telehealth schemes some of which have been led by community matrons.

Telehealth coaching

Health coaching has been defined as an interactive role undertaken by a peer or professional individual to support a patient to be an active participant in the self-management of a chronic illness (Lindner et al. 2003). In particular, it addresses the encouragement a person with an LTC may require to support behavioural change in adherence to medication, weight loss or dietary changes, physical activity and blood monitoring for example. Support may be offered and received via the Internet, by email or over the telephone. Telephone Health Coaching (Telecoaching) has been shown to be effective in lowering cholesterol in patients with heart disease where the 'patients are coached to know their risk factor levels, the target level for their risk factors, and how to achieve the target levels for their risk factors' (Vale et al. 2003 p. 2776). Telecoaching has been shown to support healthy behaviour change in older people using the telephone and email (Bennett et al. 2005) and is being tested in the management of diabetes (Young et al. 2007).

In their review, Lindner et al. (2003) stated that despite limited literature, health coaching has great potential in enhancing self-management in chronic illness. Further research needs to address the mechanisms that make coaching successful (including the focus of the intervention, the mode of delivery, and the characteristics of the coach), providing guidelines for evidence-based practices, and facilitating its integration into routine healthcare.

Virtual wards

The concept of the virtual ward was developed in Croydon Primary Care Trust (South London) in 2006. Led by community matrons, virtual wards care for vulnerable patients living at home who have long-term health conditions and run the highest risk of unplanned admission to hospital (see Croydon NHS Trust Virtual Ward case study (Lewis 2006)).

Virtual wards use the systems, staffing and daily routine of a hospital ward to provide care management in the community; the term 'virtual' is used because there is no physical ward building:

patients are cared for in their own homes (Lewis 2006). This 1-year pilot study at Croydon PCT has cost around £68,000; however, it is expected to save Croydon PCT £1.5 million, suggesting that virtual wards are cost-effective (NHS 2009).

The Virtual Wards pilot study has sparked the development for other innovative uses of technology to improve patient care. One concept is the use of location-based virtual notes where hospital staff leave short digital messages at appropriate locations, such as patient's bed, so that intended staff can pick up the messages later (Dahl 2006). The concept has been trialled in Norway, with results reporting that location-based virtual notes have the potential to improve information exchange between hospital workers (Dahl 2006). This would be an interesting concept to extend to community-based services with the virtual notes situated within the person's home.

Telemedicine

In an attempt to define Telemedicine, Sood et al. (2007) carried out an extensive literature review that produced 104 peer reviewed definitions of Telemedicine and concluded that 'it is a branch of e-health that uses communications networks for delivery of healthcare services and medical education from one location to another. It is deployed to overcome issues like uneven distribution and shortage of infrastructural and human resources' (Sood et al. p. 573). They also went on to discuss the promise of numerous benefits of Telemedicine including improved access to services, diminished inequalities in care, lower costs – particularly transport costs, and improved quality and efficiency of services. Telemedicine offers advantages to those communities that are very rural and a long way from major health centres in that specialist opinion can be sought without the patient having to travel long distances for consultation.

One of the major criticisms of Telemedicine is often directed towards that of acceptability to patients. However, as early as 2000 when remote communication technologies such as video conferencing, use of webcams and Skype (a software application that allows users to make voice calls over the Internet) were not as advanced, a systematic review of 32 studies of patient satisfaction with Telemedicine found that tele-consultation was acceptable to patients in a variety of circumstances, though firm conclusions were limited by methodological limitations of the studies included in the review (Mair and Whitten 2000).

Telehealthcare integration

The Telecare Services Association (TSA) has developed a Code of Practice for use by Telecare service providers to ensure quality standards for service delivery and identifies the need for protocols to be established that build confidence in the whole Telecare solution (which may include Telehealth monitoring), the equipment, and the remote monitoring and response elements (TSA 2009). Beech and Roberts (2008) cite an example where Telehealth systems for monitoring a person's vital signs must be linked to systems and protocols for providing assistance when required.

Activity monitoring

Lifestyle monitoring systems (LMS) typically make use of passive infrared (PIR) movement detectors in the key rooms of a house that are triggered as a person moves around their home and provide a chart of activity via the Internet. Data from the sensors are gathered by the controller and sent via an integral mobile phone to a web server. Family members and professionals can log on to a password protected website to view an activity chart, the advantage being that lifestyle monitoring systems need no input from the person who is being monitored.

This type of system has been mostly used to support people with dementia and their carers whilst healthcare professionals use the system for assessment and planning care. The system highlights what a person is still able to do for themselves in the familiarity of their own home, which is often more than expected. These systems are simple to install, there are no video cameras. The system is radio-based and there is no wiring. All that is required is a mains power socket in the person's home, and Internet access by the professional or carer (Just Checking 2010).

Generally, activity monitoring systems do not provide alerts and are not connected to call centres to raise an alarm, though these can be integrated in some systems.

Despite several commercial systems being available, there have been relatively few studies aimed at evaluating monitoring systems (Barnes et al. 1998, Glascock and Kutzik 2006, Sixsmith et al. 2007). In an evaluation of the activity monitoring 'Just Checking' system carried out by the Care Services Efficiency Delivery (CSED) (2008), stand-alone lifestyle monitoring systems that do not link to a call centre, have been shown to be cost-effective. Though this was a relatively small evaluation with only 21 participants, cost savings were shown of up to £120,400. A cost-benefit analysis of the same system carried out by Warwickshire County Council in 2006, estimated that if half an hour of home care could be saved for 150 people then net annual savings of £33,528, or 2730 hours of home care could be made (Warwickshire County Council 2006). Case study 6.1 (with kind permission of Just Checking) provides an example of how the system can be used.

Case study 6.1 Activity monitoring – supporting independence

Mrs Bowler lives in private retirement flat where she moved some years ago. She has moderate dementia and doesn't always recognise her daughter who calls a couple of times a week in her lunch hour (she works close to her mother's home). Mrs Bowler has two home care calls a day – breakfast and teatime. Mrs Bowler is a very private person. Her daughter says she has never been someone who has sought much social contact. She doesn't like someone coming in and out of her house that she doesn't know and finds the home care visits intrusive. There are several concerns regarding Mrs Bowler:

- The home care staff report that Mrs Bowler was not eating when they went in.
- Her daughter often finds her asleep in the chair in the lounge at lunchtime and wonders if she is up a lot in the night and tired in the day.
- The care manager is considering putting in third home care visit at lunchtime, though Mrs Bowler is not keen on this.

The monitoring charts show
Mrs Bowler gets up just after 7 a.m., uses the bathroom, goes into the lounge and then into the kitchen where she spends half an hour or so. The time in the kitchen is repeated at lunchtime, and again in the evening, and correlates to mealtimes. Home care call comes in at 8.30, by which time it looks as if Mrs Bowler has already had breakfast and doesn't want to eat again. Typically in the evening she was eating after the home care call. Regular visits to the bathroom help to confirm that Mrs Bowler is eating and drinking. In the night, movement in the bedroom and bathroom as Mrs Bowler gets up to go to the toilet, but she returns to bed – she is not using any other rooms in the house.

Section 2

There are periods of activity and periods of quiet. Often there was a period of quiet after lunch, when Mrs Bowler would doze in the chair, and this was the time when her daughter usually came in. Her daughter was surprised at the level of activity in the day, she thought her mother was much more inactive than the charts show.

At the weekend, the door was not used at all, and Mrs Bowler did not receive a home care visit. Once this had occurred for several weekends the care manager took action with the care agency that had not been providing the agreed care package.

Outcomes

Reduced home care from two to one visit a day, more independence for Mrs Bowler, saving 3.5 hrs per wk × £13.60 = £47.60 = £2475 p.a.

Home care call emphasis changed to showering and changing clothes two times a week (daughter noticed her mother was not changing her clothes).

The system provided objective information about missed home care visits.

-With kind permission of Just Checking

> ## Points for reflection
>
> - Could a lifestyle monitoring system be useful to support people with other LTCs? Think about how and when it could be used.
> - What are the ethical implications to consider with this type of technology?

Further activity monitoring development

Lifestyle monitoring systems

Fuzzy ambient intelligence (Martin et al. 2007) is an example of a third generation system where a customised sensor network is installed within a person's home. The sensors detect a person's movements and their use of furniture and household items, for example the cooker, kettle, toilet, the intelligent device then analyses the movements to answer questions, such as, 'is the person eating regularly?' The lifestyle monitoring system (LMS) provides long-term trend patterns of the user's behaviour, to enable the intelligent system to detect any abnormal patterns of behaviour (Martin et al. 2007). Systems like this are now available such as 'ADLife' (Tunstall 2010) which is designed as an early warning system to provide information about the person's activities of daily living and combines the benefits of a Telecare system. The device is useful for care providers as it provides a summary of the user's data, so that even providers with limited expert knowledge can analyse the data.

Porteus and Brownsell's (2000) field trial of an LMS with 22 participants found that 80% were either very or fairly satisfied with the LMS and 70% thought that if they needed help the LMS would detect this and automatically call for help (even though this would only be possible if the LMS were linked with a Telecare system) and 64% of carers believed that the LMS was more effective than the existing community alarm system. A combination of Telecare and lifestyle monitoring can ensure that systems are in place to alert relatives and professional staff to changes in individual behaviour that might indicate a need for medical attention which if left unattended may require hospital admission; this system is, therefore, of interest in managing LTCs.

Intelligent monitoring within care facilities

Similar systems to Just Checking also exist for use within residential and nursing care homes. The MyAmego (MyAmego 2010) system is an intelligent nurse call system that has been developed specifically for people with cognitive impairments and dementia.

A wireless system is set up in the care home that can detect special fobs which are worn by the resident and pagers that care staff wear. Information about the relative location of residents and staff is transmitted to a personal computer (PC) within the home via a simple web interface. This can enable staff to be alerted should residents enter any identified risk areas in real time; for example, exits, kitchen areas, stairs, other residents' private rooms. It is customisable so that each resident can have their own personalised care programme or profile set-up that allows them a degree of independence by the creation of 'safe zones' within their environment without the constant need for intrusive monitoring or 'shadowing' by staff. This can enable staff and residents to engage in the development or more meaningful occupations that could improve the quality of care experienced.

At the moment little evidence exists of the efficacy of such systems apart from anecdotal accounts. Case study 6.2 gives such an account.

Section 2

Case study 6.2 Intelligent monitoring – a vital bridge between own tenancy and care

Background

Opened in January 2009, Madelvic Square is a new waterfront housing development in Edinburgh. Created by Edinburgh City Council and NHS Lothian, in partnership with Cairn Housing Association, it aims to deliver a Housing Support Service to older people with varying impairments and support needs, including dementia. Accommodation consists of seven two-bedroom flats and seven one-bedroom flats – all with living room, kitchen and shower room. All flats are accessible by lift and the building enjoys a communal roof garden. A warden is on site seven days a week from 8 a.m. to 10 p.m., providing assistance and meals. Overnight cover is provided remotely by Edinburgh's Community Alarm Service.

Independent living for longer

The residents of seven of the flats have high-care needs, such as blindness and cognitive impairment. These residents have elected directly, or through relatives holding power of attorney, to take advantage of the MyAmego monitoring system. "MyAmego passively monitors risks and mobility, to alert staff when assistance is required – thereby allowing these residents both to participate in community living and enjoy the full safety of their own homes," said the development's Occupational Therapist, Paddy Corscadden. "It also allows us to be proactive in identifying potential problems associated with lack of movement and lack of normal activity such as toilet visits." With MyAmego in operation, people who otherwise were within a month of care home entry, can remain independent at Madelvic Square. "Indeed, one of our high-care residents actually came out of a care home to live with us", said Donna Fleming, Edinburgh Council's Telecare Projects' Manager. "An essential feature of MyAmego is its ability to provide activity reports, for both internal review and care commission inspection - where," Donna was proud to report, "it ticked all the boxes for better care delivery."

-By kind permission of MyAmego

Points for reflection

- What are the benefits to the residents of this type of AT?
- What might be the risks in using a system like this?
- How might consent for use of a monitoring system like this be obtained from residents?

Summary

Activity monitoring systems such as lifestyle monitoring and intelligent monitoring systems typically make use of PIR movement detectors in the key rooms of a home/care environment that are triggered as a person moves around their environment and provide a chart of activity via the Internet. This can be done within an individual's own home, supported living accommodation or within a residential care facility. It affords the opportunity for relatives or care staff to be proactive rather than reactive in identifying potential problems or areas of risk for the person within in their environment.

Environmental controls and communication devices

Environmental control systems (ECS) encompass an area of AT designed to:

> ...help people with a severe physical disability to maintain or increase independence by giving them the means to operate electrical ... home security, communication and domestic appliances. (Medical Devices Agency 1995)

ECS have very close development links to home automation and 'smart homes' that have evolved over recent decades. Whereas the focus on home automation is on the mainstream intelligent automatic control of the environment, environmental controls (EC) can provide environmental accessibility solutions for people with specific LTCs or disabilities to operate aspects of the home.

Section 2

How do environmental control systems work?
ECS work on the principle that the user provides the *input* (via a 'switch') to the system *processor* (a computer) that provides an *output* in the user's environment (the 'peripheral', for example a domestic appliance). Within this three-part process, careful consideration needs to be given to the way the input is created by the user. The type of switch chosen depends on the ability of the user to activate/deactivate it. The skilled assessment for appropriate switches that make best use of the existing movement of the individual is essential for any ECS to be of value.

There are many types of switches available that can vary considerably in size, touch/texture or pressure sensitivity. Examples of switches include large button, pillow (soft to the touch), highly coloured or contrasting, chin, sip and puff to name a few. ECS switches can also be triggered by tongue movements, eye blinks and eye gaze.

Augmentative and alternative communication devices

Augmentative and Alternative Communication (AAC) is a term used for a range methods that can assist individuals that have limited or absent verbal and/or non-verbal abilities. The purpose of AAC is to enable the participation of children and adults with severe communication difficulties within their social, work and educational environments. Some ECS may have communication devices built into them depending on the particular product.

AAC can range from facial expressions, gestures, signing (for example British Sign Language) (which are usually described as unaided) to aided solutions that can involve the use of high tech such as adapted computers or electronic speech systems (Communication Matters 2010). As with an EC it is imperative that the person can use the equipment and this means ensuring that the interface between the user and the communication device are well matched. Similar assessments for relevant switching methods may be required depending on the degree of the communication difficulty.

In 2008, the Bercow Report reviewed what steps needed to be taken to transform provision of the experiences of children and young people with speech, language and communication needs. Identified within its key recommendations was the need for Primary Care Trusts (PCTs) and local authorities to work jointly in the surveillance and monitoring of the needs of children and younger people, particularly at key transition points. PCTs were identified to deliver this monitoring function up to the age of five.

Accessing specialised electronic AT equipment

In terms of accessing both ECS and AAC a wide variation of routes exist. For example, although an AAC Referral Pathway may exist in one area or region this may not be replicated elsewhere. A number of regional specialist centres exist; for example, Access to Communication and Technology, which is a specialist NHS assessment and review service in the West Midlands, or the charity ACE Centres in Oxford and Oldham. Professionals working in these specialist teams are well placed to carry out the complex assessments required before equipment or systems can be recommended. These teams can include occupational therapists, speech and language therapists, teachers, assistive technologists, clinical scientists, rehabilitation engineers, technical instructors and nurses.

Complex needs are likely to require complex team assessments that lead to unique solutions for many of the individuals that require this kind of AT. An example is given in Case study 6.3.

Section 2

Case study 6.3 Anthony

My name is Anthony. I'm 40 years old. I broke my neck when I was 15 and was paralysed at the C5 level. This means I have no movement or feeling below chest level. It also means my hands and wrists are paralysed. I have use of my biceps, but not triceps. So, I can bend my arms, but not straighten them. All my muscles, below my neck, are quite weak.

Above my neck, most people say that I'm *too* active! My jaw muscles get too much exercise. I have a very lively mind, and there isn't much that I'm not interested in - business, psychology, science, art, music, everything really. I like to spend time with my old friends and I like to travel and meet new ones.

I use my computer a lot - for communication, entertainment and research. I'm also the one who sorts out the computers of friends and family when they go wrong. I have to confess to being a bit of a 'gadget freak'. I can use the excuse, that because of my disability, technology can be extremely useful, but a bit of fun does no harm as well.

I'm not employed, but I do test specialised disabled equipment and attend exhibitions, to demonstrate it to people.

I live in a large bungalow in the West Country. It's on a steep hill, but luckily there have been very few structural modifications, just a couple of ramps. I'm very keen to keep my home as a 'normal' house. Any specialised equipment has to really earn its place, and preferably has to be installed 'invisibly'. I share the house with my parents, who have also been my carers since my accident, so I have to remember it's their home as well. I am in the process of arranging separate carers at the moment. Combined with the use of AT, I'm hoping to, at least maintain, if not improve, my level of independence.

To get around, I use a wheelchair, which to the surprise of many, is an incredibly capable form of transport, as long as you don't have a stair obsession! I use two different wheelchairs, both electric. One is lightweight and manoeuvrable, which is great for visiting friends, or travelling. The other is slightly more robust, but is safer if I'm out on my own, as it's more stable and has greater battery life. I also have a four-wheel drive 'outdoor' wheelchair, which lets me get out onto the hills, which I love.

I'm much more physically able during the day, when I'm sat up in my wheelchair. I can use joysticks, type and use a computer trackpad. I can feed myself, answer phones, use remote controls, etc. Obviously, there are many things I can't do for myself - washing, dressing, cooking, and a long list of others, but generally, that doesn't bother me. I want to be able to do as much as possible, but I know my limitations and I don't believe in militant independence. If someone wants to help me with something, that's fine with me.

At night, things become much more difficult for me. Almost all of my movement becomes useless, as I no longer have the assistance of gravity, to help me. That means all I can move is my head. I don't sleep very much, so before assistive technology arrived, nights were pretty boring, but now, thankfully, that has changed.

There are a couple of problems I would like to be solved. Firstly is when people come to the front door. I can't get to the front door quickly and I couldn't open it, even if I got there in time. Secondly, when I'm in bed, getting to the door is impossible. So, from either my bed, or my living room, if someone comes to the door, I want to be able to see who they are, talk to them and let them in. The solution has to be totally safe and reliable. Also, as with my other equipment, the solution needs to be as invisible as possible.

Points for reflection

- What are your thoughts about Anthony and his lifestyle?
- Does his story surprise you in any way?
- Would you consider Anthony as a 'typical' user of AT?
- If not, who would you consider to be a typical user of AT?
- Explore the potential of environmental control systems.
- What solutions can you find that might be useful for Anthony?

Whole system demonstrators

In line with proposals set out in the White Paper 'Our Health, Our Care, Our Say' (DH 2006), the DH set up a funded 2-year project to find out how technology could help people manage their own health whilst maintaining their independence. The Whole System Demonstrators (WSD) trial is focused around Telecare and Telehealth and is believed to be the largest randomised controlled trial (RCT) of Telecare and Telehealth in the world. As a result much is riding on the evaluation of this project expected in 2011.

The project aimed to recruit up to a total of 6000 participants from three demonstrator sites in Cornwall, Kent and the London Borough of Newham. Alongside the project a WSD Action Network (WSDAN) was developed to provide updates, disseminate findings and provide resources/materials from what had been learnt to share with other services undertaking similar projects.

The trial has required a high degree of planning and coordination in order to overcome significant barriers. For example, Johnson (2009: 9) has identified there have been difficulties at several levels. At the service user level barriers appeared to relate to demographic variables, social support levels, trust issues and personal practices. At the provider level issues around capacity, skills and attitudes have been highlighted. Finally, at the system level there have been difficulties with joint working and information sharing. Issues around successful uptake and recruitment to the relevant sample groups have also been identified. These challenges have been embraced as opportunities to identify key learning points regarding executing a RCT and speedy implementation of service level changes.

One evaluation theme to be undertaken by the Nuffield Trust (no date) will be highly relevant as it will investigate the impact of Telecare and Telehealth on the use of NHS and social services, and the associated costs and whether ATs pay for themselves, over what time period, and in which individuals.

The Newham whole system demonstrator trial

As previously mentioned, the London Borough of Newham is one of the trial sites. This followed a successful bid to participate from Newham Council and Primary Care Trust. Around 1600 local people are taking part and are trialling either Telecare or Telehealth systems in their homes. Specifically, it is anticipated that the trial will enable Newham to understand to what extent the integration between health and social care and these technologies can:

- promote people's long-term health and independence;
- improve quality of life for people and their carers;
- improve the working lives of health and social care professionals;
- provide an evidence base for more cost-effective and clinically effective ways of managing LTCs.
  Source: Newham Whole Systems Demonstrator 2010.

The following two case study examples (Case studies 6.4 and 6.5) adapted from the Newham Whole System Demonstrator website (with kind permission) illustrate the issues and potential benefits for service users with LTCs in using Telecare and Telehealth.

Case study 6.4   Newham Whole System Demonstrator Telecare

The problem

One Sunday night in December 2008, 74-year-old Ruby was washing her hands in the bathroom. When she reached out to pick something up she noticed that there was a problem with her left hand, she couldn't bend her fingers. She phoned the emergency services and an ambulance was dispatched. Ruby had had a stroke. For example, if a stroke damages the part of the brain that controls how limbs move, limb movement will be affected.

The need

Ruby's stroke affected the right side of her brain, which in turn affected her mobility, resulting in her needing additional carer support around the home. Ruby also suffers from arthritis and bradycardia.

Ruby has a strong support network of friends, but despite this added support, because Ruby lives alone, her main concern is what if an emergency situation arises where she needs urgent attention and nobody is around to help.

The answer

The hospital was willing to discharge Ruby into her own care six weeks after her stroke because she had been placed on the Telecare trial. The technology in her home is aimed at raising a call for help in emergency situations.

The method

Ruby now has a variety of different alarms and sensors fitted in her home, such as: sensors to remind her to turn off the water and the lights if they are left on, a flood detector in the kitchen and bathroom, heat detector in the kitchen, radio pull cord in the bathroom, a medication dispenser, a carbon monoxide (CO) detector and a pendant she wears around her wrist.

The equipment

Medication dispenser

Automatically dispenses medications and provides audible and visual alerts to each time medications should be taken.

Heat detector

Provides additional protection against the risk of fires in rooms where smoke detectors are unsuitable, for example kitchen.

Flood Detector

Provides early warning of potential flood situations.

CO detector

Detector warns of dangerous CO levels. The unit provides an immediate alert when dangerous emissions are detected.

The outcome

"Telecare has made such a difference to me. I used to leave the water and lights on and the windows open, sometimes I would even leave the cooker on. But now Telecare reminds me to turn all of these things off," said Ruby.

"Once I forgot to take my medicine because my sister was visiting from America, and the medicine dispenser started beeping. I was thinking to myself "What is going on? Then I heard my phone ringing and I knew it was the Telecare team. They asked me if I'd taken my tablets and advised me to take them right away."

"I am confident because I have Telecare. If anything should happen to me, I can press my pendent and it's ok, help is there."

-Ruby Forde-Alexander

Points for reflection

- Think about patients that you have come into contact with in the past that have LTCs similar to Ruby's. Was Telecare being used to support these patients? If so, how? If not, think about how Telecare could be used to support them.
- Explore the range of Telecare sensors and monitors that are available. How might these be used to support individuals with a wide range of health and social care needs?
- How might existing Telecare equipment be used in alternative ways, other than those originally intended? Refer to Dawn's case study on the Newham WSD website as an example (see 'Resources').
- Explore the case study and video examples identified on the Newham WSD website. What are the wider benefits of using Telecare for example from the point of view of informal carers such as family members?

Section 2

Case study 6.5 Newham Whole System Demonstrator Telehealth

The problem

Ahmed is self-employed as a screen printer and has had diabetes for a number of years. Initially, Ahmed did not take his condition seriously despite urgings from his GP, which resulted in his condition worsening and in Ahmed having a below-the-knee amputation and he now walks with the assistance of a prosthetic limb. People with diabetes have high levels of glucose in their blood because the body cannot use it properly. Insulin is a hormone produced by the pancreas and helps the glucose to enter the cells where it is used as fuel for energy so we can work, play and generally live our lives.

The need

Ahmed was diagnosed with diabetes 18 years ago and has been battling with his condition for the past ten. At the end of 2008, his health deteriorated so much that he lost all feeling in his body from the neck down and was hospitalised. Ahmed's health has since stabilised but he is concerned about his health deteriorating again.

The answer

Ahmed was the first person to start the Telehealth trial and has been on the trial since November 2008. The Telehealth system is aimed at giving him the tools he needs to help manage his own health at home with the supervision of health professionals.

The method

Using Telehealth, Ahmed is able to take his own blood pressure, weight, pulse and blood sugar readings each day. The readings are taken with special equipment which is linked to a set-top box connected to his television. The results, which Ahmed can view on his television, are automatically uploaded to a team of healthcare professionals who view them daily.

The equipment

Set-top box

Small, unobtrusive unit connected via the TV. The unit stores vital signs data.

Blood pressure monitor

Daily blood pressure readings are updated into the set-top box.

Body weight scales

Fluctuations in daily weight readings can indicate health problems.

Pulse oximeter

Measures blood oxygen levels and heart rate.

Blood glucometer

Measures blood sugar levels.

The outcome

Ahmed is now playing a much more active role in the management of his own health and is more conscious of any changes in his readings.

"I'm monitoring my diabetes three times a day... I do three readings... I get my weight checked, then I do my blood pressure and glucose. I am always aware of what is happening about my health."

"This is a thing that can help. Nobody wants to go to the hospital on a regular basis and stay away from home. It's best to be at home."

"A year ago my blood pressure was fluctuating a lot, it was on the higher side. I received a call from the Telehealth nurse to call an ambulance or go to the hospital or see the GP immediately. I called the ambulance... I'd had a minor stroke. I'd say that my life was saved because of Telehealth. I am aware that someone is taking care of me, that is the most important thing about Telehealth." Getting the advanced warning may have saved him from something more major.

–Ahmed Rizwan

Points for reflection

- Telehealth clearly has an important role in enabling individuals to manage their LTCs effectively at home. What might be the implications for nursing practice in using a Telehealth approach?
- Explore the range of Telehealth applications. What range of LTCs might be supported both now and potentially in the future?
- Explore the case study and video examples identified on the Newham WSD website. What are the wider benefits of using Telehealth for example from the patient, family and professional perspectives?

Ethical issues

As with many new interventions, AT has the potential to be of benefit to people and there is the acknowledgement that it offers many advantages and possibilities for people with LTCs, in particular. However, there is also the potential for misuse and there are concerns about the use of AT by service users, professionals, families and carers; that it is too intrusive; that it can be used to restrict freedom; or that it is used inappropriately and may cause more harm than good.

The four basic principles that guide moral deliberation in ethics are equally applicable when considering the use of AT.

The principles are:

- Non-maleficence
- Beneficence
- Justice
- Respect for patients' autonomy
  (*Source*: Pellegrino et al. 1989)

The principles defined

Non-maleficence simply means 'do no harm'. Is the use of AT in danger of doing more harm than good? For example, if a person has dementia, would the installation of AT lead to more confusion or distress? It will involve a balance between avoiding harm and respecting decisions, dignity, integrity and preferences.

Beneficence means striving consciously to be 'of benefit' to the person, to aim to do good. It involves finding the balance between risk tolerance and risk aversion. There may be a dilemma between beneficence, and safety and independence, for example. Consider the use of the safer walking/wandering technologies where a person with dementia may be 'tagged' to enable them to be found quickly using a GPS (Global Positioning Satellite) location device if they become lost. Who benefits? It may be the person with dementia themselves, their carer or care home staff. It may be all three, the point is that AT can enable people to live with and manage risk in new ways that have not been possible previously.

Autonomy refers to respecting the person's rights to things like self-determination, privacy, freedom, and choice. This should include informed consent, which needs to be voluntary, competent and include sufficient information about the proposed technology to enable the person and/or their family to make a choice. Healthcare professionals have a responsibility to maximise decision-making and AT can have a considerable role to play in enabling this; for example, through the use of communication aids that support users in expressing their opinion and choice about their healthcare.

Justice means treating everyone fairly. For example, providing equal access to technology, and including what the Mental Capacity Act calls freedom in making 'eccentric or unwise decisions'(DH 2005d). If someone lacks capacity to make a decision about using AT, anything that is done, or any decision that is made on their behalf, should be the least restrictive of their basic rights and freedoms. Consider what does 'least restrictive' mean? For example, what is the least restrictive – using a locator or tagging device or moving someone into residential care? AT can be used to support people to live in the environment that they would prefer to live in for as long as possible.

It is important that practitioners can articulate why they have made a decision and be able to document the decision regarding the use of AT within a particular context for an individual service user. The use of a supported decision-making tool to manage the process of choice, assess the potential impacts of any risk associated with the AT, and provide documentation of actions and decisions is considered good practice (DH 2007b).

Workforce design, education and training

Training needs

It seems that some evidence is now emerging of the benefits and cost-effectiveness of the use of Telecare and Telehealth. However, it appears that generally knowledge of AT amongst healthcare and social care professionals is low. Brownsell and Hawley reported in 2004 that fall monitoring equipment is not considered routinely in the care package for older people after a fall, and that staff's knowledge of assistive devices is basic. The staff recruited for this study were also unaware of what fall detectors are, the research evidence to support their use, the target market for the devices and financial information related to the devices. The authors found this finding surprising as the experiences and consequences of falls in the older population are high on the political agenda. However, the staff recruited in this project included a wide range of service providers including commissioners and care provider managers and although these members of staff are part of the care plan, they do not necessarily need in-depth knowledge of AT, as it is the staff who develop the intervention care plan – the practitioners – who need the greatest level of knowledge. Their research suggested that education is needed for the practitioners who provide AT to enable people with LTCs to get the correct support to continue living independently.

A study carried out in a residential home, using a quasi-experimental, non-equivalent group design to examine staff perceptions of job satisfaction after increased technology support for people with dementia found that staff members' job satisfaction and perceived quality of care improved in comparison with the control group (Engstrom et al. 2005). The technology included individualised corridor alarms, fall detectors, sensor-activated nighttime illumination and Internet communication. The authors suggest that the improvement in scores for the experimental group may have been linked to the benefits of continuing education which has also been shown to increase job satisfaction for staff. However, this study only had 33 participants, was non-randomised and had a significant dropout rate of 44% at 12 months.

Hanson et al. (2007) conducted 22 focus groups in three different regions in England to explore the extent to which older people, carers and professionals consider Telecare to be a potentially valuable service. They suggest that the differences in opinions they found between regions and groups were partly dependent on whether the supply of Telecare services is seen as a rapid response to an individual crisis or as a preventative service for access by everyone. A general lack of knowledge was felt to be an influencing factor on how valuable the service was seen to be for both older people and professionals, both groups confirming they came to the research out of curiosity and to find out more about Telecare.

Likewise, Orton (2008) found inconsistency in Occupational Therapy practice in AT services and poor rates of referral into services, such as social alarm services, through a lack of knowledge of the benefits of such systems.

This research raises concerns relating to the Government's ambitions for mainstreaming Telecare to support people with LTCs in their own home, which may be problematic unless the deep-rooted perceptions of the devices are eliminated though training and education. Doughty (2009: 27) describes the different types of training that are required across a Telecare team including:

- *Awareness:* To make all health, social care and housing frontline and management staff aware of the technology and its potential.
- *Prescription:* This requires a greater knowledge of individual items of technology and how they may be used to manage the risks and unmet needs identified during the assessment process.
- *Home survey:* To help staff to identify practical technology and safety issues within the home.
- *Installation:* The setting up of the Telecare unit including the physical location, attachment and programming of individual sensors, and the information provided to the service user and his or her family or informal carers.

- *Alarm handling:* Aimed at staff at the monitoring centre in dealing with the different types of alarms generated by Telecare equipment in the field and in accordance with locally agreed response protocols.
- *Physical response:* The processes required for the mobile physical response offered in the event of an emergency.

Doughty (2009) goes on to state that there are major gaps in training available via accredited courses for Telecare staff. These findings are supported by an earlier survey of 350 healthcare practitioners (FAST 2005) that highlighted the lack of education and continuing professional development opportunities in AT for experienced staff from a range of professional groups including occupational therapists, physiotherapists, speech and language therapists, rehabilitation engineers and nurses.

A qualitative study carried out at Coventry University (Ward et al. 2009) on workforce development needs regarding AT within a primary care trust found there was a need for staff to:

- recognise that AT can help a service user with a need;
- know what AT can help, what AT is available, and also know about alternatives to AT;
- know how to assess and select the correct AT to meet the need;
- know how to access and provide the AT within the service context;
- have knowledge and skills that inform clinical reasoning and support decision-making about AT;
- know where to go for information – be aware of sources of support and advice, be able to access information and advice.

The study identified that the most pressing training needs for staff from a range of healthcare professional groups (including community matrons, occupational therapists and physiotherapists) in relation to AT were:

- The purpose and benefits of AT through general awareness raising education
- The assessment and selection of appropriate AT to meet the user's needs
- The methods of referral and processes used to access and provide AT such as Telecare

It was also indicated that this education should also include service managers and commissioners of services.

Health and social care staff must be aware of the possibilities, choices and benefits that AT can offer to a service user with an LTC in order to support the service user, carer and their families to make an informed choice about the use of AT.

A technological future?

As providers begin the move away from the *provision* of services and equipment towards the increasing *personalisation* of care, it is critical that new practitioners have an increased awareness of the potential contribution that AT can make to health and social care that will complement their range of interventions or suggested solutions to meet service user's needs. Education and training in AT beyond that of preregistration will be needed so that employers can be sure that their workforce has the required knowledge and skills to implement AT solutions. This education will need to include all levels of staff from support workers through to clinical specialists, managers and commissioners of services.

There is a growing emphasis on the empowerment of service users to obtain direct payments (to pay for equipment, adaptations and services), control of their own personal care budgets and utilisation of the 'retail model' to purchase an increasingly affordable and available range of AT much of which is being produced for mainstream consumer consumption. As a result, the role of the practitioner will need to embrace that of a resource for impartial information and advice, appraisal of AT products or systems and signposting to key resources and AT services such as Telecare. Therefore, within person-centred assessments it is imperative that practitioners are able to consider potential AT solutions within their interactions with individuals, families and carers.

Ethics around the use of AT is an area that practitioners will need to revisit to ensure that their practice is sound, risks are appropriately assessed and consent processes are carefully implemented. The wider ethical implications of remote monitoring of individuals needs to be considered and planned for, as will the storage of increasing amounts of data that may potentially be produced. This sensitive data will need to be stored securely by effective gatekeepers. Examples from the US show a healthcare system that is increasingly dominated by large corporations that offer end users control over their health, social care and well-being data. The Microsoft HealthVault (2010) and Google Health (2010) are two systems that enable individuals and families to manage their personal health records (PHR) and then decide how and when they want this to be shared with medics or other professionals. These examples epitomise an unprecedented level of empowerment and control of individuals that breaks the mould on organisations and services that might to attempt to offer a one-size-fits-all approach to its customers. Far from being a US phenomenon, it is notable that HealthVault, originally launched in the US in 2007, has now been introduced into Germany (eHealthEurope 2010) by Siemens and further roll out to the United Kingdom could be considered by future governments (ZD Net UK 2009). Indeed, the NHS (in England) are currently introducing Summary Care Records (SCRs) with an NHS Chip and Pin Smartcard that will allow access to an individual's health information by healthcare staff anywhere in England and individuals can look at and amend their own SCR at a secure website called HealthSpace (www.healthspace.nhs.uk) (NHS 2010).

Intelligent home automation linking to digital TV and mobile technology as a primary means to access information and services including health and social care services is also expanding. 'Looking Local' is a national portal offering access to local government and relevant related services on digital interactive TV, mobile phones, kiosks and Internet-enabled consumer electronics such as the Nintendo Wii. It is available on all Sky, Virgin and broadband connected Freeview boxes, so almost half of all households (13 million homes) have access to real time, interactive government services. The Looking Local website gives an example of how this interactive service can be used: 'Mrs. Smith, 76 years old, who does not have PC – and doesn't want one – can use her TV remote to find out when her next community centre session is, book online for the lunch and order transport to the centre. After which she can confirm her doctor's appointment, and order her repeat prescription' (Looking Local 2010). All of this is possible today and new services are being developed. However, as was emphasised earlier, much of the uptake of these new services will be dependent on technology aware health and social care professionals that can signpost service users and their carers to these services, and be able to use this interface themselves to communicate and interact with service users via this media.

Further developments in robotics with the advent of exoskeletons to enhance or replace lost movement and electronic prosthetic limbs are all part of the continuum of AT that may transform the way of life for people with long-term health conditions. Smart clothing and worn sensors that can replace some of the monitoring sensors used currently within Telecare and Telehealth monitoring are being developed. Internal sensor diagnostics, for example sensors that can be embedded within

Section 2

a sticking plaster or chips that can be swallowed may further revolutionise the monitoring of vital signs and health conditions. The possibility of virtual worlds that can enable people with LTCs and disabilities to experience and 'take part' in activities that they may no longer be able to do along with the development of 'virtual friends' to alleviate social isolation and depression are thought-provoking. This may seem too far into a technological future but development is already happening in these areas. The idea of robotic assistance to help people is not new and the technology exists to provide robots to carry out rehabilitation and some personal care activities. The question to consider is: What is acceptable? Where do we draw the line? Although technologically possible, that does not mean that it is the right thing to do.

Technology is firmly shaping the future of health and social care from the delivery of information about an individual's health to the emergence of more sophisticated portable devices to monitor individuals. There is a rapid drive to harness innovative AT within the market place to push the point of healthcare delivery to the home through the development of new products and manufacturers are increasingly involving end users in the design and usability testing of these products to ensure that they are inclusive of user's needs. A decrease in hardware size and an increase in mobility and connectivity, advances and improvements in access to digital communication, telemonitoring and videoconferencing with health and social care professionals will enable the management of people with LTCs away from the acute care setting.

AT will probably never replace the need for human contact but it can help by improving workflow and making manual and routine tasks more efficient. It also offers people with LTCs, their families and carers, choice and empowerment in how they live their lives and are supported to live with their condition.

Conclusion

This chapter has provided an overview of ATs that are currently available, how they work and examples of their use within a broad range of health, social care, and community and home settings. It is important to take into consideration that the aforementioned technology already exists and is making a contribution to how care is being delivered in contemporary health and social care services and the choices that people can make in the way they are supported.

References

Advanced Care Technologies Programme (2010) Telecare and Assistive Technology Glossary. Available at: http://www.actprogramme.org.uk/content/134/telecare-assistive-technology-glossary (accessed 26 April 2010).

Barlow, J., Singh, D., Bayer, S. and Curry, R. (2007) A systematic review of the benefits of home telecare for frail elderly people and those with long-term conditions. *Journal of Telemedicine and Telecare* **13**, 172-179.

Barnes, N., Edwards, N., Rose, D. and Garner, P. (1998) Lifestyle monitoring-technology for supported independence. *Comput Control Eng* **9**, 169-74.

Beech, R. and Roberts, D. (2008) *Research Briefing 28: Assistive Technology and Older People*, p. 2-12. London: Social Care Institute for Excellence.

Bennett, J., Perrin, N., Hanson, G., Bennett, D., Gaynor, W., Flaherty-Robb, M., Joseph, C., Butterworth, S. and Potempa, K. (2005) Healthy aging demonstration project: Nurse coaching for behaviour change in older adults. *Research in Nursing and Health* **28** (3), 187-197.

The Bercow Report: A Review of Services for Children and Young People (0–19) with Speech, Language and Communication Needs (2008). Available at: http://www.dcsf.gov.uk/bercowreview/docs/7771-DCSF-BERCOW.PDF DCFS Publications Nottingham. (accessed 5 October 2010).

Birmingham City Council Housing Department (1997) In: Brownsell, S.J., Bradley, D. A., Bragg. R., Catlin, P. and Carlier, J. (2000) Do community alarm users want telecare? *Journal of Telemedicine and Telecare* **6**, 199–204.

Blackhurst, A. and Lahm, A. (2000). Foundations of technology and exceptionality. In: J. Lindsey (ed) *Technology and Exceptional Individuals*, 3rd edn., pp. 3–45. Austin, TX: Pro-Ed.

Brownsell, S., Bradley, D., Bragg, R., Catlin, P. and Carlier, J. (2000) Do community alarm users want telecare? *Journal of Telecare and Telemedicine* (**6**), 199–204.

Brownsell, S. and Bradley, D. (2003) *Assistive Technology and Telecare: Forging Solutions for Independent Living*. Bristol: The Policy Press.

Brownsell, S. and Hawley, M. (2004) Fall detectors: Do they work or reduce the fear of falling? *Housing Care and Support* **7** (1), 18–24.

Brownsell, S., Blackburn, S. and Hawley, M. (2008) An evaluation of second and third generation Telecare services in older people's housing. *Journal of Telemedicine and Telecare* **14**, 8–12.

Care Services Efficiency Delivery (CSED) (2008) Assistive Technology (AT): Efficiency Delivery: Supporting Sustainable Transformation: Staffordshire (Cannock) – Case Study. Available at: http://www.dhcarenetworks.org.uk/_oldCSEDAssets/atstaffordshire.pdf. (accessed 23 May 2009).

Communication Matters (2010) *Focus on. . .What is AAC?* Available at: www.communicationmatters.org.uk. (accessed 5 October 2010)

Dahl, Y. (2006) You have a message here: enhancing interpersonal communication in a hospital ward with location-based virtual wards. *Methods of Information in Medicine* **45** (6), 602–9.

Department of Health (DH) (1999) *Royal Commission for Long-term Care With Respect to Old Age*. London: HMSO.

Department of Health (DH) (2000) *The NHS Plan*. London: HMSO.

Department of Health (DH) (2001) National Service Framework for Older People. Available at: http://www.dh.gov.uk/prod_consum_dh/groups/dh_digitalassets/@dh/@en/documents/digitalasset/dh_4071283.pdf (accessed 24 April 2010).

Department of Health (DH) (2005a) Green Paper: Independence, Wellbeing and Choice. Available at: http://www.dh.gov.uk/en/Publicationsandstatistics/Publications/PublicationsPolicyAndGuidance/DH_4106477 (accessed 13 March 2010).

Department of Health (DH) (2005b) National Service Framework for Long-term Conditions. Available at: http://www.dh.gov.uk/prod_consum_dh/groups/dh_digitalassets/@dh/@en/documents/digitalasset/dh_4105369.pdf (accessed 24 April 2010).

Department of Health (DH) (2005c) Building Telecare in England. Available at: http://www.dh.gov.uk/prod_consum_dh/groups/dh_digitalassets/@dh/@en/documents/digitalasset/dh_4115644.pdf (accessed 13 March 2010).

Department of Health (DH) (2005d) *Mental Capacity Act*. London: HMSO.

Department of Health (DH) (2006) *Our Health, Our Care, Our Say*. London: HMSO.

Department of Health (DH) (2007a) *Putting People Frst: A Shared Vision and Commitment to the Transformation of Adult Social Care*. London: HMSO.

Department of Health (DH) (2007b) *Independence Choice and Risk*. London: HMSO.

Department of Health (DH) (2008a) The Darzi Report: High Quality Care for All. Available at: http://www.dh.gov.uk/en/Publicationsandstatistics/Publications/PublicationsPolicyAndGuidance/DH_085825 (accessed 24 April 2010).

Doughty, K., Lewis, R. and McIntosh, A. (2000) The design of a practical and reliable fall detector for community and institutional care. *Journal of Telemedicine and Telecare* **6** (1 suppl.) , 150–154.

Doughty, K., Monk, A., Bayliss, C., Brown, S., Dewsbury, L., Dunk, B., Gallagher, V., Grafham, K., Jones, M., Lowe, C., McAlister, L., McSorley, K., Mills, P., Skidmore, C., Stewart, A., Taylor, B. and Ward, D. (2007) Telecare, telehealth and assistive technology – do we know what we are talking about? *Journal of Assistive Technologies* **2** (1), 6–10.

Doughty, K. (2009) Improving the quality of telecare services – the role of audit and training. *Journal of Assistive technologies* **3** (1), 24-28.

eHealthEurope (2010) First European Deal for HealthVault. Available at: http://ehealtheurope.net/news/5599/first_european_deal_for_healthvault (accessed 4 May 2010).

Engstrom, M., Ljunggren, B., Lindqvist, R. and Carlsson, M. (2005) Staff perceptions of job satisfaction and life situation before and 6 and 12 months after increased information technology support in dementia care. *Journal of Telemedicine and Telecare* **11**, 304-309.

Foundation for Assistive Technology – FAST (2005) Assistive technology an Education, a Career, a Partnership. Available at: http://www.fastuk.org/pagedocuments/File/workforce_and_self_care/AT%20Education%20v5.pdf (accessed 2 October 2009).

Foundation for Assistive Technology – FAST (2006) Self Care in Assistive Technology – Choice, Risk and Independent Living. Available at: http://www.fastuk.org/atforumactivities/serviceuserparticipation.php (accessed 26 April 2010).

Gatward, J. (2004) Electronic assistive technology: benefits for all? *Housing, Care and Support* **7**. 4 December 13-17.

Glascock, A. and Kutzik, D. (2006) The impact of behavioural monitoring technology on the provision of health care in the home. *J Univers Comput Sci* **12**, 59-79.

Google Health (2010) Google Health Homepage. Available at: http://www.google.com/intl/en-GB/health/about/index.html (accessed 4 May 2010).

Great Britain Parliament (1990) NHS and Community Care Act (Act of Parliament) London: HMSO.

Griffiths, R. (1988) *Community Care: Agenda for Action*. London: HMSO.

Hanson, J., Percival, J., Aldred, H., Brownsell, S. and Hawley, M. (2007) Attitudes to Telecare among older people professional care workers and informal carers: a preventative strategy or crisis management? *Universal Access in the Information Society* **6** (2), 193-205.

Johnson, S. (2009) In Telecare Services Association, Annual Report 2008-9, Telecare and Telehealth in Action. Available at: http://www.telecare.org.uk/files/47961/FileName/TSAAnnualReportMay2009.pdf. (accessed 5 October 2010)

Just checking (2010) Just Checking – Supporting Indepenence of People with Dementia. Available at: http://www.justchecking.co.uk/ (accessed 18 March 2010).

Lewis, G. (2006) Case Study: Virtual Wards at Croydon Primary Care Trust. Available at: http://www.networks.nhs.uk/uploads/06/12/croydon_virtual_wards_case_study.pdf (accessed 14 May 2009).

Lindner, H., Menzies, D., Kelly, J., Taylor, S. and Shearer, M. (2003) Coaching for behaviour change in chronic disease: a review of the literature and the implications for coaching as a self-management intervention. *Australian Journal of Primary Health* **9** (2, 3), 1-9.

Looking Local (2010) National Portal for Local Government and Related Public Services. Available at: http://www.lookinglocal.gov.uk/site/ (accessed 4 May 2010).

Mair, F. and Whitten, P. (2000) Systematic review of studies of patient satisfaction with telemedicine. *British Medical Journal* **320**, 1517-1520.

Martin, T., Majeed, B., Beum-Seuck, L. and Clarke, N. (2007) A third-generation Telecare system using fuzzy ambient intelligence. *Studies in Computational Intelligence* **72**, 155-175.

Medical Devices Agency (1995) Environmental control systems. An evaluation. *Disability Equipment Assessment* No. A414. Norwich: HMSO.

Microsoft HealthVault (2010) HealthVault Homepage. Available at: http://www.healthvault.com/ (accessed 4 May 2010).

MyAmego (2010) MyAmego Homepage. Available at: http://www.myamego.co.uk (accessed 3 May 2010).

Newham Whole System Demonstrator (2010) WSD Trial. Available at: http://www.newhamwsdtrial.org/wsd-trial (accessed 28 April 2010).

National Patient Safety Agency (2007) Slips, Trips and Falls in Hospital, the Third Report from the Patient Safety Observatory. Available at: http://www.npsa.nhs.uk/nrls/alerts-and-directives/directives-guidance/slips-trips-falls/ www.npsa.nhs.uk (accessed 25 August 2009).

National Health Service (NHS) (2010) National Service Frameworks and Strategies. http://www.nhs.uk/NHSEngland/NSF/Pages/Nationalserviceframeworks.aspx (accessed 24 April 2010).

NHS National End of Life Care Programme (2009) Virtual Community Wards for Patients in Croydon. Available at: http://www.endoflifecare.nhs.uk/eolc/CS250.htm (accessed 22 September 2009).

NHS (2010) *Changes to your health records* [Leaflet]. London: NHS Publications.

Nuffield Trust [no date] Evaluation of the Whole System Demonstrator Project. Available at http://www.nuffieldtrust.org.uk/projects/index.aspx?id = 294 (accessed 24 April 2010).

Oliver, D. (2004) Prevention of falls in hospital inpatients. Agendas for research and practice. *Age and Ageing* **33**, 328–300.

Orton, M. (2008) Factors that may be considered by occupational therapists during the assessment of clients for assistive technology and whether it permeates through to the eventual prescription. *Journal of Assistive Technologies* **2** (1), 11–22.

Pellegrino, E., Thomas, M. and David, C. (1989) *For the Patient's Good: The Restoration of Beneficence in Health Care.* Oxford: Oxford University Press.

Porteus, J. and Brownsell, S. (2000) *Using Telecare: Exploring Technologies for Independent Living for Older People.* Kidlington, Oxon: Anchor Trust.

Richardson, S. (2009) Falls Technology: Medical Applications on the iPhone. Available at: http://www.profane.eu.org/newsletters/pdf/ProFaNE_NL_Volume02_Issue02.pdf?sid = 36a6c015f60 3457e313299f85fb921d5 (accessed 13 May 2009).

Royal Commission for Long-term Care (1999a) *With Respect to Old Age.* London: The Stationary Office Limited.

Royal Commission for Long-term Care (1999b) *With Respect to Old Age: Research Volume 2.* London: The Stationary Office Limited.

Sixsmith, A., Hine, N., Neild, I., Clarke, N., Brown, S. and Garner, P. (2007) Monitoring the well-being of older people. *Top Geriatr Rehabil* **23**, 9–23.

Sood, S., Mbarika, V., Jugoo, S., Dookhy, R., Doarn, C., Prakash, N. and Merrell, R. (2007) What is telemedicine? A collection of 104 peer-reviewed perspectives and theoretical underpinnings. *Telemedicine and eHealth* **13** (5), 573–590.

Spetz, J., Jacobs, J. and Hatler, C. (2007) Cost effectiveness of a medical vigilance system to reduce patient falls. *Nursing Economics* **25** (6), 333–8, 352.

Technology-Related Assistance for Individuals with Disabilities Act of 1988. Report. House of Representatives, 100th Congress, 2nd Session. Available at: http://www.eric.ed.gov/ERICWebPortal/search/detailmini.jsp?_nfpb=true&_&ERICExtSearch_SearchValue_0=ED303016&ERICExtSearch_SearchType_0=no&accno=ED303016 (accessed 5 October 2010)

Telecare Services Association (2009) Telecare Code of Practice. Available at: http://www.telecare.org.uk/files/47734/FileName/TSACodeofPracticeExecutiveSummary.pdf (accessed 26 April 2010).

Tunstall (2010) ADLife – An Activities of Daily Life (ADL) Monitoring Solution. Available at: http://www.tunstallhealth.com/assets/Literature/ADLife%20solutions%20for%20web.pdf (accessed 18 March 2010).

Vale, M., Jelinek, M., Best, J., Dart, A., Grigg, L., Hare, D., Franz, C., Ho, B., Newman, R. and McNeil, J. (2003) Coaching patients on achieving cardiovascular health (COACH) a multicenter randomized trial in patients with coronary heart disease. *Arch Intern Med* **163**, 2775–2783.

Wanless, D. (2002) *Securing Our Future Health: Taking a Long-term View: Final Report.* London: HM Treasury.

Wanless, D. (2004) *Securing Good Health for the Whole Population: Final Report.* Norwich: HMSO.

Ward, G., Fielden, S. and Jackson, E. (2009) *Assistive Technology Workforce Development: Using Assistive Technology to Support a Falls Care Pathway. Project Report.* Health Design and Technology Institute, Coventry University, Coventry.

Warwickshire County Council (2006) An Evaluation of the Just Checking Telecare System for People with Dementia. Available at: http://www.justchecking.co.uk/downloads/pdfs/trial_results.pdf. (accessed 18 August 2009).

York Health Economics Consortium at York University/Scottish Government (2009) Evaluation of the Telecare Development Programme. Available at: http://www.jitscotland.org.uk/action-areas/telecare-in-scotland/telecare-publications/ (accessed 18 August 2009).

Section 2

Young, D., Furler, J., Vale, M., Walker, C., Segal, L., Dunning, P., Best, J., Blackberry, I., Audehm, R., and Sulaiman, N. (2007) Patient engagement and coaching for health: the PEACH study – a cluster randomised controlled trial using the telephone to coach people with type 2 diabetes to engage with their GPs to improve diabetes care: a study protocol. *BMC Family Practice* **8**, 20.

ZD Net UK (2009) Tories Pledge to 'Dismantle' NpfIT. Available at: http://www.zdnet.co.uk/news/it-strategy/2009/08/11/tories-pledge-to-dismantle-npfit-39710784/ (accessed 4 May 2010).

Resources

Access to Communication and Technology (2010) Homepage. Available at: http://www.actwmids.nhs.uk/

ACE Centre Oxford (2010) Homepage. Available at: http://www.ace-centre.org.uk/index.cfm?pageid=8C5D2633-3048-7290-FE27E5C59A39AECFandCFID=35485342andCFTOKEN=fe978ce9f5e28939-2203791E-3048-7290-FEAA2A35F62A9E96

ACE Centre North (2010) Homepage. Available at: http://www.ace-north.org.uk

Birmingham Own Health Available at: http://www.birminghamownhealth.co.uk/

Comment: Birmingham Own Health is an innovative collaboration between Birmingham East and North Primary Care Trust, NHS Direct and Pfizer Health Solutions. People with diabetes, heart failure or other long-term cardiovascular conditions receive regular telephone-based coaching from highly experienced care managers.

Croydon NHS Trust (2010) Virtual Ward Case Study. Available at: http://www.dhcarenetworks.org.uk/_library/croydon_virtual_wards_case_study.pdf

Foundation for Assistive Technologies (FAST) Available at: http://www.fastuk.org

HealthSpace Available at: www.healthspace.nhs.uk

The Housing Learning and Improvement Network (LIN) Available at: http://www.dhcarenetworks.org.uk/IndependentLivingChoices/Housing/

Comment: The Housing Learning and Improvement Network (LIN) is the national network for promoting new ideas and supporting change in the delivery of housing, care and support services for older and vulnerable adults, including people with disabilities and long-term conditions.

Justchecking Available at: http://www.justchecking.co.uk

MyAmego Available at: http://www.myamego.co.uk

Newham Whole System Demonstrator (2010) Cases Studies. Available at: http://www.newhamwsdtrial.org/case-studies

Telecare Services Association Available at: http://www.telecare.org.uk

Tunstall Available at: http://www.tunstallhealth.com

Further reading

Cook, A.M., Polgar, J.M. and Hussey, S., M. (2008) *Cook and Hussey's Assistive Technologies: Principles and Practice*, 3rd edn Missouri: Mosby Elsevier.

Pain, H., McLellan, L. and Gore, S. (2002) *Choosing Assistive Devices: A Guide for Users and Professionals*. London: Jessica Kingsley.

Chapter 7

Risk and Empowerment in Long-term Conditions

Annette Roebuck

Learning objectives

By the end of this chapter, the reader will be able to:

- Identify the impact of societal, cultural and individual views of risk upon the risk assessment and management process for people with LTCs
- Discuss how the current emphasis on empowerment within health and social care affects the way that risk is viewed and managed for this client group
- Utilise a range of clinical reasoning styles within an empowerment framework to reflect upon how to empower people with an LTC in the risk assessment and management process

Introduction

Think back to your routine this morning; for many people this would include getting up, washed and dressed, eating breakfast and getting ready to go out. Unless it was a very unusual day it is unlikely that the concept of the risks associated with these activities crossed your mind, and it is even more unlikely that other people or circumstances would have prevented you from carrying out these basic activities of daily living because they were deemed too risky. Reading the morning paper, however, would probably have brought the topic of risk to your attention, for risk is a ubiquitous topic within modern Western society. A glance through the paper may include subjects ranging from crime, national security, and the latest health scares being debated with regard to the risks that they pose to the general population. As a health professional, you may well have made a few comments on the health scare, and your view may have differed from that in the paper or that of your family or friends. For most people, risk could therefore be argued to have both implicit and personal components as well as explicit and socially/culturally determined components. Thinking of the number of different health-related scare stories that have hit the headlines in recent years, it is not surprising that risk

Long-term Conditions: A Guide for Nurses and Healthcare Professionals, First Edition. Edited by S. Randall and H. Ford.
© 2011 Blackwell Publishing Ltd. Published 2011 by Blackwell Publishing Ltd.

assessment and management have taken an increasingly central role within the framing of health and social care services. There are many books written on these topics (see 'Further reading'), it is advisable to refer to some of these to gain a fuller understanding of the way that risk is understood and managed within these cultures. The purpose of this chapter is to give the reader a brief overview of key concepts and help them to think about ways of framing the decisions that are made when working with people with LTCs.

For people with LTCs who are often in and out of contact with health and social care services at different points in their disease process, everyday activities such as those outlined above may be subject to a potentially bewildering range of advice and restrictions. Since risk perception is affected by a multitude of factors including culture, the risk management procedures that a person experiences may vary greatly depending upon the setting they are in. Walking independently to the bathroom to wash and dress before taking the morning tablets may be deemed acceptable in the home setting, yet be deemed risky within the hospital setting. In addition to familiar everyday activities, people are also often required to undergo more complex specialised interventions that involve an element of risk in hospitals, GP surgeries or clinics. Numerous professionals will be making their clinical judgements on the risks involved, and the person on the receiving end of this advice will be living with the decisions made, and may well be adhering to the advice long after the person who gave it has forgotten all about it. In order for professionals to manage risk effectively, it is therefore vital that they understand the factors that impact upon this decision-making process, and utilise frameworks to enable them to work with people to manage risk in a way that maximises, rather than unnecessarily restricts quality of life.

Risk in context – the bigger picture

Risk cannot be avoided – it is an integral part of our everyday lives. Going downstairs to make breakfast may result in a trip and an injury, and yet the vast majority of us would still include this in our familiar daily routine. When going on holiday, some of us may weigh up the various risks involved – whether to fly or to drive, where is a safe or exciting holiday destination. Here the risks are associated with conscious decision-making and choices. Risk itself is a multifaceted concept, and the ways in which we define and address risk are context-dependent (Mythen and Walklate 2006).

Within healthcare, definitions of risk usually include the following elements:

- *Hazards:* Anything that may cause harm.
- *Harm*: The adverse effect of a hazard.
- *Likelihood:* The chance that a hazard may cause harm, usually quantified in terms of high or low probability.
- *Uncertainty:* An inherent difficulty in determining how serious or likely a risk is to occur.
- *Assessment:* Hazards can be quantified and assessed.
  Source: Haynes and Thomas 2005; Department of Health (DH) 2007; Carson and Bain 2008

The factors influencing the way risk is viewed within health and social care include the individual concept of risk as well as the cultural, political, economic, managerial and societal perspectives. Such factors are not static but evolve over time (Crowe and Carlyle 2003). Against this backdrop, current UK policy places patient/client/service user empowerment and control at the heart of the personalisation agenda (Taylor Gooby 2008a; Taylor Gooby 2008b). This requires health and social care professionals to support people to make informed choices about the care that they receive, and empower them to take everyday risks to meet their needs and wishes (DH 2007).

Wider views of risk and empowerment

When we consider risk, we often think of the circumstances affecting ourselves or those around us. Rarely do we consider the wider context, and yet our own personal views of risk are shaped either consciously or subconsciously by the society in which we live. These views change over time, and are dependent upon the environments in which risk is viewed. The society in which we live also helps to define what is or isn't a hazard, the likelihood of it harming us, how we should react when faced with the perceived harm, and who should be making the decisions (see the example below on societal views of smoking). Current views on risk and empowerment within health and social care are relatively recent, and it takes time for people and cultures to change (Schein 2010). Therefore, within organisations there may be differences between the espoused values on risk that are written within policy documents and the values put into action by staff. It is important for practitioners to appreciate the range of perspectives and how they may have originated to enable an effective approach to risk management to be adopted and articulated. Risk can be categorised and viewed in multiple ways. For the purposes of this chapter, it has been divided up into the way that groups view the topic from societal, government and cultural perspectives (Lupton 2008), and the way that individuals view and frame risk (Wilkinson 2008).

Group views – society and government

From a societal perspective, the nature of the threats we face within Western society has changed dramatically with increasing industrialisation and globalisation. Earlier societies faced risks as a result of threats from nature (for example famines or natural disasters). Natural risks were predominantly addressed by means of local knowledge about weather patterns or farming methods for example, or by religious beliefs. The amount of knowledge in each area was relatively limited; experts knew a lot about the topic, and were often trusted although the actual amount of influence they had over events was relatively limited. Nowadays humans have much more influence and control over the environment and those living in it. Threats posed by human actions such as terrorism, global warming, and pandemics are far more complex and require many more experts to help us to frame and understand how we should deal with the risks associated with them (Giddens 1991; Beck 1999). However, increased globalisation means that health and social care professionals will be working with individuals from a wide variety of cultural backgrounds: the way in which LTCs are viewed by different cultures, and consequently the associated risk perceptions from them may vary (McGuigan 2006). The government perspective sees risk as being framed in terms of how the government controls individuals. In recent times in Western society, there has been a shift away from a paternalistic approach with those in power making decisions on behalf of individuals, towards individual empowerment (Taylor Gooby 2008a; Taylor Gooby 2008b). Now the emphasis in Western society is upon individuals being encouraged to take control and responsibility for their own actions. Once people have been made aware of risks by experts they are expected to manage these responsibly and people who fail to do so face societal approbation (Lupton 2008). People with LTCs are likely to be at the forefront of some of the policy changes linked to these shifts, since they are most likely to be those that need to access money and resources to support them with health and social care.

At the point of writing, the societal discourse on risk is dominated by recognition of the global uncertainties that face us on a daily basis. A societal view of health risks includes the idea that some groups of people are more 'at risk' than others, or may pose a risk to others. People with LTCs may be considered vulnerable and in need of additional support or advice (for example flu vaccination programmes) or as a potential cause of harm to others (for example people with HIV/AIDS). Society often relies upon expert opinion to determine the best course of action to take in both scenarios. However, experts often give widely differing opinions as to how to manage these threats, and scientists or politicians have been known to add to problems rather than relieve them. Faced with conflicting views, lay members of the public may be mistrustful of expert opinion and be uncertain as to whom they should turn to. Where cause and effect can be linked to human actions rather than forces of nature, it is also human to attach blame, and we live in a society where media coverage often focuses upon which experts are responsible for causing a particular situation (Lupton 2008). Experts may be in a situation where they fear litigation and blame, and in turn, may be worried as to the potential repercussions of any actions they may take. However, all of us are both experts and lay people in different spheres of our lives. We gain our information about topics from numerous sources in society – from friends and family, our own experiences and we learn to read media reports with some scepticism as we recognise inaccuracies in areas in which we have some expertise. People, therefore, react to societal influences of risk in complex ways (Lupton 2008) and whilst media images may fuel the fears of professionals, it does not necessarily follow that such fears are accurate.

People with LTCs often face uncertainties at many stages of their contact with services – from the early stages where a diagnosis may be unclear, to later stages where treatments and prognosis may also be subject to different opinions (Lorig et al. 2000). They may have received advice and treatment from a bewildering variety of health and social care professionals in a number of different settings. Each individual will have their own journey and their views of services will be based upon all of the influences outlined above. Where experiences have been positive, people may be trusting of the professionals with whom they engage in the risk management process; where experiences have been less positive, this may require more work. You may not be the professional who was the cause of the negative experience, but you may be seen as being part of the same group of experts and will have to re-establish trust. Health and social care professionals are not immune to this process – previous negative experiences or fear of litigation may impede the risk management process. A relationship of trust and good communication between parties is essential to protect both service users and professionals. Where this is not present, it becomes more difficult for service users to disclose information that may affect decision-making in the risk management process, and the decisions taken may in turn affect the levels of risk experienced.

Group views – health and social care cultures

Just as the contemporary view of risk within wider society has developed, so too has the view of risk within specific subgroups or cultures. Health and social care has become increasingly politicised, and the current climate is that of a market economy, with providers within both the private and public sectors competing over limited resources within a society that increasingly seeks to attach blame when things go wrong (Flynn 2008). Balanced against this, however, is the recognition that in health and social care, a crucial driver is also the need to ensure that people are supported to live their lives to the full, and that risk management needs to balance both risks and benefits. The key stated principles behind risk management in health and social care at the time of writing are:

- People have the right to live their lives to the full as long as this does not stop others from doing the same.
- Independence, well-being, and choice are the concepts that should underpin decision-making in risk management.
- People should have support plans that enable them to manage identified risks in ways that best suit them.
- Person-centred approaches should be adopted for everyone.
- Supported decision tools should be used to assess and manage risk.
- People who have limited capacity to make decisions (for example because of mental health problems, learning disability) have the same rights to choice and independence, but additional mechanisms may need to be utilised to support decision-making.
- Where decisions are made on behalf of people who lack capacity, these must be in their best interests and with the least restriction – lack of capacity on one area does not mean a lack of capacity to make all decisions.
- Informed choice also includes the option to choose 'unwisely'.
 Source: DH 2007

The DH 2007 document 'Independence, Choice and Risk' includes a tool that supports this approach to risk assessment by examining the person's perceptions as to what is important in their life, what is working well at the moment and what could be improved. People are then asked to identify risks. The views of family or carers are sought, and any discrepancy in views are recorded. People are also given the opportunity to outline ways in which organisations may need to change in order for the risk to be managed more effectively (DH 2007). Many of the questions address areas that are covered in assessments outlined in the table below (see Table 7.1), but here the focus is firmly upon the perspective of the client. Staff completing the tool are asked to consider the following amongst other things:

- The communication requirements of the person to ensure that questions are presented in a way that is meaningful (for example use of Braille, picture communication aids for people with a learning disability or language problems).
- Options that may address risk such as environmental adaptation, use of assistive technology (AT), opportunities for learning new skills, finding support networks, and so on.
- Quality of life outcomes including factors such as reducing social isolation or exclusion and ensuring dignity and recognition of diversity.

The factors identified within the tool are closely aligned with the difficulties that people with LTCs face on a daily basis (Anderson and Bury 1988; Lorig et al. 2000; Kielhofner 2008). The tool may, therefore, be considered to be an excellent way of matching the needs of people with LTCs to the requirements of the risk assessment and management process.

In practice, however, this may be easier said than done. As a cultural group, people working in health and social care may have been socialised to view risk as a factor to be feared and avoided, rather than viewing risk as a potential opportunity to enhance quality of life (Carson and Bain 2008).

Section 2

Table 7.1 Overview of risk.

Client level	Organisational level – health and social care
• Clinical assessments (for example, Waterlow scale for assessing risk for pressure sores, falls assessments, Derby scale for assessment of nutritional needs) • Specific departmental risk assessment tools • Care programme approaches • Safe guarding vulnerable adults procedures • Multi-agency public protection arrangements (MAPPA) • Mental Health Act (1987) • Valuing People Now White Paper (DH 2009)	• Commission for Social Care Inspection standards (CSCI) • NHS standards – controls assurance standards • Local authority overview and scrutiny committees • Clinical negligence scheme for trusts (CNST) requirements for insurance purposes • National Patient Safety Agency (NPSA) reporting mechanisms • Health and safety executive requirements • Modernisation and clinical governance requirements • Multidisciplinary and multi-agency assessment arrangements • Integrated reactive (complaints/incidents) and proactive (risk assessment) procedures

Source: NPSA website, Haynes and Thomas 2005, DH 2007, National Patient Safety Agency, http://www.Judy-waterlow.co.uk.

Organisations that fear litigation may find it difficult to facilitate the level of service user control that is outlined above, and staff working in such organisations may find barriers to enacting the above principles. As discussed previously, people with LTCs could be argued to be particularly vulnerable to the organisational impact of risk management since they are often in contact with so many different areas of the health and social care markets, and these do not always have a unified approach to risk. A quick overview of the types of processes that impact the way that risk is viewed when considering a person in contact with these organisations gives an idea of the scale of the problem. These may include examples as shown in Table 7.1.

Depending upon the organisation that they are dealing with, people with LTCs may find themselves having different levels of control over decision-making in risk situations. Reduced levels of control are not in keeping with the patient-centred approach and empowerment principles within current policies. Nor are they in keeping with the governmental and societal moves towards individuals taking responsibility for their own actions. There may, therefore, be a discrepancy between the expectations that a person with an LTC has in terms of how they should be involved in risk management, and what actually occurs. Studies in America, a culture well versed in the litigation culture, concluded that whilst precipitating factors for being sued included adverse outcomes and mistakes in care provision, people only tended to actually sue when they were unhappy with the communication style or attitude of the doctor providing the care (Haynes and Thomas 2005). It could, therefore, be argued that failure to empower service users within the risk management process in itself increases the risk of litigation or complaints against an organisation.

Understanding the culture in which risk is being addressed, and putting forward arguments that are in keeping with the values inherent within that culture may enable staff to put the empowerment values outlined above into action. For cultures that are already taking a person-centred approach to risk, this may be no more than making explicit links between actions and policy. For cultures that are fearful of litigation, this may involve an approach that articulates the point that fear of litigation far outweighs the likelihood of it occurring (DH 2007), and that adopting a person-centred approach may reduce the risk of complaints or litigation, and hence the risks to the organisation.

Case study 7.1 Fred

Fred is an 85-year-old man with Chronic Obstructive Pulmonary Disease (COPD). He was conscripted in the army towards the end of the Second World War, and although he had never previously smoked, the government issue ration packs included cigarettes. Fred soon took up the habit as most of his colleagues were smokers, and smoking was recognised to help with the stress of warfare. His friend Bill had heard some rumours about smoking being linked to health problems, and he stopped smoking, but Fred argued that if it really were dangerous, the army wouldn't issue them with cigarettes. After the war, Fred got married, had a couple of children, and continued to smoke up to 30 cigarettes a day. Over the years, Fred experienced a number of bouts of bronchitis. He started to notice that some papers were running articles linking smoking to chest problems, but experts were also arguing that smoking wasn't harmful, so he decided that if the experts couldn't agree, then it couldn't be too much of a problem. Over the years, the articles in the papers increasingly warned people against smoking, and the cigarette packets started to carry government health warnings. Fred and his mates at the local pub would sometimes complain about the way the government kept putting tax onto cigarettes every time there was a budget. By now, Fred was suffering with chronic bronchitis and emphysema. He had regular admissions into hospital during the winter months when he often developed chest infections. Whilst he had been able to smoke in hospital during his first admissions, this became increasingly difficult as smoking was first banned from the main ward, and was then banned completely. He was also finding that nurses, doctors and his family were nagging him about giving up smoking, and he started to wonder if there was something in the health warnings after all. Fred tried to give up smoking on a number of different occasions, but found this almost impossible. After retirement, his health had continued to deteriorate, and a visit to the pub was his main hobby. Every time he went to the pub, he'd be offered a cigarette and his resolve would go out of the window. Although he was dreading the ban on public smoking, he thought it might help him to give up the habit. However, the smoking ban hit Fred hard as his local pub closed down, and he could no longer get out to visit his friends. His wife worried about him, health professionals nagged him, so he promised to give up smoking. By now, Fred needed oxygen at home to address his increasing breathlessness associated with the COPD, and he had been warned that as smoking near oxygen was very dangerous, he would only be issued the tanks on the understanding that he did not smoke. He had limited access to cigarettes, but every time his friend from the pub dropped in, and his wife went out, Fred would be persuaded to have a cigarette with him. They sometimes joked that it was like the war again – hiding from the enemy and waiting to get blown up!

Section 2

Points for reflection

- Identify the changes in government policy in relation to smoking in the scenario.
- Consider the impact of the policy changes on Fred's perceptions of risk.
- How do the policy changes affect Fred's health and quality of life?
- How does Fred view the professional's assessment of smoking-related risks?
- Who influences Fred in his decisions about smoking?
- Why does Fred hide the fact that he has an occasional cigarette?
- What are the health risks associated with continued smoking?
- Read the section on individual views of risk below, and make links between this scenario and the ways that individuals judge risk.

Consider practice environments you have been in either as a practitioner or service user

- What government or departmental policies are you aware of that have affected the way that risk is viewed in the practice environment?
- What are the benefits and risks associated with people following these policies?
- What are the benefits and risks associated with people not following these policies?
- Does everyone always follow official risk policies, and if not, why not?

Individual views of risk

So far the discussion has focused upon the way in which groups frame and respond to risk, and work of this nature is generally informed by disciplines such as sociology and anthropology. In contrast, individual views of risk are informed by psychology, and here the discourse is preoccupied with how people estimate the probability that an adverse incident or hazard will affect them, and how they respond to perceived threats (Wilkinson 2008). The terms that are used such as 'likelihood' are ones that are frequently used within risk assessments in health and social care. The first problem that professionals face is that although many of our risk management systems are based on this skill, on the whole, human beings are pretty poor at estimating probabilities. We tend to base our decisions upon whether a risk is known or unknown, new or old, and whether we have control over it (Wilkinson 2008). A newly qualified member of staff making a decision about a patient diagnosed with an uncommon condition in a community setting may well judge the associated risks very differently from an experienced member of staff who is based in hospital with all the associated resources. There are also differences in the way that lay people and experts judge risk. In sectors where actuarial tables exist to help explain the probability of an event occurring, experts tend to judge risk in line with scientific evidence, whilst lay people tend to base their decisions on the factors above. Thus, a person working in an accident and emergency setting may think twice about purchasing a motorbike where the risk of serious injury is eight times higher than that of other road users, whilst a young person living with diabetes may hesitate to eat a chocolate bar when blood sugars are high, but then happily hop onto a motorbike to buy a banana instead. Even when the rate of risk is known to an individual, human beings tend to judge risks to be high *for other people in society*, but low for themselves (the *optimistic bias approach*) – the young motorcyclist may have some awareness of accident statistics from the cost of the insurance premiums, but assume that the accident will not happen *to them*.

The difficulty in estimating probability from a lay and expert perspective needs to be considered from another angle when we think about LTCs. Unlike insurance companies, health and social care professionals rarely have access to uncontested actuarial data. Instead, evidence-based practice requires practitioners to access and evaluate information on topic areas in an environment where information proliferates at an incredible rate (Taylor 2007). That information is now often available to patients/service users/carers, many of whom take an active and specialised interest in their condition. In this situation, who is the expert and who is the layperson? Each could argue to hold specialist information – the professional who is able to read and evaluate information from the perspective of their own academic discipline, and the patient or carer who is able to read and interpret information according to their own experience. In some cases too, the patient may have access to far more information on the topic than a hard-pressed practitioner who is expected to know about a wide variety of conditions and interventions. Despite their best intentions, neither party is likely to be able to give a wholly objective assessment of the level of risk.

Some of the answers to the areas addressed above are already implicit within risk assessment and management procedures outlined in the section 'Group views: health and social care cultures'. Since we only see the risks we have active knowledge on, the more varied the background of those involved in assessment, the more likely it is that a balanced view of risk will be achieved. Multidisciplinary and multi-agency risk assessments/plans that include the person as an active participant in the process are recognised to be good practice (DH 2007), and there is a good fit between these types of processes and the wider empowerment agenda that may help to prevent some of the communication issues raised above.

Case study 7.2 Mrs Amber

Mrs Amber is 39 weeks pregnant and has been an insulin-dependant diabetic for 8 years. She has been receiving close monitoring of her and her baby's well-being currently under joint care from a consultant obstetrician and a diabetologist at her local hospital. During the last few months, Mrs Amber has had regular observations of her blood glucose control via blood tests, and ultrasound scans to assess the growth and well-being of her baby. Her family is very supportive of her and she has remained very active, working part-time as a hairdresser until 34 weeks pregnant.

Mrs Amber was admitted to the antenatal ward for induction of labour the following morning. The admission procedure was performed by a student midwife who completed the appropriate documentation and admission observations. On admission, her clinical observations of pulse, blood pressure and temperature were all within normal parameters, so too was the monitoring of the baby's welfare via cardiotocograph recordings. She had been managing her own diabetes extremely well for the last 8 years; however, during her pregnancy she had occasionally experienced a few hypoglycemic attacks due to the increased demands from her developing pregnancy. The early shift had just finished receiving handover from the night shift when at around 7.30 a.m. one of the student midwives called for assistance as it appeared that Mrs Amber was having a severe hypoglycemic episode.

Section 2

The medical team was summoned and after receiving a bolus dose of intravenous glucose administration via peripheral cannulae, Mrs Amber proceeded to make a swift recovery. On questioning, Mrs Amber informed the staff that she always self-administers her insulin at 6.00 a.m. as she is normally up early to 'sort' her husband out before he goes off to work. She then eats her breakfast half an hour after giving herself the injection. She had brought her own insulin in, and administered it as normal. She had then asked for breakfast, but had been informed she would need to wait for the trolley to come at 8.00 as the ward was not allowed to keep food on the premises. Following this incident an adverse incident form is completed as per hospital protocol.

Points for reflection

- How much did the hospital clinical assessments incorporate an individualised view of risk?
- What assumptions regarding the management of the risks associated with diabetes did
  (a) Mrs Amber make?
  (b) hospital staff make?
- How did the hospital risk assessment policy relating to storage of food impact risk in this case?
- What expectations does the service user have in terms of involvement?
- How do the approaches of each map to the principles in DH documentation?
- How have the approaches to risk impacted the way in which the organisation may be viewed?

Consider practice environments you have been in either as a practitioner or service user

- What clinical assessments have you experienced?
- How did they link to the principles outlined in the bullet points in Table 7.1?
- How much power did the recipient of services have in the risk management process?
- What factors may have helped or hindered empowerment within the culture you were in?

Summary

How risk impacts daily personal lives and professional lives has been examined. Wider views of risk have been compared to different group's views. The latter have included society and government as well as health and social care cultures. Finally, the chapter has focused on an individual's views of risk. Links have been made throughout to individuals with LTCs. Links between these aspects of risk and how we then balance them as professionals are illustrated in Figures 7.2-7.8.

Empowerment

Within the United Kingdom, there has been an increasing move towards increased control and choice for users of health and social care (Daly and Roebuck 2008; Taylor Gooby 2008b). Policy drivers such as 'Independence, Choice and Risk' (DH 2007) emphasise the need to empower service users to have more choice and control. But what does the concept of empowerment really mean in practice? Empowerment has its roots within movements such as social justice and advocacy where certain social groups (for example women, ethnic minorities and those with disabilities) were seen to have unequal access to resources and measures needed to be taken to address inequality. A concept analysis undertaken by McCarthy and Freeman (2008) identified a number of components associated with the term and these included the following:

- A disadvantaged population.
- *Agency:* Empowerment needs to be claimed by the individual not conferred by others.
- Empowerment includes the ability to make decisions and carry out the actions associated with these decisions.
- Empowerment is an ongoing process.
- Empowerment is associated with self-efficacy, competency and an internal locus of control.
- Equality of access to resources.
  Source: McCarthy and Holbrook Freeman 2008

As we have seen above, concepts are complex since they mean different things to different people in different settings, and also depend upon whether we think as an individual or as part of a group. The authors included in the concept analysis (McCarthy and Holbrook Freeman 2008) often varied in the way in which they defined and operationalised empowerment. People with LTCs interact with a multitude of different professions and agencies in a variety of environments, and will therefore experience different views of empowerment. Where differences in viewpoints are not recognised or acknowledged, this may have a negative impact upon communication within the risk management process, which in turn may increase the risk to individuals or organisations. It is, therefore, important that practitioners are able to reflect upon the impact of the empowerment agenda when considering risk, and utilise this knowledge to inform their decision-making.

To consider empowering someone, there first needs to be recognition that an organisation or person has power over someone or something and can, therefore, make choices that affect the individual or object. Power may come in many forms but definitions usually include concepts such as having knowledge to make informed decisions and choices. Thinking of our own lives, there are some decisions that we have the power to undertake alone (for example what to have for breakfast), some that we may take with permission from others (an example may be using money from a joint account to buy a new car), and some that we do not have the power to undertake (passing a new law to make it a legal requirement to provide chocolate for all employees for example!). The power to make these decisions may change over time: going into hospital may mean that the decision as to what to have for breakfast is restricted for example. Power can, therefore, seen to be held by some people who decide how, when or where they will share the decision-making process. Implicit within this is an understanding that there are power differences (Laverack 2005).

For many of the older people currently both accessing and providing services for people with LTCs, expectations and values are based around a generational view of the welfare state with the individual as a passive recipient of care, and power/knowledge held by those in authority (Daly and Roebuck 2008). That view of service provision resulted in a 'one-size-fits-all' economy. People with an LTC were usually offered health or social care services that were based upon decisions made by commissioners or managers, and their individual needs and circumstances were often ignored (Lorig et al. 2000). This started to change in the 1990s with the NHS and Community Care Act 1990 where a more personalised concept of care provision was introduced. The personalisation agenda shifts the service user from being a passive recipient of care to an active agent determining their own future. Direct payments and individual budgets have been introduced to enable people to determine and manage their own social care so that individual needs and aspirations may be met. A similar scheme to enable people with LTCs choose and manage their healthcare needs in a similar fashion is also being piloted. Such moves require changes not only in the markets that support care, but also in the way that individuals take responsibility for their care provision. The personalisation reforms in health and social care are relatively recent and not without controversy. It needs to be recognised that not everyone in health or social care will want to take control of the decision-making process. Some people may be less concerned with choice and more with the quality of services that are offered (Taylor Gooby 2008a; 2008b). Since the life stories of people with LTCs are complex and involve having to cope with many changes as health status alters, there may also be times when additional choice may be perceived as a burden rather than a blessing (Anderson and Bury 1988). However, a recent survey of people with LTCs indicates that four out of five people welcome the opportunity to take an active role in treating their condition, and that people are growing ever more comfortable with this as the years go by (DH 2009). There is, therefore, some evidence to suggest that the empowerment agenda is having a perceived impact upon the way in which healthcare professionals interact with patients/service users, with a shift towards shared responsibility and power in the decision-making process. However, for power sharing to occur, individuals need to have access to information on which to base their decision; the same survey indicates that not everyone received information. See Table 7.2.

When people did need advice, the type of advice sought was specific to their condition in 54% of cases, and general health advice in 45% of cases. The people they tended to seek advice from were predominantly the GPs (47%), followed by practice nurses (15%), hospital doctors (11%), and therapists (6%) as outlined in the chart below. Hospital nurses were asked for information in 3% of

Table 7.2 Summary of information identifying information given to people with LTCs.

	Hospital care plan provided	Instructions on taking medication in hospital	Instructions on how to manage condition in hospital	Instructions on how to make a complaint about care	Support on how to understand information given	Information on training courses to manage self-care skills
Percentage (%) of clients receiving the information/ support	42	60	47	7	66	23

Source: Based on DH Survey (DH 2009).

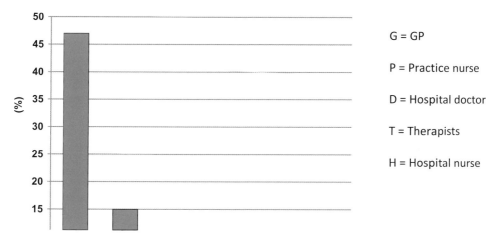

Figure 7.1 Sources of advice for help with LTCs. (DH 2009.)

cases. When people did receive advice this was seen to be helpful in terms of taking an active role in the management of their condition in 90% of cases. See Figure 7.1.

Given that information was generally well received and acted upon by patients, it is worth reflecting that in many of the areas outlined above, the majority of patients did not get access to the information that may have empowered them to take more control over their care and associated decisions. This may suggest that professional groups other than doctors also need to consider their role in the information giving and empowerment process. However, as the discussions relating to risk show, there are often many factors at governmental, societal, cultural, and individual level that affect how decisions are made, and this applies equally to the empowerment agenda.

Traditionally, power within healthcare has been held by doctors, and GPs and hospital doctors have been seen as powerful, trusted professionals (Department of Health 2009; Sheaff 2009)). In recent times, changes to policy and contractual arrangements has seen a shift in power away from doctors and towards healthcare managers within the health service. Nurses and other professionals allied to medicine, however, have generally not gained in power during this process (Sheaff 2009). Despite having professional frameworks that emphasise client centredness and empowerment as core values of the professions (College of Occupational Therapists 2005; Nursing and Midwifery Council 2008), these groups in general have not had a large impact in terms of shaping the healthcare system and empowering patients (McCarthy and Holbrook Freeman 2008).

Empowerment can be a powerful tool in successful risk management, safety and quality of care (Busch 2003; Beason 2005). However, in order to empower others it could be argued that professional groups need to understand the concept of empowerment and apply it to themselves in order to take full advantage of the policy drivers that support empowerment within risk assessment. They are then more likely to be in a position to empower service users.

Empowerment models and reasoning within the risk management process

Thus far, two complex concepts have been explored, namely risk and empowerment. Current policies link the two and provide assessment tools to help frame information collection as well as outlining

Section 2

good practice such as multidisciplinary and multi-agency assessments (DH 2007). However, the discussion above also highlights that policy changes do not automatically result in an immediate change in practice. The complexities of societal, cultural and individual perspectives on risk and empowerment may result in differences between stated values and values in action. Different professionals involved in the risk management process may view risk in different ways. The expectations that people with an LTC may have in relation to how they wish to be involved in risk assessment may change at a different pace to the institutions that provide services. It is clear that there is an increasing need for health and social care professionals to put into practice the empowerment and personalisation agendas when considering risk. What is not so clear is how individual practitioners who themselves may not be in a particularly powerful position within the health or social care hierarchy deal with such situations in such a way as to serve the needs and wishes of the patient/service user, themselves and the institution that they work for.

Ultimately, risk management requires a decision to be made (Carson and Bain 2008). The decision needs to take into account factors related to risk and empowerment, and to communicate findings in a way that meets the requirements of the parties involved. This will include the service user and family, as well as the organisations that collate information on risk outlined in Table 7.1. For professionals, decisions involve a process of clinical reasoning and the ability to consider a problem from multiple perspectives generally improves the quality of the decision made. The use of decision aids or models can be useful in that they give a simplified representation of complex information that identifies the key components and the relationships between them (Kielhofner 2008; Trevena et al. 2008).

A model that incorporates empowerment and risk within the context of clinical decision-making is, therefore, proposed to enable the practitioner to consider and discuss issues raised in a structured way.

Empowerment model

Many different models of empowerment exist and the reader is encouraged to read around this area to find one that suits their individual worldview of the concept. When doing so, it is however important to reflect that for true empowerment to occur, practitioners need to help to create the circumstances that enable service users to take control over the decisions that affect their lives, if they so choose (Laverack 2005). Empowerment is seized by the service user, and not conferred by the practitioner. When the choices concerned relate to risk however, duty of care requires practitioners to ensure that all elements have been considered, and a balanced view of risks and benefits have been considered prior to a decision being made. In order for these decisions to meet the requirements of both the risk and empowerment agendas, the practitioner needs to have the reflective skills to recognise the power that they hold, and a means of balancing the perspectives of different professional groups and service users.

A model that has been used to map the level of empowerment of health and social care services is that developed by Arnstein (1969). Arnstein proposed that services could be charted according to how much control citizens had over the decision-making process. Services were seen to be controlling (manipulation), tokenistic (giving information or consulting people without really giving them any power to effect change), working in partnership (equal power sharing in the decision-making process), or giving citizens power (citizens having the control over the decisions made). The model is not uncontested, but it does provide a guide to framing just who has the power within a decision-making

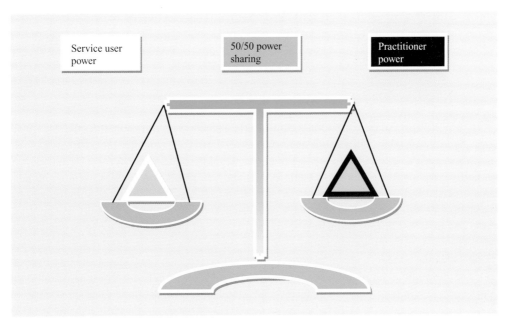

Figure 7.2 Balancing power during risk and decision-making.

process. Whilst empowerment is an acknowledged underlying principle of risk management, it is also acknowledged that organisations need to manage and ensure equitable distribution of resources (DH 2007), and, therefore, decisions will sometimes be complex. Not all situations will result in a patient or service user having equal power sharing in the final decision (for example, if the resources required to empower one service user in turn disadvantaged several other service users). However, if patients/service users are truly to be empowered, there needs to be, as a minimum requirement, the opportunity for them to affect the outcome of the decision made. If their say in the decision-making process is less than 50%, then they can always be overruled. By starting with the principle that within the risk assessment process power is shared at the very least on an equal level (50/50), empowerment is more likely to be achieved. Figure 7.2 is based on the work by Arnstein (1969), and represents how empowerment may be viewed during risk and decision-making. The scales may show the balance of power tipping towards or away from the service user, depending on the dynamics present within the decision-making process. Where service users and professionals have equal power in the decision (partnership working), the scales are balanced, and this degree of power sharing may be a goal of professional practice for professions that aspire to empower service users (Carr 2004; Kielhofner 2008).

The personalisation agenda is likely to increasingly tip the scale towards people with LTCs in the future since this is a group of people that is often in need of long-term support or interventions, and who are, therefore, in a position to access individual budgets, direct payments or health budgets. In situations where the service user holds the budget and can choose where to source personal care or health interventions from, practitioners are no longer the key decision-makers when it comes to risk management. Professionals may be unprepared for the shift in power, and may not know how best to react to the changed relationship with the service user (Daly and Roebuck 2008). In such situations, ineffective communication between parties may increase the risk to both service user and the organisation, and therefore it is important for practitioners to be able to explicitly explore power and effectively communicate their decisions.

Case study 7.3 Laura

Laura is an 18-year-old girl with moderate learning disabilities and a congenital heart defect. She lives with her family and attends a special school. Both Laura and her family are keen that she should eventually move into a place of her own, but recognise that she will need ongoing support to achieve this. Laura has explored her options with the transitions team, and her family have sorted an individual budget to help Laura to achieve her ambition. Both the school and the social worker have had some concerns regarding Laura's physical health as she tires easily and does not always want to stop to rest. They feel that an initial move to supported living may be a better option for Laura.

The individual budget is allocated and Laura and family recruit two support workers to help Laura to move into a flat of her own. The first couple of weeks went reasonably well, but then Laura contracts influenza and is admitted to hospital with complications. During her stay in hospital, Laura is adamant that she wishes to return to her flat as soon as possible, but is tired when managing basic tasks such as washing and dressing. Staff at the hospital are concerned about Laura's ability to cope once she returns home, and arrange a case conference. During the case conference, hospital staff and Laura's social worker express their concerns and raise the issue of supported living again. Laura and her family become quite angry at this suggestion. They argue that Laura had been prevented from doing many of the normal routine jobs, such as making herself a drink whilst she has been on the ward, and that sitting around all day has contributed to her lethargy. They are worried that the longer she stays in hospital, the greater the chance she has of becoming deskilled. They are happy to use some of the money that had been put aside to help Laura to go on holiday to pay for additional support until Laura is feeling stronger, and feel that Laura is not being given a fair chance at independent living. They also feel that staff are unprepared for the fact that it is now Laura and her family who are making the decisions, and are trying to use the opportunity of the hospital admission to take back control. Staff argue that they have genuine concerns regarding Laura's physical condition, given the heart defect. Laura repeatedly reminds people that she wants to go back to her flat, and becomes distressed. The case conference ends acrimoniously without a decision being agreed to, and Laura's family put in a formal complaint to the hospital.

Points for reflection

- What are the potential risks and benefits to Laura should she return to her flat?
- What are the potential risks and benefits to the organisations involved in this scenario should Laura return home?
- Who holds the power in the risk decision-making process?
- Does the balance of power change on admission into hospital?
- How could the situation be resolved?

> ## Consider practice environments you have been in either as a practitioner or service user
>
> - How empowered did you feel in the setting?
> - What factors may have affected your feelings of being in control?
> - As a practitioner, how empowered do you feel when you change roles to being a service user (for example when going to a GP appointment)?
> - At what points in the treatment process is empowerment and risk explicitly addressed, and at what points are these issues implicit?

The degrees of service user empowerment may be easy to discern when risk is explicitly on the agenda. For example, the forms that hospitals use to judge risk when a service user is admitted onto a ward often focus on the hospital view of what constitutes a risk factor, without giving an opportunity for the service user to give their view as to how the environment may put them at risk. For community settings where the service user is in their own environment for extended periods, there may be greater emphasis on individual choice. In hospital settings where turnover may be more rapid and the differing needs of a number of people have to be balanced, individual risk assessments may be more difficult to achieve, and consequently, empowerment may be reduced. However, it is often the implicit attitudes to empowerment that are present in the small day to day encounters that may prove to have the greater effect on the service user (Ramcharan 1997). This may be particularly problematic when people have chronic conditions that expose them to frequent judgements by others on their capacity to undertake tasks (Bury 1988). Long-term, repeated exposure to negative attitudes to risk can undermine an individual's self-efficacy (*power within*) and belief of their sense of control over their own life. A subtle way in which practitioners who have some decision-making and authority (*power over*) with service users may inadvertently increase risk is by imposing a top-down approach to risk management. By imposing their expert ideas as to what they believe are the most important risk factors (*hegemonic power*), they may create a situation where the service users feel powerless to challenge the decisions and are compelled to hide their actions from those that they feel will judge them (Laverack 2005), just as Fred increased his risk by smoking near his oxygen tanks (Case study 7.1).

Clearly, therefore, empowering people with LTCs to have a positive and active perspective on risk if they so choose, is a complex process that is present during every interaction with professionals. The current emphasis on empowerment requires practitioners to change their patterns of thinking, and as with all habits, this is not always easy to achieve. The sophisticated interplay of factors requires a sophisticated model of reasoning to enable practitioners to take the best-judged action in a specific context (Walter et al. 2004; Walter and Emery 2005; Higgs et al. 2008). Utilising a clinical reasoning framework that links the particular issues faced by people with LTCs with those associated with risk and empowerment will make it easier for practitioners to become conscious of the factors that impact their decision-making. Many different reasoning styles have been proposed, but common emergent themes that are particularly relevant to the consideration of risk include scientific reasoning, narrative reasoning, pragmatic reasoning and ethical reasoning (Carter and Robinson 2001; Carr 2004; Walter et al. 2004; Davidson et al. 2008; Higgs et al. 2008). Each of the reasoning styles is examined and

Section 2

the factors that help or hinder empowerment are summarised in boxes. The style of the box indicates either a factor that facilitates or a factor that hinders empowerment, as follows (Figure 7.3):

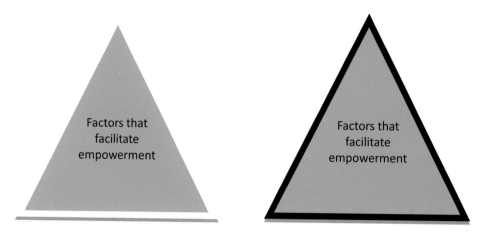

Figure 7.3   Key to factors that facilitate or hinder empowerment.

Scientific reasoning, risk and empowerment in LTCs

Scientific reasoning is used to understand the condition that is affecting the individual, and is based on hypothetico-deductive reasoning models. It helps individuals to assess probabilities, and as such has many links to the ways in which individuals consider risk. Practitioners use their knowledge of medical conditions to gather cues relating to the condition. These are used to form a hypothesis as to what the key problem areas are, and what the best intervention may be. For example, a practitioner speaking to a service user who has COPD and who is complaining of tiredness and increased breathlessness following a cold may hypothesise that the person is developing an acute infection that requires a course of antibiotics. In the past, scientific knowledge was seen to be the domain of the expert, but the shift towards empowerment has seen a move towards sharing of this knowledge. Expert-patient programmes, access to the Internet, and an expectation on the part of many service users to be an active participant in the management of their condition means that many people are either well informed about their condition, or have the opportunity to become so if supported by professionals. Service users with a vested interest in keeping up to date with the latest developments affecting them may have accessed information that is both current and relevant to the practitioner. Such changes may create challenges for staff who are used to being the guardians of knowledge. Some practitioners may be concerned that by discussing factors relating to conditions/risk, they are increasing an individual's anxiety. Research suggests, however, that if practitioners are able to explore scientific information and risk with service users, it reduces anxiety, helps individuals to plan their lives and manage risk in day-to-day situations (Moore et al. 2002). Discussions also help to identify any differences in interpretation of scientific material that may

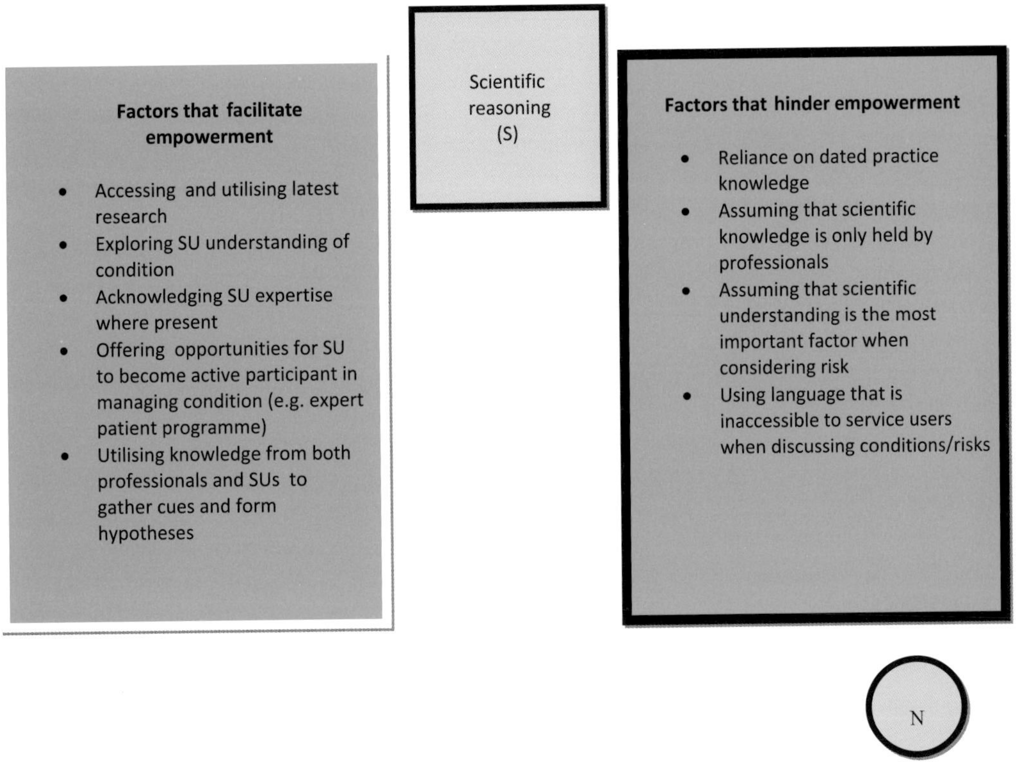

Factors that facilitate empowerment	Scientific reasoning (S)	Factors that hinder empowerment
• Accessing and utilising latest research • Exploring SU understanding of condition • Acknowledging SU expertise where present • Offering opportunities for SU to become active participant in managing condition (e.g. expert patient programme) • Utilising knowledge from both professionals and SUs to gather cues and form hypotheses		• Reliance on dated practice knowledge • Assuming that scientific knowledge is only held by professionals • Assuming that scientific understanding is the most important factor when considering risk • Using language that is inaccessible to service users when discussing conditions/risks

Figure 7.4   Scientific reasoning, risk and empowerment.

have occurred between professional and service user (Walter et al. 2004; Walter and Emery 2005; Davidson et al. 2008), but these benefit the most when risk is discussed in formats that are meaningful to the service user. This may also include the way in which risks are framed – some people find it harder to understand percentages and may find it easier to understand risk if words such as low, medium or high risk are used (Moore et al. 2002; Trevena et al. 2008). The scientific reasoning factors that may empower or disempower service users during risk assessment are shown above (Figure 7.4).

Narrative reasoning, risk and empowerment in LTCs

Scientific reasoning is a form of reasoning that most practitioners are familiar and comfortable with because it deals with facts and theory relating to conditions and interventions that are perceived to be relatively certain (Carter and Robinson 2001), but it is only a part of the picture. An LTC creates challenges for the individual. It forces them and those around them to face an uncertain future, and to constantly juggle with the risks associated with everyday activities as their condition changes. A person with Parkinson's disease, for example, may have to constantly weigh up the risks of doing even a relatively simple task such as making a hot drink, given that they may suddenly 'freeze' (Pinder 1988). If the condition progresses, then the types of roles and activities undertaken may need to be reviewed and renegotiated. Despite these challenges, the condition does not define person, and

Section 2

the story of people with LTCs can often be viewed as one of interrupted narratives, with people seeking to maintain normal interests and roles in spite of the condition (Anderson and Bury 1988, Kielhofner 2008). Lives may be put on hold as people enter hospital, or during a deterioration in condition but are then resumed or redefined when situations stabilise (Carr 2004). The way that risk is viewed in one setting may well be inappropriate in another. Therefore, there needs to be a mechanism for understanding not only the condition, but the person it affects, and the environments and occupations which that person undertakes as they move through life.

Stories can be powerful and provide an illuminating glimpse into the person's life in ways that nothing else quite does (Mattingly and Hayes Fleming 1994; Higgs et al. 2008)). They enable us to make sense of human experience in terms of understanding motives (Kielhofner 2008), and they may also help us to understand other sources of information that the service user may access and value as they develop their own interpretation of risk. If we can understand what motivates people to act and who they are influenced by, we are more likely to be able to understand the ways in which they are likely to judge and act upon risk. Narrative reasoning, therefore, can be a powerful tool within risk assessment and empowerment. It requires the practitioner not only to find a way to understand the meaning of the experience from the individual's perspective, but also to consider the other actors within the story, and how they may help the storyline to develop. Other actors include family, friends, colleagues, all the professionals involved in the client's journey, and the settings within which various chapters of the story are played out. Practitioners who are involved in a chapter that could be entitled 'Fred goes into hospital' need to also remember that there is often a follow-up chapter entitled 'Fred returns home'. Risk, therefore, needs to be considered both in terms of the individual context, and the wider cultural and societal contexts. Failure to recognise other perspectives may lead to the practitioner's risk strategy being ignored, or inappropriately transferred from one setting to another, thus increasing risk. The factors that help or hinder this are outlined below (Figure 7.5).

Pragmatic reasoning, risk and empowerment in LTCs

In an idealised world, once the scientific and narrative aspects of the condition have been considered, service user risks would be identified, and the appropriate support provided to enable them to undertake valued activities safely, regardless of the setting. In practice, however, practitioners and services are subject to the conflicting demands of a multitude of service users. Pragmatic reasoning extends beyond the service user-practitioner relationship, and considers the wider environment in which interventions occur. This includes both a personal and practice dimension (Higgs et al. 2008).

The personal dimension includes not only the abilities of the practitioner to communicate and negotiate risk with all parties, but also an awareness of the need to do so, and the motivation to undertake the necessary discussions. As highlighted above, practitioner's communication skills are an essential component in reducing risk to service users and organisations. Practitioners require the skills to access and evaluate the latest evidence base to make scientific judgments (Taylor 2007), as well as possessing the communication skills required to effectively interact with service users to access and respond to the narrative story. Communication skills also are inherent within the need to accurately record information and decisions relating to the risk management process (Lilley and Lambden 2005). Reflective practice is an implicit part of this process of monitoring a personal skill base, and responding appropriately when skills are in need of refinement.

The practice dimension includes an awareness of the policies and procedures related to risk outlined in Table 7.1, as well as the wider context that governs clinical practice. The degree to which an

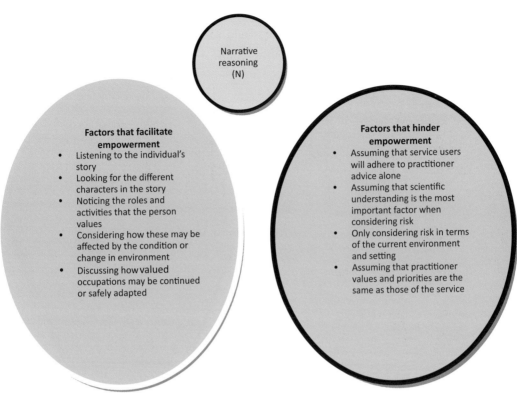

Figure 7.5   Narrative reasoning, risk and empowerment.

individual can affect policies and procedures may well be dependent upon the degree to which they themselves are empowered within an organisation. However, even if an individual cannot directly change practice, they can develop the ability to critique local practice and compare this with the empowerment principles contained within current government policy. For example, a review of risk assessment documentation used on admission to hospital may reveal a strong emphasis on scientific reasoning, with a limited emphasis placed on narrative reasoning. A practitioner may compare this with the principles contained within the DH guidelines (DH 2007) that require the service user's voice to be heard and acted upon within the risk management process. Depending upon the motivation and communication skills outlined above, the practitioner may choose to formally look for ways of changing the system (for example by volunteering to take part in risk management processes or teams) or informally decide to also listen to the service user's narrative when considering and documenting risk. See Figure 7.6.

Ethical reasoning, risk and empowerment in LTCs

Balancing all of the different factors involved in risk may appear to be an overwhelming task at times. Rogers (Rogers 1983), however, simplified this somewhat by arguing that clinical reasoning overall terminates in an ethical decision that projects itself over the entire process. Ethical principles are embedded within professional codes of practice and encompass the following:

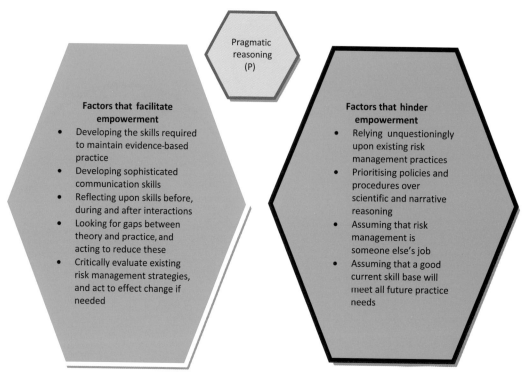

Figure 7.6 Pragmatic reasoning, risk and empowerment.

- *Autonomy:* Enabling people to decide freely and independently.
- *Beneficence/non-malificence:* Striving to do good, and not doing harm.
- *Veracity:* Being truthful.
- Confidentiality.
- *Justice:* Fair distribution of resources, dealing according to individual merit.
- *Morals:* Addressing issues of capacity to consent, choice, etc.

The issues discussed in relation to risk and empowerment in LTCs have touched upon each of these areas, and whilst in practice it may not be so easy to always see the risk decision in purely ethical terms, aspiring to do so may make some of the decision-making slightly less complex. See Figure 7.7.

Bringing all the factors together

The individual, societal, cultural and governmental views of risk impact the way that we view choices when undertaking valued activities. For people with an LTC, the activities are often affected by changes in their health circumstances or by their environment. They may well mix with a wide variety of professionals who will consciously or unconsciously affect their attitude to risk taking, and facilitate or restrict their opportunities to take part in valued activities or roles. However, the empowerment agenda currently influencing health and social care policy means that service users are no longer passive recipients of services, but have the opportunity to actively determine their own support

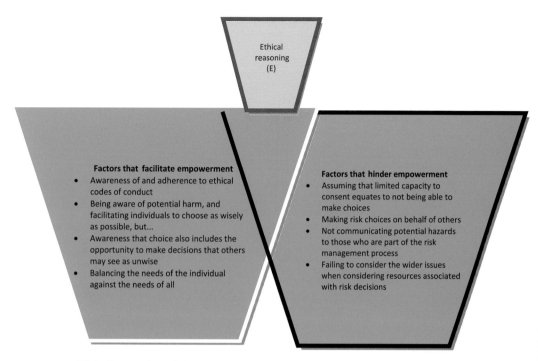

Factors that facilitate empowerment
- Awareness of and adherence to ethical codes of conduct
- Being aware of potential harm, and facilitating individuals to choose as wisely as possible, but...
- Awareness that choice also includes the opportunity to make decisions that others may see as unwise
- Balancing the needs of the individual against the needs of all

Factors that hinder empowerment
- Assuming that limited capacity to consent equates to not being able to make choices
- Making risk choices on behalf of others
- Not communicating potential hazards to those who are part of the risk management process
- Failing to consider the wider issues when considering resources associated with risk decisions

Ethical reasoning (E)

Figure 7.7 Ethical reasoning, risk and empowerment.

mechanisms. Whilst the discussions relating to clinical reasoning have focused upon the practitioner, it must be remembered that service users too may well be utilising all of the above reasoning styles, skills and information. Each party involved in making decisions, whether professional, service user, or relative may, therefore, bring these elements to the decision-making process. Each party may also bring practices that facilitate or hinder empowerment as outlined in Figure 7.8 below.

Practitioners may take into account the degree of service user voice heard within each of the reasoning styles and weigh up how much of a say the person with the LTC has within the risk decision made. If the scales are tipped towards others within the discussions (whether professionals, relatives or others), and the service user has not indicated that they want someone else to make the decision at this time, the practitioner may need to reflect on whether strategies outlined above need to be introduced to address the imbalance.

Conclusion

Whether a formal risk assessment or an informal decision as to what a service user may be supported to do during everyday activities, a decision-making process that takes into account all of these factors is more likely to result in both a well-reasoned, balanced decision, reducing the risk to the service user. Processes that include good communication tend to result in more satisfied participants, thus reducing the risk to the organisations involved. Living with an LTC is in itself often a struggle that requires energy, time and resources. Time spent on battling poor risk management processes may use up resources that could be better utilised on more valued activities. A reflective practitioner,

Section 2

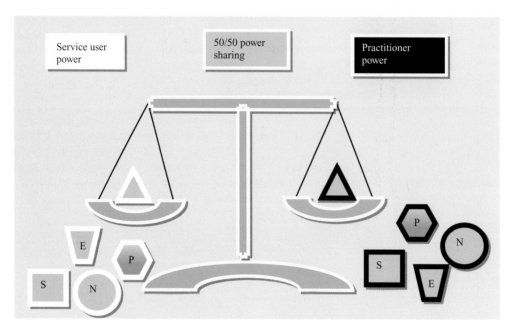

Figure 7.8   Balancing power during risk and decision-making using a range of reasoning styles.

with good knowledge of risk, empowerment and LTCs, who is able to effectively facilitate risk could, therefore, be argued to not only reduce risk, but to also enhance quality of life.

Acknowledgements

I would like to thank my colleague Dawn Suffolk, BSc (Hons) RM, RGN, for her case study contributions to this chapter.

References

Anderson, R. and Bury, M. (eds) (1988) *Living with Chronic Illness*. London: Unwin Hyman Ltd.

Arnstein, S. (1969) A ladder of citizen participation. *Journal of American Institute of Planners* **35** (4), 216.

Beason, C. (2005) The nurse as investor: using the strategies of Sarbanes-Osley corporate legislation to radically transform the work environment of nursing. *Nursing Administration* **Apr–Jun** (29), 171.

Beck, U. (1999) *World Risk Society*. Cambridge: Polity Press.

Bury, M. (1988) Meanings at risk: the experience of arthritis. In: R. Anderson and M. Bury (eds) *Living with Chronic Illness*. London: Unwin Hyman Ltd.

Busch, R. (2003) Empowering patients to direct their healthcare. *The Case Manager* **Nov–Dec** (14), 62.

Carr, S.M. (2004) A framework for understanding clinical reasoning in community nursing. *Journal of Clinical Nursing* **13** (7), 850–857.

Carson, D. and Bain, A. (2008) *Professional Risk and Working with People*. London: Jessica Kingsley.

Carter, M.A. and Robinson, S.S. (2001) A narrative approach to the clinical reasoning process in pediatric intensive care: the story of Matthew. *Journal of Medical Humanities* **22** (3), 173–194.

College of Occupational Therapists (2005) *Code of Ethics and Professional Conduct* [Green/White Paper]. London: College of Occupational Therapists.

Crowe, M. and Carlyle, D. (2003) Deconstructing risk assessment and management in mental health nursing. Journal of Advanced Nursing **43** (1), 19.

Daly, G. and Roebuck, A. (2008) Gaining independence: an evaluation of service user's accounts of the individual budgets pilot. *Journal of Integrated Care* **16** (3), 17-25.

Davidson, P., Digiacomo, M., Zecchin, R., Clarke, M., Paul, G., Lamb, K., Hancock, K., Chang, E. and Daly, J. (2008) A cardiac rehabilitation program to improve psychosocial outcomes of women with heart disease. *Journal of Women's Health (2002)* **17** (1), 123-134.

Department of Health (DH) (2009) *Long-term Health Conditions* [Green/White Paper]. London: DH.

Department of Health (DH) (2007) *Independence, Choice and Risk: A Guide to Best Practice in Supported Decision Making* [Green/White Paper] London: DH.

Flynn, R. (2008) Health and Risk. In: G. Mythen and S. Walklate (eds) *Beyond the Risk Society*. Berkshire, England: Open University Press.

Giddens, A. (1991) *Modernity and Self-Identity*. Cambridge: Policy Press.

Haynes, K. and Thomas, M. (eds) (2005) *Clinical Risk Management in Primary Care*. Oxon, UK: Radcliffe Publishing Ltd.

Higgs, J., Jones, M. A., Loftus, S., and Christensen, N. (eds) (2008) *Clinical Reasoning in the Health Professions*, 3rd edn. Amsterdam, Boston, Heidelberg, London: Elsevier Limited.

Kielhofner, G. (2008) *Model of Human Occupation: Theory and Application*, 4th edn. Baltimore, Philadelphia: Lippincott, Williams and Wilkins.

Laverack, G. (2005) *Public Health: Power, Empowerment and Professional Practice*. Basingstoke, UK and New York, USA: Palgrave Macmillan.

Lilley, R. and Lambden, P. (2005) *Making Sense of Risk Management: A Workbook for Primary Care*, 2nd edn. Oxon UK: Radcliffe Publishing Ltd.

Lorig, K., Holman, H., Sobel, D., Laurent, D., Gonzalez, V. and Minor, M. (2000) *Living a Healthy Life with Chronic Conditions*. Colorado USA: Bull Publishing Company.

Lupton, D. (2008) Sociology and risk. In: G. Mythen and S. Walklate (eds) *Beyond the Risk Society*. Berkshire, England: Open University Press.

Mattingly, C. and Hayes Fleming, M. (1994) *Clincial Reasoning: Forms of Inquiry in a Therapeutic Practice*. Philadelphia: F A Davis Company.

McCarthy, V. and Holbrook Freeman, L. (2008) A multidisciplinary concept of empowerment: implications for nursing. *Journal of Theory Construction and Testing* **12** (2), 68.

McGuigan, J. (2006) Culture and risk. In: G. Mythen and S. Walklate (eds) *Beyond the Risk Society*. Berkshire: Open University Press.

Moore, J., Ziebland, S. and Kennedy, S. (2002) People sometimes react funny if they're not told enough: women's views about the risks of diagnostic laparoscopy'. *Health Expectations: An International Journal of Public Participation in Health Care and Health Policy* **5** (4), 302-309.

Mythen, G. and Walklate, S. (eds) (2006) *Beyond the Risk Society*. Berkshire, England: Open University Press.

National Patient Safety Agency (2010) Available at: www.npsa.nhs.uk (Accessed 7 January 2010).

Nursing and Midwifery Council (2008) *The Code: Standards of Conduct, Performance and Ethics for Nurses and Midwives* [Green/White Paper]. London: Nursing and Midwifery Council.

Pinder, R. (1988) Striking balances: living with Parkinson's disease. In: R. Anderson and M. Bury (eds) *Living with Chronic Illness*. London: Unwin Hyman.

Ramcharan, P. (1997) *Empowerment in Everyday Life: Learning Disability*. London: Jessica Kingsley.

Rogers, J.C. (1983) Clinical reasoning: the ethics, science and art of reasoning. *American Journal of Occupational Therapy* **37** (9), 601-616.

Schein, E.H. (2010) *Organisational Culture and Leadership*, 4th edn. San Francisco: Jossey-Bass.

Sheaff, R. (2009) Medicine and management in English primary care: a shifting balance of power? *Journal of Social Policy* **38** (4), 627.

Taylor Gooby, P. (2008b) Assumptive worlds and images of agency: academic social policy in the twenty-first century. *Social Policy and Society* **7** (3), 269-280; 269.

Taylor Gooby, P. (2008a) Choice and values: individualised rational action and social goals. *Journal of Social Policy* **37** (2), 167-185.

Taylor, M.C. (2007) *Evidence Based Practice for Occupational Therapists*, 2nd edn. Oxford: Blackwell Science Ltd.

Trevena, L., Barratt, A. and McCaffery, K. (2008) Using decision aids to involve clients in clinical decision making. In: J. Higgs, M.A. Jones, S. Loftus and N. Christensen (eds) *Clinical Reasoning in The Health Professions*. Amsterdam, Boston, Heidelberg, London: Elsevier.

Walter, F.M. and Emery, J. (2005) Coming down the line - patients' understanding of their family history of common chronic disease. *Annals of Family Medicine* **3** (5), 405-414.

Walter, F.M., Emery, J., Braithwaite, D. and Marteau, T.M. (2004) Lay understanding of familial risk of common chronic diseases: a systematic review and synthesis of qualitative research. *Annals of Family Medicine* **2** (6), 583-594.

Waterlow, J. Pressure Ulcer Risk Assessment and Prevention. *The Waterlow Scale*. Available at: Judy-waterlow.co.uk (Accessed 10 January 2010).

Wilkinson, I. (2008) Psychology and risk. In: *Beyond the Risk Society*. Berkshire: Open University Press.

Further reading

Labonte, R. and Laverack, G. (2008) *Health Promotion in Action: From Local to Global Empowerment*. Hampshire: Palgrave Macmillan.

Lloyd, M. (2010) *A Practical Guide to Care Planning in Health and Social Care*. Berkshire: Open University Press.

Section 3

Care Management

Chapter 8

Care Coordination for Effective Long-term Condition Management

Sue Randall

Learning objectives

By the end of this chapter, the reader will be able to:

- Consider how long-term conditions (LTCs) are having an impact on healthcare not only in the United Kingdom, but also across the world.
- Have some knowledge about the effects of LTCs across a multicultural society.
- Consider how theoretical frameworks and service delivery models have been developed to enable healthcare professionals to care effectively for individuals with LTCs
- Have an understanding of care coordination as a key role of nurses in facilitating seamless care for the patients in their care, and how this impacts other healthcare professional roles
- Identify relevant resources for readers to explore through self-study.

Introduction

This chapter explores aspects of care coordination for individuals with LTCs. Although it considers demographic changes in terms of the growing number of elderly and the impact this is likely to have on the numbers of individuals with LTCs, there is also consideration that having an LTC is not simply the domain of the elderly. The transition of children into young adulthood and the movement from children's to adult services are also mentioned. The chapter examines some policy drivers, models for managing individuals with LTCs, and consider the patient journey and integrated care pathways. The impact of services such as intermediate care and community matron services will also be examined in relation to care coordination.

Long-term Conditions: A Guide for Nurses and Healthcare Professionals, First Edition. Edited by S. Randall and H. Ford.
© 2011 Blackwell Publishing Ltd. Published 2011 by Blackwell Publishing Ltd.

Population contexts in England, Scotland, Wales and Northern Ireland in relation to LTCs

An LTC can affect an individual at any age. Some people are born with conditions which will last a lifetime, for example cystic fibrosis. Others may develop conditions at a young age, such as asthma. A condition such as multiple sclerosis (MS) typically affects those aged between 20 and 40 at diagnosis. As a natural part of ageing, when cells are not able to replicate themselves, a large percentage of individuals start to develop LTCs. With LTCs affecting almost every age group, the task for healthcare professionals to meet individual's specific needs is big. Effective coordination is one part of helping individuals with an LTC to live their lives. The changing population will have an impact on the way healthcare professionals work in the future.

The effective management of chronic conditions is the greatest challenge facing healthcare systems in the 21st century (WHO 2002). As reported elsewhere, the population of those over 75 in England will be 8.2 million by 2031 (DH 2008a). As health policy is different across all areas of the United Kingdom, it is necessary to assess the implications for Wales, Scotland and Northern Ireland too. In Wales, the older population is expected to grow by 11% by 2020, with another estimate that 75% of those over 75 experiencing at least one LTC, with 78% of all health service expenditure connected to LTCs (Welsh Assembly Government 2007). In Scotland, there are 2 million individuals with an LTC, with the LTCs collaborative programme highlighting Chronic Obstructive Pulmonary Disease (COPD), asthma, diabetes, and coronary heart disease as requiring particular attention (Scottish Government 2009). The Scottish Government have introduced a national indicator to highlight individuals over the age of 65 who are admitted as emergencies two or more times per year. It should be noted that admittance as an emergency may be the result of a fall and non-LTC related, although fractures may be the result of osteoporosis. This indicator reflects the priority of improving the health of over 65s in addition to more proactive care and managing conditions in the community (Scottish Government 2009). In Northern Ireland, it is projected that the over-65 population will total 350, 000 by 2023 compared to 266, 000 in 2002 (Department of Health, Social Services and Public Safety: DHSSPS 2005).

Black and minority ethnic (BME) populations and LTC risk

As an increasingly multicultural society, the United Kingdom health services need to be able to effectively coordinate care for individuals for whom English may not be the first language, or who may not read, write or understand English at all other than through family members or interpreting services. Thorne (2008) notes the importance of culture as a powerful factor in establishing values, beliefs, expectations and attitudes to illness. The UK census of 2001 (ONS 2006) recorded individuals over the age of 65 within the groups shown in Table 8.1.

The health needs of individuals from minority ethnic groups vary too from those of the indigenous population. According to Diabetes UK (www.diabetes.org.uk), the prevalence of diabetes in the white indigenous population is around 2.4%, whilst in some BME groups, this figure can be three to five times higher. Consider the following:

- Diabetes risk is six times greater for South Asian populations than Europeans.
- Diabetes risk is three times more likely for Black African and African-Caribbean populations (DH 2001a).

Table 8.1 Percentage of individuals over 65 per ethnic group.

Black Caribbean	11%
Black African	2%
Indian	7%
Pakistani	4%
Bangladeshi	3%
Chinese	5%

Source: 2001 census.

There is a strong association between diabetes and the development of renal disease. South Asian and African-Caribbean populations have a three times greater risk of developing renal failure than their White counterparts (Fehally 2003). Similarly, there is a strong correlation between Type 2 diabetes and coronary heart disease in Black African, African-Caribbean and South Asians, although a 2004 study found that despite a high prevalence of diabetes, stroke, hypertension and end stage renal disease among UK born African people, lower coronary heart disease mortality was noted (Abbots et al. 2004).

Coronary heart disease (CHD) alone is known to be a cause of very high mortality, particularly in individuals of South Asian origin, with levels reaching 50% higher than the general population (Bhopal 2000). Mortality from CHD is dominant in all BME groups in the United Kingdom (Gill et al. 2004), although to a lesser extent amongst Chinese and Caribbean groups. Death from stroke is much higher in African-Caribbean population than other ethnic groups (Gill et al. 2004).

Although deaths from cancer are lower in the BME population, deaths from nasopharyngeal and liver cancers are higher:

- Caribbean migrants have three to five times higher rates of liver cancer than that of individuals born in the United Kingdom.
- Mortality from mouth cancers is five to ten times higher in East African groups who are now resident in the United Kingdom compared to rates in England and Wales
  Grulich et al. 1992

Being aware of the health needs of minority ethnic populations, and potential barriers to them accessing services such as religious and cultural beliefs and language barriers will assist the health-care professional to coordinate care, by providing non-discriminatory practice with improved health outcomes.

Summary

In summary then, all four countries in the United Kingdom face a challenge from a growing elderly population, which respective governments in England, Scotland, Wales and Northern Ireland are tackling via various policy initiatives. Consideration has then been given to minority ethnic populations, whose risk factors for certain LTCs are high. Care and treatment for all needs to be culturally sensitive and delivered according to the individual's wishes.

Section 3

Having considered the population context, the chapter now explores care coordination in more detail.

Care coordination

In a systematic review of mainly American literature around care coordination, the Agency for Health Care Research and Quality (AHRQ: 2007) found 40 definitions of care coordination, and having reviewed these, produced their own:

> Care coordination is the deliberate organisation of patient care activities between 2 or more participants in a patient's care to facilitate the appropriate delivery of health care services. Organising care involves the marshalling of personnel & other resources needed to carry out all the required patient care activities and is often managed by the exchange of information among parties responsible for different aspects of care.
> *Source*: (AHRQ 2007: v)

Through the systematic review, AHRQ found five common elements of care coordination. These are:

1. Several agencies, including patients are usually involved.
2. Care coordination is necessary when agencies are dependent on each other to carry out different activities in a patient's care.
3. For these activities to be carried out effectively and in a coordinated way, each participant needs adequate knowledge about their role and role of others and available resources.
4. In order to manage all required patient care activities, agencies rely on two-way communication of information.
5. Integration of care has the goal of facilitating appropriate delivery of healthcare services without undue repetition.

The case studies later in the chapter highlight the complexities of care coordination. It is not uncommon for care to be poorly coordinated and for communication to breakdown between parties. Suggested ways of improving care coordination are as follows:

● Identification and assessment of the need for coordination of services, as without effective assessment opportunities could be missed in meeting the needs of individuals with LTCs, or conversely duplication may occur.
● Role identification of those individuals/agencies involved must be defined; care should be planned with goals set and with review dates; communication should be effective - through face-to-face, electronic or telephone means.
● Coordination should be implemented with a key worker to ensure continuity, such as community matron; coordination should be evaluated to establish strengths and barriers.

Individuals who may coordinate care are shown in Figure 8.1.
Care coordination can occur across a time continuum. For example, discharge from an acute ward might mean a discharge package being implemented within a relatively short period of time,

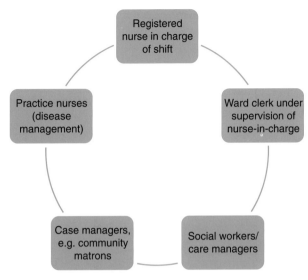

Figure 8.1   Individuals who may coordinate care.

where services need to be restarted rather than a new package organised. In the community, care coordination may take place over a period of weeks, months or years as relationships between healthcare staff and patients are often for longer terms.

Figure 8.2 shows where coordination can occur.

In Case study 8.1, there are examples of coordination within teams, for example community matron and district nursing; between community and acute settings, for example between community matron and consultant cardiologist; and lastly between and also across teams in different agencies, for example health and social care agencies.

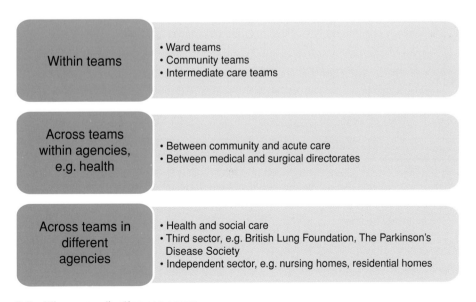

Figure 8.2   Where coordination can occur.

Case study 8.1 David Smith

Mr David Smith (name has been changed to maintain confidentiality) was referred to the community matron service by a fax message from the patient's General Practitioner (GP). David had a number of co-morbidities, and his wife was struggling to care for him. His medical condition was complex and unstable, and was the main reason for his frequent, unplanned admissions into hospital. Mr Smith's co-morbidities were:

- Diabetes (insulin dependent)
- Diabetic retinopathy
- Essential hypertension
- Chronic kidney disease stage 4
- Left ventricular failure
- Ischaemic heart disease
- Prostate cancer

A phone call to Mr Smith was made and an appointment was arranged next day with David being informed of the nature and purpose of the community matron visit. A full physical assessment was undertaken, and an assessment of current provision of services and areas of concern for David and his wife was made. It transpired that when David was unwell, his wife would dial 999 automatically as it gave her a sense of security.

The community matron planned weekly visits to monitor David's physical health needs and liaise with the GP and cardiology consultant about possible changes in management plans.

In addition, as David's diabetes was particularly unstable, which had an effect on his kidney function, with the agreement of Mr Smith he was referred to the community renal and diabetic team for a review of his condition.

There were minimal aids and adaptations in the home which could assist Mr Smith in maintaining his independence. A referral was made, therefore, to the community occupational therapist department to assess Mr Smith for further bathing aids, as he had only a bath seat which the carers were finding difficult to position Mr Smith safely on. Further, grab rails were required in the bathroom. Mr Smith would benefit from a backrest to support him sitting upright in bed to improve his lung expansion at night and a commode for easy access to the toilet downstairs as a bucket was used to improvise for a toilet.

A referral was made to the benefit advice team to review Mr Smith's benefits as he was in receipt of the attendance allowance but could be entitled to other benefits that might pay for some of his care.

A request was made to social services for a review of his package of care with the view to it being increased that included respite care that will give Mrs Smith a break from the caring role, a key pad safe that will enable carers to gain access to his home and someone to sit with David during the day once a week so that his wife can go shopping.

The district nursing team was already visiting weekly to administer injections as Mr Smith was finding it increasingly difficult to attend his surgery due to his co-morbidities. The district nurse had called to administer the above medication, but since neither David nor his wife heard the doorbell she left a note requesting that David get in touch with the service. Mrs Smith was having difficulty getting in touch with the district nursing messaging service as the telephone lines were engaged. The community matron was able to make a telephone call to the district nurse team responsible for his care, thus taking this pressure off Mrs Smith and allowing her husband to get his treatment. The installation of a key safe would prevent this situation happening again.

On assessment of Mr Smith's toes, it was found that his feet had not been treated by a chiropodist that year, as his co-morbidities made it difficult for him to travel in a taxi to attend his appointment. A request was made to the community chiropodist for David for his feet to be assessed and treated in his home.

It was important that Mr Smith's care package was assessed as soon as possible so that Mrs Smith felt supported in caring for her husband as there was a real risk of him being admitted into hospital due to the family support breaking down. Following a detailed discussion on the phone to the duty officer at the local social services department, a visit by a social worker was arranged within a week. All other referrals mentioned above were made and a referral form was sent by fax, which was followed up by a phone call to confirm that the recipient agencies had received the referral to assess Mr Smith. The plan was also communicated to the GP by fax for inclusion in Mr Smith's notes.

The package of care set-up increased the number of visits by home care staff from one visit a day to three visits daily. The aim of the increased support was to provide sustenance to the home by visiting at lunchtime to assist with preparing a light lunch and help in getting Mr Smith into bed at night. David and his wife made the decision to pay for a carer privately to visit weekly to sit with him so that Mrs Smith can go shopping or visit a friend for a couple of hours. The carer was employed by the care agency already in place but the care was paid for by David. Amongst her duties was to carry out light household chores and read to David from some of his favourite novels as he had enjoyed reading for many hours before his eyesight had deteriorated as a result of his diabetes.

On receipt of the referral form and a phone call to the diabetic and renal community team, a diabetic specialist nurse visited Mr Smith with a dietician to assess and review his condition. The occupational therapist had carried out an initial assessment within two weeks of the referral to the service, and had made arrangements for the necessary aids and adaptations to be put in place. The chiropodist made contact with Mr Smith and offered an appointment within a six-week time frame. The above services are still visiting Mr Smith. The community matron remains the single point of contact and case manager, in order to identify when further changes may be needed in Mr Smith's health or social care management plan. Currently, there is a reduction in unplanned admissions since case management was started.

Points for reflection

- How has life changed for Mr and Mrs Smith since the introduction of case management?
- What skills has the community matron shown in managing Mr Smith's case?
- How could personal budgets help Mr and Mrs Smith?
- Consider the time required to coordinate the care of Mr Smith.
- What means of communication have been used by the community matron to ensure that David's care is effectively coordinated?

Section 3

The chapter now considers the patient's journey across the health system, and how effective coordination of that journey is vital for the patient's quality of life.

Patient journey

For individuals with LTCs, services often fall down across boundaries, for example between primary (community) services and secondary (acute) care and vice versa (Edwards 2008). Current services are fragmented, accessed in any number of ways, ad hoc and often resulting in unnecessary hospital attendances (Metcalfe 2005). A suggestion for improving chronic care management is that the patient remains fully at the centre of all care decisions so that experiences are positive and consider their needs, values and preferences as patients (WHO 2005). Care needs to be coordinated, and with ease of access to services which are local, integrated and consistent. It has been noted that despite the growth in individuals with chronic disease, the education of healthcare professionals has failed to keep pace with the complex care needs of individuals with LTCs (WHO 2005). The ability to treat patients with single disease processes is routine, but preparation for coordinating care and educating patients is inadequate (Partnerships for Solutions 2002). Further discussion of this accompanies the National Service Framework (NSF) section below.

In Case study 8.2, Mrs Paul's journey from hospital to home, and back to another hospital and finally to a hospice shows the complex nature of the patient journey, as experienced by one individual with multiple co-morbidities. The care coordinator in this case is a community matron, whose role will be discussed in more detail later in the chapter.

Case study 8.2 Cynthia Paul

Cynthia Paul is a 76-year-old African-Caribbean female (all names have been changed to protect the patient and their family's confidentiality). The named patient was referred to the community matron service by the Community Rheumatoid Arthritis Nurse Consultant. The referral form stated that Mrs Paul has had three unplanned admissions into hospital in the past month.

The referrer was concerned that Mrs Paul had possibly reached the end stage of her disease process, and therefore required sequenced and coordinated care at home. Mrs Paul's suffered from a number of co-morbidities:

- Hypertension
- Chronic kidney disease stage 4
- Atrial fibrillation
- Rheumatoid arthritis
- Malignant neoplasm of the left breast (a total mastectomy had been carried out)
- Diabetes mellitus Type 2
- Crohn's disease
- Heart failure

On receiving the referral, the family were contacted about an appointment, but the community matron was informed that Mrs Paul had been readmitted to hospital. Contact was made with the hospital ward to liaise with the community matron about discharge plans for Mrs Paul.

On discharge, the community matron visited, meeting Mrs Paul, her husband and niece. Mrs Paul's husband was her sole carer supporting Mrs Paul with personal hygiene needs, cooked meals, and carried out household duties. A privately paid cleaner visited once weekly to assist with household duties. There were minimal aids and adaptations in the home which consisted of grab rails in the shower and bathroom and a stair rail from the bedroom to the lower floor.

A top-to-toe physical examination was carried out. At this visit, it became clear that Mrs Paul had numerous appointments to attend at different clinics, which was a big worry to Mr and Mrs Paul, as she was not well enough to attend:

- 2 week review by GP
- Weekly visit to the warfarin clinic
- 2 week review at the community rheumatoid nurse clinic
- Monthly visit to diabetic clinic at a local hospital
- 6 weekly appointments at the renal unit of another hospital

The outcome of the community matron's first assessment was:

- To effectively coordinate Mrs Paul's care by working with the GP, hospital consultant, renal outreach nurse and any other service that the matron deemed was required to improve Mrs Paul's quality of life.
- To support Mr Paul in caring for his wife at home, the matron took Mr Paul onto the caseload as he too had multiple co-morbidities.
- To note her most recent blood sample results taken and note any changes that may be present from previous results.
- To arrange a case conference with Mrs Paul's family present and inviting various agencies that the matron felt would be able to offer assistance in improving Mrs Paul's quality of life at home and a coordinated management plan.

A case conference was arranged at the hospital. Those in attendance were Mr and Mrs Paul, Mrs Paul's niece, the renal consultant, two renal outreach nurses, a social worker and the matron. Apologies were given by community nursing team and the community occupational therapist.

The outcome of the case conference and the management plan for Mrs Paul was as follows:

- It was acknowledged that Mrs Paul was in the end stage disease process of her heart failure and renal function. As a result of this, she will be treated conservatively rather than being treated by renal dialysis.
- A management plan will be put in place to manage Mrs Paul's increasing breathlessness, which involves titrating her diuretic medication which the community matron will review.
- The social worker was asked to make a referral to the occupational therapist to assess for further aids and adaptation in the home that will maintain Mrs Paul's independence and improve her quality of life. An assessment will be made to put a package of care in place that included offering Mrs Paul assistance with personal hygiene and a sitting service in the evening so that Mr Paul can have a break from caring. The private carer Mrs Paul had in place would be asked to assist with meals and ironing alongside her cleaning duties as she was more than capable of carrying out these additional chores.

Section 3

- A concern was raised by the community matron regarding the frequent visits to various clinics that Mrs Paul attended. During the discussion, it was suggested that Mrs Paul be referred to the community diabetic and renal specialist team headed by a consultant, which would reduce the need for her to attend a clinic at her GP surgery.
- The community matron would refer Mrs Paul to the domiciliary wafarin clinic, for blood to be taken at home.
- The district nurses would be asked to visit Mrs Paul at home to administer injections weekly rather than Mrs Paul attending the GP surgery to have the medication administered.
- The community matron would visit twice weekly to monitor Mrs Paul's condition and coordinate her care.

On return from the case conference, referrals were made to the warfarin domiciliary team, and the diabetic/renal specialist team in the community with support letters. A follow-up telephone call was made to each discipline to discuss Mrs Paul's case further and to improve communication between the services.

Equipment Loans was contacted by the matron to order a backrest for Mrs Paul which would assist Mrs Paul remaining up right in bed and becoming less breathless, as a hospital bed was declined following a discussion with Mr and Mrs Paul.

The community matron had been informed that Social Services would be putting in a package of care as a matter of urgency but there had been no assessment made by Social Services. Two letters were written by the matron for these services to be established.

Despite an initial stabilisation in Mrs Paul's condition, a routine visit by the community matron found Mrs Paul's condition had deteriorated. Following a discussion with the specialist renal nurse and the consultant, Mrs Paul's diuretic medication was increased with the view of arranging a planned admission to the hospital for a review by the consultant. This admission, though planned, resulted in Mrs Paul being taken to the hospital dealing with emergencies rather than the renal unit, as the ambulance staff were very concerned when they collected Mrs Paul. She was admitted.

Discussions took place, initiated by the community matron, with the staff and medical teams, including the renal team at the other hospital about future management and end-of-life care. In discussion with Mrs Paul's family, she was moved to a hospice having been placed on the Supported Care Pathway (end of life). Mrs Paul passed away peacefully, surrounded by her family and friends. Mrs Paul's family asked for the community matron to be mentioned by name at the funeral service.

In closing, Mrs Paul's and her family's quality of life was improved by the timely assessment, suitable referrals to other agencies, and coordination and monitoring of the community matron service.

Points for reflection

- Is the role of the community matron useful?
- Who is it useful for? Consider patients, families and professionals.
- Why is it helpful to those groups you have identified?
- What might the consequences be for patients and their families and other professionals without the community matron as single point of contact?

Section 3

Table 8.2 Hours spent caring.

Hours spent caring	Percentage of carers (%)
19 hours or less/week	68
20–49 hours/week	11
50 + hours/week	21

Consideration of the effect of caring on family members who care is also key and effective coordination will assist the whole family unit. This chapter continues by considering the needs of carers.

Family carers

Case study 8.1 highlights some of the issues which are pertinent for healthcare professionals to consider in terms of carer's needs. The 2001 census reported that there are 5.67 million carers in Great Britain. Of those, 5.2 million are in England and Wales (ONS 2006) and 500, 000 in Scotland (online census results). Female carers make up 58% and male carers, the remaining 42%. The hours of caring range as follows (see Table 8.2):

Recognition of the key role played by carers has been acknowledged. In 1994, The Carers (Recognition and Services) Act (Great Britain Parliament 1994) set out new rights and a clear legal status for carers. The inclusion of an assessment of their ability to care and to continue caring was to be made available at the time the patient is being assessed for community care services. This was followed in 2004 by The Carers (Equal Opportunities) Act (Great Britain Parliament 2004), which brought in the following three main changes:

1. Duty on councils to inform carers in certain circumstances of their right to assessment of needs.
2. When assessing a carer's needs, councils must take into account whether the carer works or wishes to work.
3. A facilitated cooperation between authorities in relation to the provision of services that are relevant to carers.

Latterly, there has been the publication of The Carers Strategy (DH 2008b): carers at the heart of 21st century family and community, and followed up by the Commission on Carers 2007–2009 (DH 2009b). This is a 10-year cross government strategy which aims to ensure that carers have increased choice and control, and are empowered to have a life outside caring. The key messages are:

● Carers will be respected as expert care partners and will have access to the integrated and personalised services they need to support them in their caring role.
● Carers will be able to have a life of their own alongside their caring role.
● Carers will be supported so that they are not forced into financial hardship by their caring role.
● Carers will be supported to stay mentally and physically well and treated with dignity. Case study 8.1 shows how support for Mr and Mrs Smith allowed Mrs Smith to go shopping, thus receiving a break from her caring role.
● Children and young people will be protected from inappropriate caring, and have the support they need to learn, develop and thrive, to enjoy positive childhood and to achieve against 'Every Child Matters' outcomes.

Section 3

The rationale around strengthening support for carers can be seen in various literature themes. An individual's physical and psychological well-being can be improved by cohesive family relationships (Frude 2010). Illness is considered a family affair by Wright and Leahey (2000), so that the family can be influenced by an illness or can themselves influence the illness and suffering of the individual in a positive manner. Such influence is recognised in the NSF for Long-term Conditions (DH 2005) and The Carers Act (Great Britain Parliament 2004). The latter acknowledges that informal carers are at risk of burnout, hence the requirement that carers have their own assessment. That healthcare professionals are aware of this is key in signposting carers to help and in assisting them to gain coordinated care, which can benefit the individual with an LTC and the carer.

Although carers can derive considerable satisfaction from their caring role (Brennan 2004) through realising the positive contribution they make, there is also evidence which highlights that extended caring can negatively impact the physical and emotional well-being of carers (Pinquart and Sorrenson 2003). Aitken (2009) suggests that carers are determined to keep promises made to patients, but if a situation becomes unmanageable, they often feel extreme guilt. Again, the impact of such circumstances should be understood by healthcare professionals, who through their professional role of ensuring ongoing physical, emotional and practical support, can assist both patient and carer. The closeness of the relationship between patient and carer is a factor in determining the level of stress experienced by a carer (Brennan 2004), whilst in giving emotional support to their loved ones, carers are also coping with anticipated loss (Zapart et al. 2007).

Healthcare professionals have a key role to play in coordinating not only the patient journey, but also the carer's journey to ensure optimal physical and mental well-being for both parties. Part of this may involve communicating clearly. Identifying ways of sharing information with carers without breaking patient confidentiality could improve the lives of all concerned and improve the quality of healthcare (DH 2009b). An example of good practice is the Partners in Care campaign, a joint initiative between the Royal College of Psychiatrists and the Princess Royal Trust for Carers. This collaboration produced a leaflet (available at: www.rcpsych.ac.uk/systempages/gsearch.aspx?cx= 001100616363437152483%3aidnunflyavs&cof=FORID%3a9&q=partners+in+care+campaign) giving guidelines surrounding issues of confidentiality and carers.

The role of carers in managing individuals with LTCs is an important one and care coordination by healthcare professionals will be as important for the carers as it is for patients themselves.

Summary

This section has considered factors which make up care coordination, professionals who can be involved, and areas where coordination can breakdown. Case study 8.1 has highlighted how complex care coordination can be for an individual with several LTCs, and the advantages of one individual (here, the community matron) being responsible for effective coordination to ensure the best outcome for the patient and their families, and that all professionals are aware of what is going on. The importance of the patient journey, which essentially is the patient's life, is also considered in terms of coordinating care across system boundaries. The importance of involving carers in decisions and being aware of carer's needs is also highlighted.

This chapter continues by considering frameworks of care delivery.

Section 3

Frameworks of care delivery

NSFs and their impact on care

The introduction of NSFs for single conditions has been going on in England since the late 1990s (DH 2000a, 2000b, 2001a, 2001b). Although such initiatives have proved effective for individuals with a single disease, criticisms point to a deficiency for those individuals who suffer co-morbidities (more than one LTC) and those who have a single disease process which does not have its own NSF (Metcalfe 2005). For those individuals who do not 'fit' there is often fragmentation of care, commonly resulting in an acute admission (DH 2005b). As a result, the NSF for Long-term Conditions, published in 2005 (DH 2005a) is seen as a more generic document. Although it is written for neurological conditions, the principles for care and treatment are intended to guide care for anyone with an LTC. The principles or quality requirements are shown in Table 8.3.

Policy is often considered a 'dry subject', but as it directly influences healthcare organisations and ultimately patients it is worth reading. Documents such as the NSFs are available on the government websites (see 'Further reading') and can be accessed as executive summaries, which are shortened versions containing the key points. As such, they are a 'friendly' way to access current information. With change in the UK government in 2010, there are likely to be changes to the aspects of health policy in the future.

Despite policy drivers such as the NSFs, there is no single recommended model for all LTCs (Lewis and Dixon 2004). To consider this statement in greater detail, some models in LTCs will now be examined.

Table 8.3   NSF long-term conditions. 2005a

Quality requirements (QR)	
QR1	A person-centred service
QR2	Early recognition and diagnosis
QR3	Emergency and acute management
QR4	Early and specialist rehabilitation
QR5	Community rehabilitation and support
QR6	Vocational rehabilitation
QR7	Providing equipment and accommodation
QR8	Providing personal care and support
QR9	Palliative care
QR10	Supporting family and carers
QR11	Caring for people with neurological conditions

Source: DH 2005a.

Wagner's chronic care model (1998)

This model, developed by Wagner and colleagues in the United States of America (USA) in 1998, has become influential and elements of it can be seen in many models from other countries across the world (see Figure 8.3). In acknowledging that a major percentage of chronic care takes place outside

Section 3

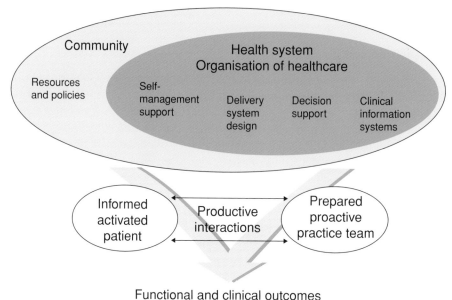

Functional and clinical outcomes

Figure 8.3 Wagner 1998. (Reproduced with kind permission of American College of Physicians: Effective Clinical Practice.)

formal healthcare settings, this model's principal aim is to provide a link between informed, active individuals who have an LTC and proactive teams of professionals.

The key principles of the model are:

- Mobilising community resources to meet the needs of individuals with LTCs.
- Creating a culture, organisation and mechanisms that promote safe, high quality care.
- Empowering and preparing people to manage their health and healthcare.
- Delivering effective, efficient care and self-management support.
- Promoting care that is consistent with research evidence and patient preference.
- Organising patient and population data to facilitate efficient and effective care.
  Source: Wagner 1998

From these principles alone, it can be seen where policy initiatives in the United Kingdom have their roots. In Lord Darzi's paper (DH 2008a), self-management is seen as a cornerstone of LTC policy (see Chapter 5 in this book), and 'patient-centred care' is a term which occurs frequently in policy. With the change in government and the new White Paper (DH 2010), the theme of patients at the heart of the NHS remains. In the United Kingdom, this requires a significant shift in the way care is delivered from a reactive, crisis led approach where individuals who have vastly differing needs have to fit into the system towards a community-based, responsive, adaptable and flexible service. In order to meet this vision set out in the White Paper 'Our Health, Our Care, Our Say' (DH 2006a), a significant whole systems change is needed. This will have implications for the workforce, which will be discussed later in this chapter.

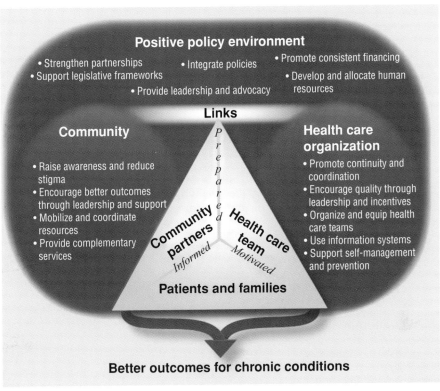

Figure 8.4   The innovative care for chronic conditions model. (Reproduced with kind permission of the WHO.)

Innovative care for chronic conditions model (World Health Organisation (WHO) 2002)

Healthcare comprises a series of systems, which are imbedded within other broader systems (Plsek and Greenhalgh 2001). The focus of this model (see Figure 8.4) is on improving care at three levels:

- Micro
- Meso
- Macro

At the micro level, patients, families, community partners, and healthcare professionals are involved. The WHO state that positive outcomes are achieved as a result of professionals being informed, motivated and working together i.e. coordination of care to benefit individuals. The micro level is supported by the meso level which comprises healthcare organisations and communities and the meso level in turn influences the macro level, but is also impacted on by the macro level which comprises policy (WHO 2002). This shows that information and actions are a two-way process, whereby issues on the ground are passed up in order to effect positive changes, but also information may be passed from government and organisational levels to be implemented on the ground.

Section 3

Essential elements for the policy environment, as shown in the Innovative Care for Chronic Conditions model, include the following:

- Leadership and advocacy.
- Integrated policies that span different disease types and prevention strategies.
- Consistent financing.
- Developing human resources.
- Legislative framework.
- Partnership working.

Arguably, health services are affected by economic climates and funding available, so the next few years are likely to be testing in health and social care, but providing effective healthcare may need to be more than 'throwing money at a problem'. Changing attitudes and ways of working may be as effective, thus requiring clear leadership and effective management as a means of keeping patients with LTCs at the heart of care. Without patients, nurses have no profession, role or even job, but nurses need to have the ability to adapt and work flexibly to ensure a new way of managing individuals with LTCs. These frameworks are ways of showing the bigger picture, all of which affect the micro level in which many health professionals and their patients coexist.

The public health model (2002)

This lesser known framework from the USA considers a broader approach to the issues surrounding LTCs. This model can be seen in a pictorial form by following the link to Singh and Ham in section 'Further reading'. It suggests the following three levels of intervention required to impact on the growing size of LTC issues:

- Population wide policies.
- Community involvement.
- Health services which include ongoing and preventative care.
  Source: Singh and Ham 2005

In English policy, the introduction of Choosing Health (DH 2004a) was a significant change in policy direction which attempted to raise the awareness of individual responsibility in managing lifestyle as a means of reducing some long-term conditions: smoking and links to COPD, sexual health (safe sex) and links to Chlamydia and possible future infertility, and alcohol (excess consumption and binge drinking) and liver diseases to name but a few.

The continuity of care model

This model of the early 1990s (see Figure 8.5) takes a linear view of health through the continuum of disease to end of life. In this respect, it may be considered easy to understand the concepts, which consider risk and suitable points at which healthcare may intervene. These are:

- Prevention
- Treatment
- Rehabilitation
- Palliative care

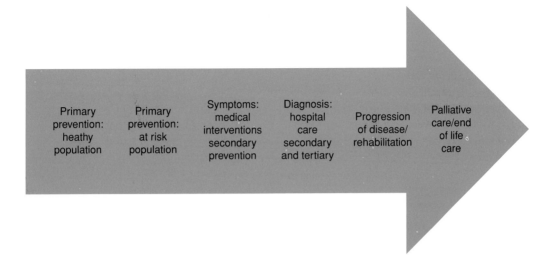

Figure 8.5   The continuity of care model.

These are all key elements within the management of LTCs and are considered to a greater or lesser extent within this text.

In a review of the effectiveness of these frameworks, Singh and Ham (2005) found limited effectiveness, although this was more often due to a lack of evaluation rather than the frameworks being known to be ineffectual. A common sense appraisal that considers the elements which are incorporated within the frameworks would suggest that the integration of biological, social, cultural, psychological and systems as well as individual influences on health are likely to be effective, although the issue of integration itself of so many elements may prove complex.

Summary

The broad frameworks consider the 'bigger picture' and how many elements need to come together to ensure that the desired outcome is effective. These broad frameworks have been reworked into service delivery models, which in essence move the theoretical frameworks into a workable model which is useful in everyday practice. The reader may be more familiar with the service delivery models, which include Kaiser, Evercare, Pfizer, and Castlefields.

The chapter moves on to consider service delivery models in more detail. This understanding should illuminate how and why services are delivered in the way that they are in order to benefit patients with LTCs.

Service delivery models

Three of the commonly cited models are Kaiser, Evercare and Pfizer which are all healthcare provider companies in the USA. Unsurprisingly, demographic changes of a similar nature to those experienced in the United Kingdom are apparent in America and these three companies undertook work to consider

Section 3

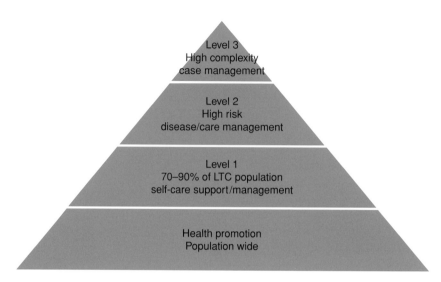

Figure 8.6   Kaiser Permanente triangle.

ways of effectively managing the growing burden of disease associated with chronic conditions (Metcalfe 2005).

There are similar characteristics in all three, but the biggest difference is in the targeted population. The Kaiser model works with the whole population, whilst Evercare and Pfizer concentrate on those who are most at risk of admission to hospital and who have the most complex health needs. This is widely shown in a diagrammatic fashion, known as the Kaiser triangle (see Figure 8.6). The whole triangle represents the Kaiser model, whilst level three is where Pfizer and Evercare efforts are concentrated. The approach of Kaiser is based on the Chronic Care Model and is concerned with working across primary and secondary care, where budgets are shared and the journey is seamless for the patient with an LTC. Although attempts have been made to introduce Kaiser in the United Kingdom and many health trusts report doing so, differences in the financial set-up of the NHS arguably prevent working to its optimum potential here. Proposed changes in the latest White Paper (DH, 2010) could have a profound effect on the way the NHS in England is run, with the potential to reduce the financial barriers to a seamless service. This may also be considered in the light of the WHO (2002) framework of the Innovative Care model where they consider consistent financing and macro level such as policy as important factors in the overall management of LTCs. It has been cited as the reason for success of the Kaiser model in the USA, that rather than in thinking and working in terms of primary and secondary care they think in terms of chronic disease as the important and major factor and care is integrated accordingly (Ham 2005).

Table 8.4, adapted from Singh (2005), gives a comparison of the key features of the three service delivery models:

The Castlefields model

One further model is the Castlefields model (also known as Unique), which was developed by a practice in the North West of England, with an overall aim of case managing those at highest risk. Criteria included disease severity and risk of admission to hospital. Key workers were nurses working closely with social workers. The approach was around practice-based management, using

Section 3

Table 8.4   Comparison of key features of three service delivery models.

	Kaiser	Evercare	Pfizer
Overall principles	With a focus on integration, this model uses a wide range of strategies to work across primary and secondary care	Uses specialist nurses to work with those individuals who are most at risk of admission as a result of co-morbidities	Uses telephone contact to support and refer individuals who are most at risk of readmission.
Underlying principles	Unplanned admissions to hospital are seen as a failure of the system Care is given in response to individual needs Boundaries do not exist between primary and secondary care Partnership in care is essential with patients as equal partners Patients can provide their own care. Information is a fundamental requirement. Commitment and a shared vision lead to improvements in care: there is no room for coercion	Whole person approach which is individualised Care provided in the least invasive way and in the least intensive place -Primary care leads all care -Decisions are based around population data Consideration is given to adverse effects of medication and polypharmacy	-Proactive contact with high risk patients who are assessed, referred, educated and monitored. -The service is supplementary to existing services. -Self-treatment and behaviour change are encouraged.
Key actions			
Education	Education, including Internet use during hospital stays	Tailor-made education Mentorship Promotion of self-care	-Patient education supported by telephone
Target	Whole remit of care Targeted risk assessment	Using an 'assessment tool' to identify high risk individuals	-Identifying high risk patients
Care planning	Proactive management across the care spectrum Reduction of inappropriate referrals by integrated care	Proactive management in high risk patients Tailor-made care plan Medicines management	-Case finding -Assessment of patients -Proactive management of high risk patients
Staff	Partnership development between managers and clinicians High percentage of doctors in leadership positions	Specialist nurses using case management GPs extending roles to work closely with nurses	-Dedicated telephone support offered by nurses

(Continued)

Section 3

Table 8.4 (Continued).

	Kaiser	Evercare	Pfizer
	Changing place of work: GPs in A&E; consultants in GP clinics		
	Dedicated multidisciplinary rounds		
Tools	Information systems which offer reminders on patient notes	Risk assessment of IT	-Local and national guidelines incorporated into telephone software
		Sharing information across systems to improve care	
	Clinical evidence base		
Discharge	Discharge summaries available online	Single point of contact	
	Dedicated discharge planning staff (ratio1:25)		

Adapted from Singh (2005)

tailor-made holistic care plans and with a multidisciplinary approach to medicines management. All aspects spanned primary and secondary care (Lewis 2008).

Evaluation of the Evercare model in the USA demonstrated a 50% reduction in admissions to acute facilities, without detriment to health (DH 2004b). With similar outcomes noted by Kaiser, several pilot sites were set up around all three of the service delivery models (Evercare, Pfizer and Kaiser) within the United Kingdom. The evaluation of the nine Evercare sites found the following:

- Vulnerable people were effectively identified.
- It helped to provide preventative healthcare.
- Showed the potential to organise care around peoples' needs.
  Source: Boaden et al. 2005

The evaluation also highlighted that finding unmet need had the potential to increase demand for health services (Boaden et al. 2005). Nine trusts piloted the Kaiser model and one, Pfizer's telephone support system (Singh and Ham 2005).

What is clear is that many trusts have employed a variety of approaches drawing on all three service delivery models, with integration of services as well as the role of community matron and the use of case management. These are examined in more depth later in the chapter. This mixture of approaches may be representative of the NHS and Social Care Model (DH 2005b).

The NHS health and social care model

In 2005, the Government introduced the Health and Social Care Model (DH 2005b). Closer inspection reveals that it has key elements of many of the broad frameworks and service delivery models already discussed. The delivery system (middle section) is a representation of the Kaiser triangle (see Figure 8.7). The model outlines how individuals with LTCs will be identified and have their needs met.

Section 3

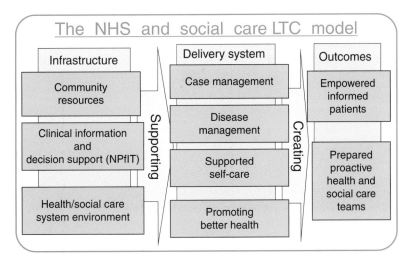

Figure 8.7   The NHS and social care long-term conditions model (DH, 2005b).

Factors which underpin the health and social care model

The bulleted points which follow about the NHS and Social Care Model (DH, 2005b) have been adapted from the work of Singh and Ham (2005). The author has expanded the points with examples of current practice issues.

- Developing a systematic approach that links health and social services, patients and carers.
- Being able to identify everyone with an LTC:
  - In general practice, this requires a system of recording and recall to offer patients regular re assessment of their ongoing conditions. This requires coordination between GP partners and practice nurses and the wider multidisciplinary team.
- Stratifying people so that care can be received according to individual needs:
  - The Kaiser triangle can help with stratification, but it may be possible for individuals to move up and down the triangle (see Figure 8.6). For example, a young woman with MS is generally at level one and self-manages her care, but when her supra-pubic catheter needs changing, this becomes an aspect of disease management which requires professional input from the District Nursing Service. Once this episode is complete, this lady is able to move back down to level one where she self-manages her condition with support from her husband (Madden 2008).
- Focusing on those individuals who are high users of secondary care services:
  - This is where variations in service delivery can become apparent. When deciding on criteria for those individuals suitable for case management, which is discussed at a later point in the chapter, it was found that some services have criteria around age. Some services specify individuals over 65 years of age, whilst other services consider individuals over 18 years of age. The rationale behind such decisions may lie with demographics. By 2031, the population of over-75s will be 8.2 million, an increase from the 4.7 million at the time of the chapter's writing. This older age group uses a disproportionate amount of NHS resources: an individual aged over 85 is 14 times more likely to be admitted to hospital than a 15–39-year-old (DH 2008a). However, LTCs are not entirely the domain of the older person; 17% of those aged under-40 have an LTC, but this is in comparison to 60% of over-65s (DH 2008). To expand on this further, an increasing number of children with an LTC are surviving into young adulthood (RCN 2007). With over 85% of children

Table 8.5   PARR data.

Risk band for readmittance predicted by PARR: 1-100 (NB: do not confuse with age ranges)	Admitted	Not admitted	Grand total of those in risk band for readmittance
40-49	261	448	709
50-59	183	201	384
60-69	86	64	150
70-79	44	24	68
80-89	34	13	47
90-99	18	1	19

with an LTC (Betz 1999) and 90% of children with a disability (Bloomquist et al. 1998) surviving into adulthood, age becomes an important issue in care coordination of such individuals. Harrison and Lydon (2008) concur in their study that there is a focus on very high intensity service users who have disabilities and cross the age spectrum.

- Using community matrons to provide case management:
  - The role and scope of community matrons is discussed at a later point in the chapter.
- Developing ways to identify people who may become high intensity service users:
  - Tools have been developed such as the PARR Tool (King's Fund, Health Dialog Analytic Solutions and New York University 2006). PARR is an acronym for Patients At Risk of Readmission.

PARR is a software tool with an easy to use interface which uses information from previous hospital admissions to predict future admissions, within the next year. Data are collated and passed on to GPs and community matrons who can then use it to check if individuals have been assessed for case management, but often staff have little or no training in its use or advantages. However, a criticism levelled at this process is that there are limitations in trying to make predictions for those who have not yet had a hospital admission (Curry et al. 2005).

Table 8.5 gives an example, based on real figures of the accuracy of the predictive nature of the data:

- Concentrate on the last box, where the risk band in the last box is 90-99% chance of readmission and then look at the figures which show that of the 19 individuals in that top risk band, 18 were actually admitted, hence a strong correlation and predictive accuracy (Wells 2007). This can be seen in a graph form (Figure 8.8).
- These data were based on the original PARR system, which since has developed into PARR 2 and PARR Combined (King's Fund, Health Dialog Analytic Solutions and New York University 2006), the latter is able to consider attendances at Accident & Emergency (A&E) which do not require admission, visits to outpatient clinics and also has the potential to link primary care data as well.
- A new tool which is being piloted at sites in the West Midlands is the BUPA Health Dialogue tool (BUPA 2010). Establish multidisciplinary teams in primary care supported by specialists.
- Developing local ways to support self-care:
  - In 2006, Birmingham Own Health was set up. This is an innovative approach to supporting individuals with LTCs and is a collaborative venture between Birmingham Trust, NHS Direct, and Pfizer Health Solutions. People with LTCs receive regular telephone-based coaching from highly experienced care managers. The approach is holistic and not just disease focused, and works to local guidelines and pathways. It supports individuals who are considered to be at level two of

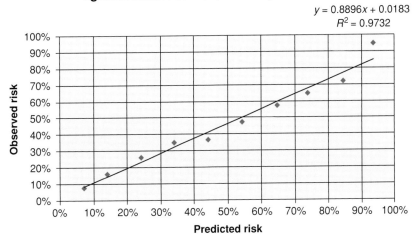

Risk of emergency admission: average predicted risk against observed risk, for ten-point risk bands

$y = 0.8896x + 0.0183$
$R^2 = 0.9732$

Figure 8.8 Graph showing correlation of emergency admissions against predicted risk.

the Kaiser triangle, and also supports those individuals who were at level three but have been 'stepped down' (Birmingham Own Health 2008).
- Expand Expert Patient Programme and other self-management programmes:
  - See chapter on self-management (Chapter 5).
- Using tools and techniques already available to make an impact. (Singh and Ham 2005).

The delivery system (middle column of health and social care model (DH 2005b))
Promoting better health and self-care
Discussion of the lower tiers of promoting health can be found throughout the chapters of this book, and self-management can be found in Chapter 5.

Disease management
Those patients represented at level two in the Kaiser triangle (see Figure 8.6) are likely to have a single condition, but which carries a high risk of complications which would be best dealt with by a multidisciplinary approach, often through the use of clinical pathways (DH 2004c). This level is often the domain of General Practice. The introduction of General Medical Services contract (DH 2004d) provides for care of specific LTCs and as such the role of the practice nurse in chronic disease management is crucial. It includes the identification, diagnosis, monitoring and management of patients in the primary healthcare environment (Carrier 2009). However, the list of conditions covered by the Quality Outcome Framework (QOF) (NHS Information Centre 2010), the annual reward and incentive programme which rewards best practice amongst GP practices, is not exhaustive, potentially leading to an inequality in attention paid to different LTCs. A means of undertaking this is the establishment of disease registers which accurately record patient information and changes, and work on a system of patient recall. An example showing the work of a practice nurse is given in case study 8.3. This allows regular reassessment of their condition to allow effective changes to be made and future planning to take place. Deterioration of condition, development of co-morbidities and inability to leave the home environment may necessitate individuals with LTCs moving up to level three of the Kaiser triangle, that of case management, which is considered next.

Case study 8.3 Practice nurse experience

For a nurse working in primary care, one role is to see patients in the nurse-led diabetes clinic. This is an annual review in addition to 3-4 monthly appointments with the GP. The appointment lasts for half an hour and a computer template has been devised for use in the clinic. This allows a structured format for the appointment and ensures all the relevant areas for review are discussed. It also allows data to be collected to fulfil QOF requirements. Occasionally, these strict targets are not appropriate for some patients. For example, tight blood glucose control may not be appropriate for a frail elderly patient who could be more at risk of hypoglycaemia with some medication and therefore more at risk of falls and other injuries.

The practice nurse saw a 52-year-old gentleman - Mr H for review of his diabetes recently. He is a manual worker in a nearby packaging company. He had been diagnosed with Type 2 diabetes in the past year. It quickly became apparent that this gentleman was finding it difficult to accept the diagnosis of diabetes. The diagnosis had been made following investigations for another problem, which had since been resolved. He did not feel unwell and normally rarely visited the doctor's surgery.

After introducing herself, Mr H was given time to express his frustration and reluctance to take medication for something he did not consider to be a problem. The practice nurse and patient briefly discussed the micro- and macrovascular complications of uncontrolled diabetes such as retinopathy, kidney disease, heart disease and stroke, but in a way that the practice nurse hoped to be non-threatening.

His blood pressure was found to be elevated at 162/96 and his weight was 93 kg, giving him a BMI (body mass index) of 32. Recent blood tests showed both his Hba1c and total cholesterol to be elevated. In listening to the patient, he disclosed that he had been suffering from recurrent penile thrush, but he hadn't seen anybody about this because he was embarrassed and also saw it as a trivial problem which was not serious enough to see the doctor about.

As part of the practice diabetes reviews, it is practice policy to always ask males if they have experienced any erectile dysfunction (ED), as this is known to affect many men with diabetes, but many are reluctant to seek help. By asking the question, this allows the question to be broached in a matter-of-fact way and allows discussion to take place. Mr H stated that he had indeed had difficulties with ED for the past few years. The practice nurse was able to give Mr H treatment for candida and explained it was probably as a result of his high blood sugar levels and should resolve as his diabetes was controlled. During the consultation, the practice nurse was also able to reassure Mr H regarding his difficulties with ED and that this may improve with better-controlled diabetes and also that treatments were also available to help.

By the end of the appointment, a good rapport had been established and the practice nurse had managed to alleviate some of Mr H's anxieties. It was agreed that Mr H would start oral medication for his diabetes, blood pressure and cholesterol. They were introduced gradually and titrated appropriately, with relevant blood monitoring carried out.

A further appointment was arranged in three months. Mr H's blood pressure, and cholesterol had improved. Although Mr H's Hba1c was better, it remained too high. Because good communication had been established, Mr H was aware of the importance of establishing good blood glucose control and agreed to take an additional agent for his diabetes. He reported that his thrush had resolved, but that ED was still a significant problem. However, now that he knew the diabetes was probably one of the causes and that treatment was available for many men, he felt encouraged that this could be improved upon. It was agreed that he would start some medication and would report back the effectiveness.

The practice nurse has seen Mr H regularly since, and he continues to do well. He understands that Type 2 diabetes is a progressive condition and that he may need to adjust his medication in the future, but because he has a good comprehension of what the various medications are for, he accepts this may be necessary.

Points for reflection

- Consider the importance of building a rapport with patients with LTCs. Why is a good rapport so important?
- How does the practice nurse move this consultation around areas which matter to this patient? (The reader may refer to Chapter 5 for further discussion.)
- How does having a system of recall for patients on the LTC register benefit the patient?

This chapter now moves on to consider the top layer of the delivery system, that of case management.

Case management

Case management has been defined as: 'the process of planning, co-ordinating, managing and reviewing the care of an individual.' (Hutt et al. 2004: 1) The term 'case management' was first used in North America in the 1950s for psychiatric patients (Lee et al. 1998). This was the principal user group addressed when case management was first introduced in the United Kingdom, although renamed care management as part of the NHS and Community Care Act (Great Britain Parliament 1990).

No one model of case management has been adopted, which means that Health Trusts are able to target their diverse populations through varied approaches and interventions (Hutt et al. 2004). According to Hutt et al. (2004), there are six core elements to case management which should apply whatever the setting. These are:

- Case finding
- Assessment
- Care planning
- Coordination and referral/intervention
- Monitoring
- Review

As discussed earlier, PARR and the BUPA Health Dialogue tools are means of finding suitable individuals for case management. Other methods include referral from members of health and social care teams. Referral criteria are established to fit with local need. Tables 8.6 and 8.7 exhibit local criteria from an urban trust, which was using two service models, hence two sets of criteria. Similarities can

Table 8.6   Example 1: criteria for case management.

Patients should be 50 years old or over and must meet two of the following criteria:

- Two recent unplanned hospital admissions in the last six months
- Older people in the top 3% of frequent visitors to GP practices
- Two or more attendances to A&E in the past 12 months
- Falls associated with dizziness and impaired mobility
- One or more LTCs:
  COPD
  Arthritis
  Asthma
  Diabetes
  Polypharmacy (four or more medicines)
- Lives alone and is dependent
- Impairment of one or major activity of their daily living
- Older people who have a total stay in hospital which exceeds more than 4 weeks in a year
- High risk patients:
  Recent exacerbation of chronic illness within the past 90 days
  Recently bereaved and at risk of medical decline
  Cognitively impaired, living alone and medically unstable
  High intensity social service package

Table 8.7   Example 2: criteria for case management.

The patient must be a resident, 18 years or over and meet the criteria of at least three of the following:

- Two or more active LTCs
- Four or more medicines, prescribed for six months or more
- Two or more hospital admissions, not necessarily as an emergency, in the past 12 months
- Two or more A&E attendances in the past 12 months
- Significant impairment in one or more major activity involved in daily living
- Significant impairment in one or more of the instrumental activities of living, particularly where no support systems are in place
- Older people in the top 3% of frequent visitors to the practice
- Older people who have had two or more outpatient appointments
- Older people whose total stay in hospital exceeded four weeks in a year
- Older people whose social work contact exceeded four assessment visits in each of the three month period.
- Older people whose prescribing costs exceeded £100 per month.
NB: There is no clarification of what constitutes older.
High risk patients

- Recent exacerbation of chronic illness within the past 90 days
- Recent falls > two falls in the past 2 months
- Recently bereaved and at risk of medical decline
- Cognitively impaired, living alone and medically unstable
- High intensity Social Service Package (15 hours or more per week)

be seen, but so can the differences. Of particular note is the difference in ages depicted in the criteria in the example. As noted elsewhere in this chapter, although the elderly population do account for a large proportion of individuals with LTCs, there is also a proportion of the population below 50, as in the case of Example 1 (see Table 8.6), who could benefit from case management. Searching out original work from Kaiser, Evercare and Castlefields shows how most trusts have a variation on the themes of the original service delivery models.

Considering the six requirements put forward on page 245 in this chapter by Hutt et al. (2004), Lewis (2008) makes a link to similarities with the nursing process, which is undertaken in primary and secondary care. The specific features which are unique to case management are:

- The intense involvement of the case manger with level three individuals.
- The number of services who are involved.
- The length of time for which case managers are involved.

Re-read the Case studies 8.1 and 8.2, to refresh the complicated scenarios which can make up case management, as demonstrated by a community matron.

Case management is noted in the USA for reducing emergency admissions to hospital (Kane et al. 2003). Hutt et al. (2004) undertook a literature review on case management and although they found some evidence that case management had a positive effect in reducing emergency admissions, it was not conclusive. Since 2004, a number of other studies in the United Kingdom have linked case management with the introduction of community matrons. A quantitative study by Gravelle et al. (2007) found that case management had no significant impact on emergency admissions and bed days. Conversely though Roland et al. (2005) found that over a period of 4–5 years admission rates and bed use fell. However, the latter study notes that it did not consider death rates, so admissions may have appeared reduced due to death and not the impact of case management. Gaffney (2009) reports reductions in admissions and bed days on 19 case-managed individuals in a small-scale study.

The quantitative studies undertaken in the United Kingdom, however, have not reproduced the results seen in the USA. There may be several reasons for this: the UK baseline of general service provision is usually higher in the United Kingdom than in the US making the impact of service innovations less marked; there are differences in the way healthcare systems are run in the US; different methodologies are used for the studies in the United Kingdom; therefore, they are not considering 'like for like'. The evidence does not show consistent reduction in hospital admission or cost savings for individuals with LTCs as a result of being case managed and/or the introduction of community matrons.

The qualitative studies undertaken in the United Kingdom are more positive. The service is reported to be effective by community matrons, patients, carers and GPs (Sargent et al. 2007, Leighton et al. 2008, Brown et al. 2008, Elwyn et al. 2008).

The qualitative studies, highlighted above, cover areas such as self-management, seeking appropriate help for exacerbations, quality of life and support. A perceived reduction in hospital admissions is reported, although not shown statistically. Fletcher and Mant (2009) report an increase in GP consultations as a result of case management, which may be accounted for by patients becoming active self-managers. All areas within the United Kingdom run their services differently; therefore, it is difficult to draw overall conclusions as the nature and composition of the population needs to be considered. This literature highlights complexities of health policies and also the complexities of how effectiveness is measured.

Section 3

Table 8.8 Domains of case management for community matrons.

A. Advanced clinical nursing skills

B. Leading complex care coordination

C. Proactively managing complex LTCs

D. Managing cognitive impairment and mental well-being

E. Supporting self-care, self-management and enabling independence

F. Professional practice and leadership

G. Identifying high risk patients, and promoting health and preventing ill health

H. Managing care at end of life

I. Interagency and partnership working

Source: NHS Modernisation Agency & Skills for Health (2005).

Case managers can be allied health professionals or social workers, but a new role emerged: that of community matron (DH 2004b).

Community matrons

A community matron has been defined as a nurse who provides advanced clinical nursing care in addition to case management to a specific group of high intensity users identified through case finding (NHS Modernisation Agency & Skills for Health, 2005). A key aspect is that the community matron becomes a single point of contact for those individuals who are at Kaiser level three and are balancing co-morbidities and all the associated agencies, appointments, medications, to name but a few that go with LTCs. In simplest terms, the community matron is the 'lynch pin' to coordinate these issues, in partnership or on behalf of the individual, easing their journey not only across primary and secondary care, but also across social care. Elwyn et al. (2008) considered the special place community matrons hold at the primary/secondary care interface which allows them to manage what Cook et al. (2000) described them as the 'care gap'.

The domains of case management for community matrons are shown in Table 8.8.

The NHS Modernisation Agency & Skills for Health (2005) suggest that case managers may work with individuals who have a dominant single condition, but still have intensive needs which require coordination. What differentiates the community matron from other case managers, in the criteria in Table 8.2, is the provision of advanced clinical nursing care. However, including advanced clinical nursing skills may cause disquiet amongst allied health professionals (AHPs), who themselves may have advanced health assessment skills and be non-medical prescribers, and yet cannot claim the 'nursing aspect'. In terms of caseload differences, individuals on a community matron caseload will have more complex clinical nursing care needs (Thunhurst and Randall 2010). This has been illustrated in the Case studies 8.1 and 8.2.

As with case management as a whole, there is no one model of community matron services. A variation on the theme can be seen in the introduction of virtual wards.

Virtual wards

The concept of virtual wards was developed by Croydon PCT in 2006 (Lewis 2007), and the innovation and creativity shown in the development resulted in the project being awarded four prizes at the Health Service Journal Awards in Nov 2006 (Lewis 2007).

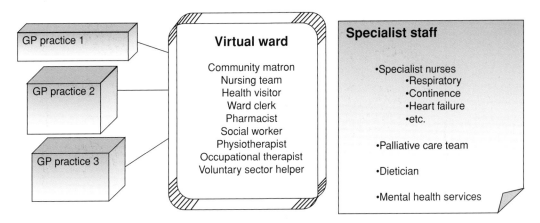

Figure 8.9   Virtual ward. (Adapted from Lewis 2007.)

Lewis (2007) describes a virtual ward as using the systems, staffing and routines of a traditional hospital ward as a means of providing case management in the community. In essence, virtual wards have the following features:

- They mimic hospital wards.
- Patients are cared for in their own homes.
- No physical ward in a building, hence the term 'virtual ward'.
- Patients are case managed by a multidisciplinary team.
- Ward team is led by a community matron.

If virtual wards are to be successful in the long-term, Lewis (2007) stresses the importance of them being embedded in GP practices. In this way, strong working relationships are established.

The following model shows how GP practices link with virtual wards, the constituent members of the virtual ward team, and how specialist nurses and teams visit patients 'on the virtual ward' as and when patient need arises (Figure 8.9):

Virtual wards have been established across the country. One such pilot is underway in Warwickshire (Murray 2009). The team show their day-to-day working in the following terms:

- Identification of new patients
- Admission pathway
- Clinical input and visiting plan
- Self-management plans
- Information leaflets
- Discharge pathways
- *Daily 'ward round'*: Teleconference call
- *Community beds*: Direct admission for virtual ward
- Intermediate care
- Social care
- Monthly retrospective meeting to discuss unplanned hospital admissions
- Evening and weekend working
  Source: Murray (2009)

Section 3

Admission criteria for virtual wards follow broad criteria such as those shown on page 246 and can be altered to suit a particular location's needs.

Impact of the community matron role

Studies which have been undertaken to consider the impact of the community matron role have considered impact from the perspective of patients, carers, GPs and community nursing teams. Overall satisfaction with the service was rated at 97% by patients and carers of the 54% who returned their postal questionnaire (Leighton et al. 2008). The comments which patients and carers offered about the service fell into three themes: service reliability and patient and carer confidence in the service, improvement of communication and coordination of care, and lastly reduction in hospital admissions as perceived by the patients and their carers.

Lyndon (2007) found that through aspects of care provided by the community matrons such as care coordination and liaison with other healthcare professionals to deliver complex care packages, diagnosis and assessment and patient and carer education on managing conditions, and recognising and acting promptly on signs of exacerbations contributed to the avoidance of hospital admissions comparable to savings of £152, 000/year. Similarly, Gaffney (2009) found that the effectiveness of the community matron service when measured across six criteria showed savings. The six service aspects considered by Gaffney were: admissions to secondary care, number of bed days, GP contacts, out of hours contacts, accident and emergency visits, and ambulance contacts. In a retrospective analysis of GP contacts (Gaffney 2009), appointments were reduced by 58%, telephone contacts by 74% and out of hours contacts reduced by 62.5%. In a qualitative appraisal, GPs considered the greatest impact of the community matron service to be around managing patients with complex needs, admission avoidance and in increasing levels of communication (Leighton et al. 2008).

Another area of cost reduction resulted from regular medication reviews undertaken by the community matrons in three rural PCTs in England (Brookes 2008). In undertaking one-to-one interviews with 72 patients and 52 carers, reviews of medication along with physical examinations were rated 'enthusiastically' (Sargent et al. 2007: 514) by those interviewed. Other areas which were valued about the role of the community matron included care coordination, education and advice, advocacy and psychological support – the latter being rated as highly as clinical care.

Overall, patients highly valued the community matron role (Wright et al. 2007). Elwyn et al. (2008) consider the community matron impact to be greatest at the primary/secondary care interface where they are able to manage the 'care gap'.

Another service which aims to plug the 'care gap' is that of intermediate care, and the chapter considers the role of this service as a means of coordinating care for those individuals with LTCs.

Summary

Service delivery models such as Kaiser, Evercare and Pfizer, along with Castlefields have been considered. Particular attention has been paid to the NHS and Social Care Model and the underpinning rationale for its creation. Consideration of identifying patients and timely interventions by appropriate personnel has been examined. In particular, the impacts of effective disease management and case management have been examined as a means of producing the desired outcomes of this model: proactive patients and prepared proactive healthcare teams.

Section 3

Other ways of working which influence care coordination

Intermediate care

Another tier of healthcare has emerged: that of intermediate care (IC), which sits between primary and secondary care (Herbert and Lake 2004). The purpose of IC is described by the Institute of Health Sciences and Public Health Research at the University of Leeds (2005) as that of firstly, avoiding inappropriate hospital admissions and secondly, enhancing independence through maximising an individual's abilities. They conclude that intermediate care should be seen as a set of bridges at key points of transition in the person's journey from hospital to home (and vice versa) and from illness/injury to recovery.

As discovered in this chapter, there are often variations in service delivery according to area, but with a base in a broad framework. IC is no different.

> ### Point for reflection
>
> - Ask about IC in your area and find out what services are on offer.
> - Would it be possible to spend a day with the IC team?

Some intermediate care services work on a 'step-up model' which prevents inappropriate hospital admissions and responds to a health crisis enabling an individual to remain in their home environment (Barton et al. 2006)). A 'step-down model' will facilitate early discharge from secondary care providing nursing and therapy services in an individual's own home (Barton et al. 2006). Some IC services have access to residential beds which can bridge a period when acute admission is not required, but a greater level of care than remaining at home is needed. For individuals with LTCs, this vital service may represent the difference between a hospital admission or not, or where admission to hospital is appropriate, timely discharge is facilitated.

Teams

Teams of staff within IC comprise: nurses, IC support workers, social workers, occupational therapists (OTs) and physiotherapists. Within the services, there may be two strands. Firstly, a health crisis team who react to a sudden short-term nursing need, which is manageable within the patient's own home, but is likely to be resolved within 7–10 days. Through this system patients are assessed within 3 hours of referral. Some areas have a facility to provide live-in carers for a week and have access to fast response social services assistance. Up to three visits/day can be provided and will include accessing equipment if required. Secondly, referrals can be made for rehabilitation at home where an individual would benefit from a rehabilitation programme involving OTs and physiotherapists, where need can typically be met in 2–6 weeks.

The emphasis here is on coordination of care across services and disciplines with the patient at the heart of a plan structured around individual needs. It is a time-limited service and coordination and referral for ongoing care may be necessary if treatment plans are not effective.

Views on benefits and challenges of IC (Barton et al. 2006) considered several aspects of care coordination:

Section 3

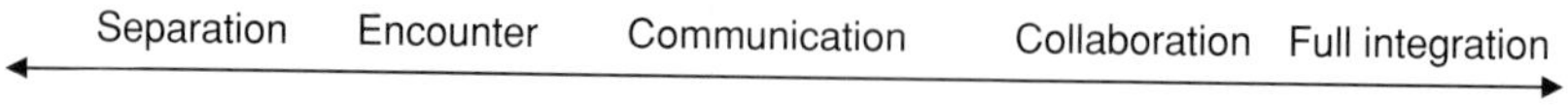

Separation   Encounter   Communication   Collaboration Full integration

Figure 8.10 Continuum of interagency working. (Adapted from Glendenning 2002.)

- The most important aspect in developing IC was effective partnership working between PCTs and social services.
- Where partnership working was poor, funding was inadequate (either due to amount or being time-limited), or there was poor recruitment of staff, care was affected.
- Lack of awareness of IC or the inability of the IC service to respond to referrals had a negative effect on other services.

A need for integrated community-based IC services to work well within a 'whole systems' context is the conclusion drawn (Barton et al. 2006). The push for integration of services is considered next.

Integration of care services

Earlier in the chapter, it was highlighted that communication and coordination can break down across boundaries and in an attempt to alleviate this difficulty in the management of individuals with LTCs (and other health problems), the concept of integrating care was introduced (DH 2006b, DH 2008a). Rosen and Ham (2008: 2) define integration as:

A single system of needs assessment, commissioning and/or service provision that aims to promote alignment & collaboration between cure & care sectors.

As a result, enhancing the quality of care, improving patient outcomes and efficiency in the use of resources are all goals of integrating services. Rosen and Ham (2008) also discuss the effects of integration in terms of a whole systems approach comprising micro, meso and macro levels as described by the WHO (see Figure 8.4).

Glendenning (2002) draws on previous work by Hudson et al. (1997, 1999) in placing integration on a continuum of interagency working (see Figure 8.10) with the lowest point noted as separation with complete autonomy of organisations, the next stage would be 'encounter', followed by 'communication', 'collaboration', and finally and optimally 'full integration', at which point collaboration is so tight that the agencies' separate identities no longer exist or matter.

Glendenning (2002) goes on to suggest that at the point of full integration, the following elements are exhibited within the relationship:

- Joint goals.
- Networks which are highly connected.
- A mutual vision of long-term obligation which does not need to be underpinned by reciprocation.
- High level of mutual trust and respect.
- Mainstream 'core' business is jointly arranged.
- Joint arrangement of strategic and operational issues.
- Management arrangements which are clear: single or shared.
- Joint commissioning at macro and micro levels.

Such considerations may seem far away if you are reading this chapter as a student nurse, but in the context of effectively managing individuals with LTCs, it is important to be aware of key aspects that are shaping patient care and also the roles of healthcare professionals.

Another tool employed to increase integration are care pathways, which the reader will see out in practice. Vecchiato (2004: 83) describes care pathways as:

integrated care strategies that offer a means of achieving better integration among practitioners, community-based services and other health and social care partners.

They can contribute better continuity of care either simultaneously (where services are delivered at same time) or sequentially (when delivered in distinct periods), and are essentially instruments which reduce improper access to hospital emergency services, inappropriate admissions or unplanned discharges.

Perceived barriers to integration

A major barrier to true integration is seen as professional identity. Indeed, Castledine (2009) talks about a new form of professional, demonstrated by disciplines concentrating on their own agendas. This is worrying as such an ethos is unlikely to have the patient at the heart of care. There is evidence to contradict, however. Hudson (2007) reports that anticipated problems with conflicting professional identities have not been seen, with team members reporting that they support each other and work well together. Issues have also been raised about roles and Basset (2006) considers the potential conflicts associated with the introduction of the community matron role as a means of increasing the effectiveness of individuals with LTCs, when considered next to specialist nurses and their roles. Basset (2006) concludes that there is a role for both whereby the specialist nurse may take a step back and act as consultant to the community matron, whose role is as a generalist. The issue of roles is further considered by Mitchell (2008) who considers that the poor integration across primary and secondary care is due to poor understanding.

Despite coordination being a fundamental skill required by healthcare professionals and particularly by nurses who are often seen as the catalyst for coordination (Abraham 2004), in a review of community nursing services in an urban PCT, Parker and Glasby (2008) found a lack of integration and coordination with services operating in silos, only communicating if required and with no consistency. As referral routes were vague, there was poor understanding amongst services of who did what, when and to whom, there was evidence of care being inconsistent, duplicated and of poor quality, despite the real commitment and enthusiasm of individuals (Parker and Glasby 2008).

In considering the use of integrated care pathways as a tool to enhance the management of individuals with LTCs, Wilson et al. (2009) highlights that they were originally developed for time-limited and predictable trajectories, and that there is little evidence of how effective they will be in LTCs where trajectories are anything but predictable. There may also be tensions as a result of patients with LTCs being effective self-managers, and also tensions caused by patient's choice which is another key concept of caring for individuals with LTCs (Wilson et al. 2009).

Already, a central tenant of care coordination is seen to be effective communication and this chapter will now consider some elements of communication.

Communication

Coordination of care requires effective communication. Kvamme et al. (2001) consider that as healthcare systems become more complex, more people will need coordinated care from both sides of the primary/secondary care interface and that communication is a crucial factor. Part of effective communication across this interface means ensuring timely and relevant high quality information is transmitted from primary to secondary care and vice versa (Werrett et al. 2001). A 'dynamic

Section 3

system of care' such as that advocated by Kaiser rather than structures which work at 'levels of care' (primary, secondary) is seen as the solution by Kvamme et al. (1998).

If asked, most nurses and other healthcare professionals would claim to be effective in communicating, and yet many complaints are as a result of poor communication (DH 2001c, Grover 2005). When working with individuals with LTCs, healthcare professionals may be working with individuals who are very knowledgeable about their conditions and competently self-manage, or with individuals who are in denial of the situation or have goals which are not in harmony with professional perceptions of care. These two situations require different types of communication. Similarly, for individuals whose first language is not English, communication will be different and may be through an interpreter. For those individuals who have lost the ability to communicate verbally, due to disease progression or loss of cognition, communication will need to change again. Such situations may also result in alterations to the services involved, continuing the requirements of skilled coordination.

In developing guidelines on MS for NICE (National Institute of Health and Clinical Excellence), the National Collaborating Centre for Chronic Conditions (2004) undertook focus groups with people with MS. Communication and its breakdown were raised as a central issue by the participants and as a result, the guidelines offered a résumé of good practice for communication. Although the example in Table 8.9 is for individuals with MS, there are many aspects which are transferable across a range of LTCs.

Not only is communication essential between professional and client, it is also essential between professionals as well, and the chapter has already examined how factors such as poorly understood roles, barriers between health sectors, such as primary and secondary care, and barriers across sectors such as health and social care can all affect the patient's journey. Over communication, checking and double checking, but in a non-threatening way, so that one professional does not appear to be checking up on another, or be seen to be mistrusting their abilities, will prevent key actions from falling through cracks. The chapter concludes by considering how new ways of working may be able to remove barriers.

Summary

Other ways of delivering effectively managed care for individuals with LTCs include the use of IC, either as a step-up or a step-down option. The importance of teamwork and the introduction of integrated teams as a means of breaking down barriers where care coordination can 'fall down' have been examined. The fundamental importance that communication plays in care coordination has also been noted.

New ways of working

The WHO (2005) considers that the shifting balance between acute and chronic health problems is placing new demands on the workforce, requiring expansion of health professionals' skills to meet the changing demands. The vision of the WHO is that skills should be reflected in five competencies that apply to all members of the workforce who care for patients with LTCs and are:

- Patient-centred care
- Partnering

Table 8.9   Principles of effective communication in a healthcare setting.

Principle (healthcare professional responsibility)	Comment
Consider the environment and possible distractions and interruptions.	Privacy and quiet are key
Consider who is present. Check whether the patient is comfortable and has the people they may wish present as well.	Think students and family
Enquire about what patient already knows.	Manage expectations
Consider the information required by the individual and the amount of information required.	Manage expectations
Weigh up risks and benefits of each piece of information being given.	Cannot withdraw information once given
Tailor-make the information to the individual. Consider: • Existing knowledge • Communication and cognitive abilities • Culture	Information is timely and relevant
Do not exceed your level of knowledge. Refer on if necessary.	Be certain of your own knowledge
Be clear about options and choices. Ensure patient can make an informed choice and understands: • Likely outcomes of the options • Risks and benefits of the options	Through both diagnosis and treatment
Re-enforce information being given: • In different medium (leaflet, tapes) • By different team member (specialist nurses) • At a follow-up appointment	Information can be forgotten
Give information about local or national agencies	Enable individuals to follow-up available help for themselves
Consider and arrange emotional support if required, particularly when giving difficult information.	Make an automatic part of the process, not an after thought
Maintain communication across all parties: write in notes, liaise with other colleagues about information imparted. Include GP.	Continuity across time and settings

Source: Adapted from The National Collaborating Centre for Chronic Disease MS guidelines (2004).

• Quality improvement
• Information and communication technology
• Public health perspective

The chapter has shown how policy themes across the United Kingdom have mirrored such ideals and Modernising Nursing Careers (DH 2006b) hoped to create a competent, flexible workforce with an updated career pathway which would prepare nurses to lead into a healthcare system that is

Section 3

changing. It also stated that care should be organised around the needs of patients and this would require nurses to work in a range of settings.

With this in mind, a trust in the West Midlands created new role named 'in - reach'. The posts were rotational in nature, taking the post holders across clinical areas which comprised primary and secondary care with the express intention of considering the patient journey, and working to coordinate their care and promote timely discharge or work with others such as community matrons and District Nursing Teams to prevent admission. By working across the following four keys areas:

- Acute admissions
- Community hospital
- Community
- IC

the post holders were able to build up new skills and consider where barriers occurred within the system and build bridges between existing services (Randall, Dignon and Mills, in press). With the implementation of Transforming Community Services (DH 2009c) continuing to go ahead following the recent change of government, most PCT provider arms will be expected to integrate with acute or mental health arms, thus offering further opportunities for role innovation.

'Our Health, Our Care, Our Say' (DH 2006a) set the vision for care outside of hospitals. The anticipated benefits of such a move in care setting are that care can be delivered in a timely fashion, and be efficient, effective, equitable, patient-centred and safe (DH 2009a). With an emphasis on providing more care in the community and reduction in acute beds, it is likely that innovative ways of working will become more apparent in the future.

Conclusion

Wherever an individual sits within the Kaiser triangle, their care needs to be coordinated to a greater or lesser degree. For those who are healthy members of the population, health promotion campaigns – delivered by healthcare professionals - are coordinated efforts such as immunisations, fit for life, etc. For those individuals with an LTC at level 1 and who predominately self-manage, may require the GP practice to order medications in a timely fashion. At disease management level 2, the practice nurse is instrumental, in partnership with GP colleagues and patients, in ensuring recall and monitoring of conditions, and preventing complications as a result, wherever possible. Following any admission to hospital, acute staff may need to coordinate an effective discharge plan, liaising with health and social care professionals, as well as patient and family members. Finally, this chapter has examined those individuals at the top of the triangle for whom co-morbidities impact their lives to a considerable degree and how effective coordination through case managers, often community matrons, can contribute to quality of life. Whether student or experienced nurse, the skills required to ensure effective care coordination for individuals with LTCs cannot be underestimated.

Acknowledgements

I would like to thank Lesley Mukwedeya and Mandy Taylor for providing the case studies for this chapter, and to the patients who consented to the use of their cases as a means of raising awareness and educating future and existing healthcare professionals.

References

Abraham, A. (2004) Lack of communication affects the care of patients and families. *Professional Nurse* **19** (6), 351-353.

Abbots, J., Hardins, S. and Cruickshank, K. (2004) Cardiovascular risk profiles in UK-born Caribbeans and Irish living in England and Wales. *Atherosclerosis* **175**, 295-303.

Agency for Healthcare Research and Quality (AHRQ) (2007) Closing the Quality Gap. Available at: http://www.ahrq.gov/clinic/tp/caregaptp.htm (accessed 12 January 2010).

Aitken, A. (2009) *Community Palliative Care: The Role of the Clinical Nurse Specialist.* Oxford: Wiley-Blackwell.

Barton, P., Bryan, S., Glasby, J., Hewitt, G., Jagger, C., Kaambwa, B., Martin, G., Nancarrow, S., Parker, H., Parker, S., Regen, E. and Wilson, A. (2006) *A National Evaluation of the Costs and Outcomes of Intermediate Care for Older People: Executive Summary.* Birmingham, Leicester: Health Services Management Centre, University of Birmingham; Leicester Nuffield Research Unit, University of Leicester.

Basset, S. (2006) *Developing Integrated Health & Social Care Services for LTC.* London: RCN.

Betz, C. (1999) Adolescents with chronic conditions: linkages to adult services. *Paediatric Nursing* **25**, 473-476.

Bhopal, R. (2000) What is the risk of coronary heart disease in South Asians? A review of UK research. *Journal of Public Health Medicine* **22** (3), 375-385.

Birmingham Own Health (2008). Available at: http://www.birminghamownhealth.co.uk/gp (accessed 2 January 2010).

Bloomquist, K., Brown, G., Perrson, A. and Presler, E. (1998) Transitioning to independence: challenges for young people with disabilities and their caregivers. *Orthopaedic Nursing* **17** (3), 27-35.

Boaden, R., Dusheiko, M., Gravelle, H., Parker, S., Pickard, S., Roland, M., Sheaff, R. and Sargent, P. (2005) *Evercare Evaluation Interim Report: Implications for Supporting People with Long-term Conditions*, pp. 45-47. Manchester: National Primary Care Research and Development Centre, Manchester University. Available at: http://www.natpact.nhs.uk/uploads/2005_Feb/Evercare_evaluation_interim_report.pdf (accessed 4 January 2010).

Brennan, J. (2004) *Cancer in Context: A Practical Guide to Supportive Care.* Oxford: Oxford University Press.

Brookes, D. (2008) An evaluation of community matron prescribing. *Nurse Prescribing* **6** (2), 67-70.

Brown, K., Stainer, K., Stewart, J., Clacy, R. and Parker, S. (2008) Older people with complex long-term health conditions. Their views on the community matron service: a qualitative study. *Quality in Primary Care* **16**, 409-416.

BUPA Health Dialogue Tool (2010) Available at: http://www.bupahealthdialog.co.uk/html/data.html (accessed 11 October 2010).

Carrier, J. (2009) *Managing Long-term Conditions and Chronic Illness in Primary Care.* London: Routledge.

Castledine, G. (2009) Let's work together. *British Journal of Nursing* **18** (20), 128.

Cook, R., Render, M. and Woods, D. (2000) Gaps in the continuity of care and progress on patient safety. *BMJ* **320**, 791-794.

Curry, N., Billings, J., Darin, B., Dixon, J., Williams, M. and Wennberg, D. (2005) *Predictive Risk Project.* London: King's Fund.

Department of Health (DH) (2000a) *National Service Framework for Coronary Heart Disease.* London: The Stationery Office.

Department of Health (DH) (2000b) *NHS Cancer Plan; a Plan for Investment, a Plan for Reform.* London: The Stationery Office.

Department of Health (DH) (2001a) *NSF Diabetes.* London: The Stationery Office.

Department of Health (DH) (2001b) *NSF for Older People.* London: The Stationery Office.

Department of Health (DH) (2001c) *Reforming the NHS Complaints Procedure: A Listening Document.* London: The Stationery Office.

Department of Health (DH) (2004a) *Choosing Health.* London: The Stationery Office.

Department of Health (DH) (2004b) *The NHS Improvement Plan: Putting People at the Heart of Public Services.* London: The Stationery Office.

Department of Health (DH) (2004c) *Chronic Disease Management: A Compendium of Information.* London: The Stationery Office.

Department of Health (DH) (2004d) *National Standards, Local Action: Health and Social Care Standards and Planning Framework 2005/06, 2007/08.* London: The Stationery Office.

Department of Health (DH) (2005a) *NSF Long-term Conditions.* London: The Stationery Office.

Department of Health (DH) (2005b) *Supporting People with Long-term Conditions. An NHS and Social Care Model to Support Local Innovation and Integration.* London: The Stationery Office.

Department of Health, Social Security and Public Safety (DHSSPS) (2005) *A Healthier Future: A Twenty Year Vision for Health and Well-being in Northern Ireland 2005-2025.* Belfast: DHSSPS.

Department of Health (DH) (2006a) *Our Health, Our Care, Our Say.* London: The Stationery Office.

Department of Health (DH) (2006b) *Modernising Nursing Careers: Setting the Direction.* London: The Stationery Office.

Department of Health (DH) (2008a) *High Quality Care for All (The Darzi Report).* London: The Stationery Office.

Department of Health (DH) (2008b) National Carers Strategy. Available at: http://www.dh.gov.uk/en/Publicationsandstatistics/Publications/PublicationsPolicyAndGuidance/DH_085345 (accessed 10 May 2010).

Department of Health (DH) (2009) *Implementing Care Closer to Home: Convenient Quality Care for Patients.* London: The Stationery Office.

Department of Health (DH) (2009b) Report of the Standing Commission on Carers 2007-2009. Available at: http://www.dh.gov.uk/prod_consum_dh/groups/dh_digitalassets/@dh/@en/@ps/@sta/@perf/documents/digitalasset/dh_107481.pdf (accessed 9 May 2010).

Department of Health (2009c) *Transforming Community Services: Enabling New Patterns of Provision.* London: The Stationery Office.

Department of Health (2010) *Equity and Excellence: Liberating the NHS.* London: The Stationery Office.

Diabetes UK (2008) Risk factors. Available at: http://www.diabetes.org.uk/Guide-to-diabetes/Introduction-to-diabetes/Causes_and_Risk_Factors/. (accessed 3 May 2010).

Edwards, M. (2008) A nursing perspective. *London Journal of Primary Care* (June), 1-3. Available at: http://www.londonjournalofprimarycare.org.uk/articles/responses/7.pdf. (accessed 11 October 2010).

Elwyn, G., Williams, M., Roberts, C., Newcombe, R. and Vincent, J. (2008) Case management by nurses in primary care: analysis of 73 "success stories". *Quality in Primary Care* **16**, 75-82.

Fehally, J. (2003) Ethnicity and renal disease: questions and challenges. *Critical Medicine: Journal of the Royal College of Physicians* **3** (6), 578-582.

Fletcher, K. and Mant, J. (2009) A before and after study of the impact of specialist workers for older people. *Journal of Evaluation in Clinical Practice* **15**, 172-177.

Frude, N. (2010) The family: a psychological perspective. In: D. Watkins and J. Cousins (eds) Public Health and Community Nursing Frameworks, *137-146.* Edinburgh: Balliere Tindall.

Gaffney, K. (2009) Becoming a community matron. *Journal of Community Nursing* **23** (1), 4-9.

Gill, P., Jai, K., Bhopal, R., Wild, S. (2004) Black and minority ethnic groups. In: A. Stevens, J. Raftery, J. Mant and S. Simpson (eds) *Health Care Needs Assessment: The Epidemiology Based Needs Assessment Reviews,* 3rd edn.

Glendenning, C. (2002) Breaking down barriers: integrating health and care services for older people in England. *Health Policy* **65**, 139-151.

Gravelle, H., Dusheiko, M., Sheaff, R., Sargent, P., Boaden, R., Pickard, S., Parker, S. and Roland, M. (2007) Impact of case management (Evercare) on frail elderly patients: controlled before and after analysis of quantitative outcome data. *British Medical Journal* **334**, 31-34.

Section 3

Great Britain Parliament (1990) NHS and Community Care Act (Act of Parliament). London: HMSO.

Great Britain Parliament (1994) The Carers (Recognition and Services) Act (Act of Parliament). London: HMSO.

Great Britain Parliament (2004) The Carer (Equal Opportunities) Act (Act of Parliament). London: HMSO.

Grover, S. (2005) Shaping effective communication skills and therapeutic relationships at work: the foundation of collaboration. *American Association of Occupational health Nurses Journal* **53** (4), 177-182.

Grulich, A., Swerdlow, A., Head, J. and Marmot, M. (1992). Cancer mortality in African and Caribbean migrants to England and Wales. *British Journal of Cancer* **66**, 905-911.

Ham, C. (2005) *Developing Integrated Care in the NHS: Adapting Lessons from Kaiser.* Birmingham: Health Services Management Centre, School of Public Policy, University of Birmingham.

Harrison, S. and Lydon, J. (2008) Health visiting and community matrons: progress in partnership. *Community Practitioner.* **81** (2), 20-22.

Herbert, G. and Lake, G. (2004) *Leading Ideas Leading Change. Developing the Intermediate Tier: Sharing the Learning.* Leeds: Nuffield Institute for Health, University of Leeds.

Hudson, B., Hardy, B., Henwood, M. and Winston, G. (1997) *Interagency Collaboration.* Final Report. Leeds: Nuffield Institute for Health.

Hudson, B., Exworthy, M., Peckham, S. and Callaghan, G. (1999) *Locality Partnerships: The Early Primary Care Group Experience.* Leeds: Nuffield Institute for Health.

Hudson, B. (2007) Pessimism & optimism in inter-professional working: the Sedgefield Integrated team. *Journal of Inter-professional Care* **21**, 3-15.

Hutt, R., Rosen, R. and McCauley, J. (2004) *Case-managing Long-term Conditions.* London: King's Fund.

Institute of Health Sciences and Public Health Research (2005) *An Evaluation of Intermediate Care for Older People.* Final Report. University of Leeds.

Kane, R., Keckhafer, G., Flood, S., Bershadsky, B. and Siadaty, M. (2003) The effect of evercare on hospital use. *Journal of the American Geriatric Society* **51**, 1427-1434.

King's Fund, Health Dialog Analytic Solutions and New York University (2006) Case Finding Algorithms for Patients at Risk of Re-hospitalisation. Available at: http://www.kingsfund.org.uk/research/projects/predicting_and_reducing_readmission_to_hospital/index.html. (accessed 2 January 2010).

Kvamme, O., Eliasson, E. and Jensen, P. (1998) Co-operation of care and learning across the interface between primary and secondary care. Experiences from 2 Workshops at the 15th WONCA World Conference 1998. *Scandinavian Journal of Primary Health Care.* **16**, 131-134.

Kvamme, O., Olesen, F. and Samuelsson, M. (2001) Improving the interface between primary and secondary care: a statement from the European working party on quality in family practice (EQuiP). *Quality in Health Care* **10**, 33-39.

Lee, D., Mackenzie, A., Dudley-Brown, S. and Chin, T. (1998) Case management: a review of definitions and practices. *Journal of Advanced Nursing* **27** (5), 933-939.

Leighton, Y., Clegg, A. and Bee, A. (2008) Evaluation of community matron services in a large metropolitan city in England. *Quality in Primary Care* **16**, 83-89.

Lewis, R. and Dixon, J. (2004) Rethinking management of chronic diseases. *British Medical Journal* **328** (7433), 220-222.

Lewis, G. (2007) Case Study: Virtual Wards at Croydon PCT. Available at: http://www.networks.nhs.uk/uploads/06/12/croydon_virtual_wards_case_study.pdf (accessed 7 January 2010).

Lewis, S. (2008) Case management. In: R. Neno and D. Price (eds) *The handbook for Advanced Primary Care Nurses.* Maidenhead: Open University Press.

Lyndon, H. (2007) Community matrons – a conduit for integrated working? *Journal of Integrated Care* **15** (6), 6-13.

Madden, H. (2008) Case study of an individual with a long-term condition. Unpublished work. Coventry.

Section 3

Metcalfe, J. (2005) The management of patients with long-term conditions. *Nursing Standard* **19** (45), 53-60.

Mitchell, G. (2008) Multidisciplinary care planning in the primary care management of completed stroke: a systematic review. *BMC Family Practitioner* **9**, 44.

Murray, M. (2009) Virtual ward pilot: North Leamington (lecture) 313 CPD, 12 Oct 2009. Coventry: Coventry University.

The National Collaborating Centre for Chronic Conditions (2004) *Multiple Sclerosis: National Clinical Guidelines for Diagnosis and Management in Primary and Secondary Care.* London: The Royal College of Physicians.

NHS Modernisation Agency & Skills for Health (2005) *Case Management Competencies Framework.* Department of Health (DH): London.

NHS Information Centre (2010) Available at: http://www.ic.nhs.uk/statistics-and-data-collections/audits-and-performance/the-quality-and-outcomes-framework (accessed 9 March 2010).

Office for National Statistics (ONS) England and Wales Census Data 2001. (2006) Available at: http//www.statistics.gov.uk/StatBase/ssdataset.asp?vlnk=7545&Pos=&ColRank=2&Rank=256 (accessed 9 May 2010).

Parker, H. and Glasby, J. (2008) The art of the possible: reforming community health services. *British Journal of Community Nursing* **13** (10), 480-486.

Partnership for Solutions (2002) Physician Concerns: Caring for People with Chronic Conditions. Johns Hopkins University, Baltimore. Available at: http://www.partnershipforsolutions.org/DMS/files/2002/physicianccern.pdf (accessed 5 January 2010).

Pinquart, M. and Sorrenson, D. (2003) Differences between care givers and non care givers in psychological health and physical health: a meta analysis. *Psychology and Ageing* **18**, 250-257.

Plsek, P. and Greenhalgh, T. (2001) The challenge of complexity in health care. *British Medical Journal* **323**, 625-628.

Randall, S., Dignon, A. Mills, N. (in press) *The impact of an in-reach nursing role for people with long-term conditions.* Journal of Nursing and Healthcare of Chronic Illness.

Roland, M., Dusheiko, M., Gravelle, H. and Parker, S. (2005) Follow up of people aged 65 and over with a history of emergency admissions: analysis of routine data. *British Medical Journal* **330**, 289-292.

Rosen, R. and Ham, C. (2008) *Integrated Care: Lessons from Evidence & Experience.* In: Report of the 2008 Sir Roger Bannister Annual Health Seminar. London: The Nuffield Trust.

Royal College of Nursing (RCN) (2007) *Adolescent Transition Care: Guidance for Nursing Staff.* London: Royal College of Nursing.

Sargent, P., Pickard, S. and Sheaff, R. (2007) Patient and carer perceptions of case management for long-term conditions. *Health and Social Care in the Community.* **15** (6), 511-519.

Scottish Census Data. (2001) Available at: http://www.scrol.gov.uk/scrol/common/home.jsp. (accessed 10 May 2010).

Scottish Executive (2009) Long-term Conditions Collaborative Programme. Available at: http://www.scotland.gov.uk/Topics/Health/NHS-Scotland/Delivery-Improvement/1835/210369 (accessed 2 January 2010).

Scottish Government (2009) Improving the Health and Wellbeing of People with Long-term Conditions in Scotland: A National Action Plan. Available at: http://www.scotland.gov.uk/Publications/2009/12/03112054/4 (accessed 11 October 2010).

Singh, D. (2005) *Transforming Chronic Care: Evidence about Improving Care for People with Long-term Conditions.* Birmingham: University of Birmingham and Surrey and Sussex PCT Alliance.

Singh, D. and Ham, C. (2005) *Improving Care for People with Long-term Conditions: A Review of UK and International Frameworks.* Birmingham: University of Birmingham and NHS Institute for Innovation and Improvement. Available at: http://www.download.bham.ac.uk/hsmc/pdf/improving_care_06.pdf (accessed 30 December 2009).

Thorne, S. (2008) Editorial: communication in chronic care: confronting the evidence in an era of system reform. *Journal of Clinical Nursing* **17** (11c), 294-297.

Thunhurst C. and Randall, S. (2010) Applied research: building the evidence base for health sector development. *International Journal of Therapy and Rehabilitation*.

Vecchiato, T. (2004) Care pathways. In: H. Nies and P. Berman (eds) *Integrating Services for Older People: A Resource Book for Managers*. Utrecht: European Health Management Association.

Wagner, E. (1998) Chronic disease management: what will It take to improve care for chronic illness? *Effective Clinical Practice* **1**, 2-4.

Wilson, P., Bunn, F. and Morgan, J. (2009) A mapping of the evidence on integrated long- term condition services. *British Journal of Community Nursing* **14** (5), 202-206.

Wells, G. (2007) *Case Finding (lecture) 313 CPD March*. Coventry: Coventry University.

Welsh Assembly Government (2007) *Service Improvement Plan 2007-2011: Designed to Improve Health and the Management of Chronic Conditions in Wales*. Cardiff: Welsh Assembly Government.

Werrett, J., Helm, R. and Carnwell, R. (2001) The primary and secondary care interface: the educational needs of nursing staff for the provision of seamless care. *Journal of Advanced Nursing* **34** (5), 629-638.

World Health Organisation (WHO) (2002) *Innovative Care for Chronic Conditions: Building Blocks for Action*. Geneva: WHO.

World Health Organisation (WHO) (2005) *The Challenge of Chronic Conditions: Preparing a Healthcare Workforce for the 21st Century*. Geneva: WHO.

Wright, K., Ryder, S. and Gousy, M. (2007) An evaluation of a community matron service from the patient's perspective. *British Journal of Community Nursing* **12** (9), 398-403.

Wright, L. and Leahey, M. (2000) *Nurses and Families*. Philadelphia: F.A. Davis.

Zapart, S., Kenny, P., Hall, J., Servis, B. and Wiley, S. (2007) Home based palliative care in Sydney, Australia: the carers perspective on the provision of informal care. *Health and Social Care in the Community* **15** (2), 97-107.

Resources

Birmingham Own Health Available at: www.birminghamownhealth.co.uk

Welsh Assembly Government Available at: www.wales.gov.uk

Scottish Executive Health Department Available at: www.scotland.gov.uk

Northern Ireland Department of Health, Social Services and Public Safety Available at: www.dhsspsni.gov.uk

Department of Health, England Available at: www.dh.gov.uk

The King's Fund Available at: www.kingsfund.org.uk

Singh D., Ham C. (2005) Improving care for people with long-term conditions: a review of UK and international frameworks. University of Birmingham and NHS Institute for Innovation and Improvement. Available at: http://www.download.bham.ac.uk/hsmc/pdf/improving_care_06.pdf:

Carers UK Available at: Helpline 0808 808 7777 www.carersuk.org

Carers Scotland Available at: www.carersscotland.org

Carers Northern Ireland Available at: www.carersni.org

Carers Wales Available at: www.carerswales.org

Crossroads Care Available at: www.crossroads.org.uk

Scotland Available at: www.crossroads-scotland.co.uk

Northern Ireland Available at: www.crossroadscare.co.uk

The Princess Royal Trust for Carers Available at: www.carers.org

Section 3

Further reading

Costello, J. (2009) *Caring for Someone with a Long-term Illness: Support for Family and Friends.* Manchester: Manchester University Press.

Robb, M. (ed) (2004) *Communication and Care.* London: Routledge.

McCabe, C. and Timmins, F. (2006) *Communication Skills for Nursing Practice.* Basingstoke: Palgrave Macmillan.

Chapter 9

Rehabilitation in Long-term Conditions

Bernie Davies and Jo Galloway

Learning objectives

After reading this chapter, the reader will have:

- Considered definitions and key concepts of rehabilitation
- Explored the role of rehabilitation in the management of long-term conditions (LTCs).
- Gained information on models and theories informing rehabilitation in LTCs
- Explained the role of interprofessional and multidisciplinary teams in rehabilitation
- Identified the principles and process of rehabilitation for people with LTCs
- Explored outcome measures and evaluation used in rehabilitation

Introduction

This chapter explores concepts underpinning rehabilitation practice in the management of LTCs. Key principles and the use of these in the rehabilitation process are discussed. The importance of teamwork and approaches to this in a variety of settings are considered. Case studies are used to illustrate the use of models in the practice, evaluation of rehabilitation and the implication of policy, ethical issues, and cultural needs for rehabilitation in LTCs.

Definitions and concepts of rehabilitation

Definitions of rehabilitation are many, varied, and often lengthy (see Table 9.1). Historically, they have not made the link between LTCs and rehabilitation explicit. However, taken together they do highlight some concepts and characteristics that are useful in explaining what rehabilitation is and considering how to go about it in relation to a range of conditions and settings. Interestingly, some

Long-term Conditions: A Guide for Nurses and Healthcare Professionals, First Edition. Edited by S. Randall and H. Ford.
© 2011 Blackwell Publishing Ltd. Published 2011 by Blackwell Publishing Ltd.

Table 9.1 Rehabilitation definitions and concepts.

Definitions	Concepts and Characteristics
Rehabilitation is an active intervention to achieve maximum function and to improve quality of life (Hoeman 2008). Rehabilitation of people with disabilities is a process aimed at enabling them to reach and maintain their optimal physical, sensory, intellectual, psychological and social functional levels. Rehabilitation provides disabled people with the tools they need to attain independence and self-determination. (WHO – http://www.who.int/topics/rehabilitation/en/) An educational, problem-solving process aimed at reducing disability and handicap (Wade 1996) The process by which an individual's movement towards health is facilitated (Dittmar 1989, Kumar 2000); Reynolds 2005) An enabling process in which sometimes communities, agencies and professionals meet the social, psychological and economic needs of the disabled person (Baker et al. 1997) An active process which seeks to reduce the effects of disease (in its broadest sense) on daily life (Greenwood et al. 1993) An active process by which those disabled by injury/ disease achieve a full recovery, or if a full recovery is not possible, realise their optimum physical mental and social potential, and are integrated into the most appropriate environment (British Geriatrics Society 2005)	Active process Autonomy Community Disabilities Education Environment Facilitation Health Holistic Independence Interdisciplinary Optimal functioning Problem-solving Process Quality of life Teamwork

rehabilitation texts, for example Kumar (2000) and Reynolds (2005), focus on explaining concepts rather than providing overarching definitions. This serves to emphasise the complex and varied nature of rehabilitation.

Nolan and Nolan (1999) suggest that with policy now addressing 'chronic illness' there is a call for rehabilitation to be reconceptualised away from a traditional focus on 'cure'. Undoubtedly, the nature of rehabilitation is indeed influenced by policy and also by history. According to Squires (2002) rehabilitation services started to develop during the 1950s following the Second World War. As a result of the large number of casualties among service personnel, military and work forces were depleted, creating a need to get the wounded fit and back into work. Healthcare and physical training staff leaving military services added to the rehabilitation workforce and the polio epidemic of the 1950s increased the numbers of people with disabilities in need of rehabilitation. Despite these early efforts, Davis and Madden (2006) identified that rehabilitation was underfunded and services lacked ownership, resulting in inadequate provision which for many failed to meet their needs. In the 1970s and 1980s increasing awareness of disability did lead to developments in rehabilitation services, though more in the community than in hospitals (Smith 1999).

Until recently, when more priority was given to rehabilitation with the introduction of the NHS Plan (Department of Health (DH) 2000) and the National Service Framework (NSF) for Older People (DH 2001), and more recently, Transforming Community Service (DH 2009a) many people thought of 'rehabilitation' as a place patients would be sent to and gave the idea little consideration beyond that. Rehabilitation was something that 'happened' in a set place for a particular length of time (Davis 2006, Jester 2007). Most commonly, it was seen as happening as part of an acute episode, such as after an accident (orthopaedic rehabilitation, for example), or in relation to age (historically 'geriatric rehabilitation') or as a short-term phase of the recovery process after a life threatening medical event (for example stroke and cardiac rehabilitation after a myocardial infarction). That it was time limited may have been reinforced by policies such as the NSF for Older People (DH 2001) which identifies re-habilitation as a function of intermediate care (IC). The purpose of IC is to support the transition from hospital care to independent living in the community. It aims to prevent the 'revolving door' scenario, where patients are discharged but then rapidly readmitted, as can often be the case for individuals with LTCs. As policy limits provision of IC services to a fixed period of 6 weeks, some may continue to view rehabilitation as a relatively short-term endeavour. However, it is now clear that rehabilitation is not only an inpatient, but also a community-based activity. In practice, as will be seen in this chapter, it may continue not just for weeks, but for months and even years. It is now argued that rehabilitation should be defined, not as a separate service, but as an underpinning philosophy (DH 2009b).

Summary

This section has presented some of the many definitions of rehabilitation that can be found within the literature. Key concepts within these definitions have been identified. These concepts are helpful in informing the practice of rehabilitation which can be summarised as a holistic process to educate, empower and advocate for individuals in order to achieve personalised goals, maximum independence and quality of life.

The role of rehabilitation in the context of managing LTCs

Rehabilitation is delivered in a diversity of settings – both within secondary care and in the community; services are similarly disparate and range from short-term intervention to longer-term support. Over recent years there has been a shift towards increased community service provision which has witnessed the development of new service models that include, for example, admission avoidance, reablement and IC. The Transforming Community Services Programme was established to support the NHS to deliver modern and responsive community services of a consistently high standard (DH 2009a), and is central to the achievement of the ambitions set out in 'High Quality Care for All' (DH 2008).

The Transforming Community Services best practice rehabilitation guide (DH 2009b) is based on a framework of 'ambition, action and achievement' and addresses what is considered to be best practice in the delivery of community rehabilitation services. The evidence-based practice component includes a number of recommended actions, examples of which are outlined in Table 9.2.

Healthcare systems currently face a number of challenges that include an ageing population, increasing prevalence of LTCs together with a significant financial challenge and rising consumer expectations. National priorities include a focus on the achievement of high quality care that is fair, personalised, effective and safe (DH 2008). There is, therefore, a significant challenge in im-proving quality in the context of limited additional investment. The Quality, Innovation, Productivity and Partnership (QIPP) challenge outlines the DH's plan to respond to the financial challenge by

Section 3

Table 9.2 Recommended actions for rehabilitation services.

Provide rehabilitation in the community	Important components of community rehabilitation services include: • Social support • Carer involvement • Physiotherapy and occupational therapy • Good links between community and hospital services • Multidisciplinary team • Acceptable and accessible premises for service users
Multifaceted rehabilitation is most effective	The most successful rehabilitation services include: • Personalised care plans • Physical and cognitive therapies • Regular practice • Proactive follow-up
Multidisciplinary teams improve rehabilitation	Six factors have been identified as having impact on how well teams work together in healthcare: • Team size • Multiprofessional composition • Good organisational support and equipment • Regular team meetings • Clear goals and objectives • Regular audit and review

Source: Adapted from *Transforming Community Services: Ambition, Action, Achievement - Transforming Rehabilitation Services* (Department of Health 2009b)

focusing on improving quality and productivity while making efficiency savings. There are a number of national QIPP work streams including one on LTCs; further information can be found at www.dh.gov.uk/qualityandproductivity.

Table 9.3 summarises some of the national priorities for healthcare, together with suggested opportunities for their achievement within contemporary rehabilitation practice of LTCs.

Table 9.3 National healthcare priorities and application to rehabilitation.

Priority area	Opportunities for Application to Rehabilitation
Patient involvement and empowerment	• Person-centred assessment • Integrated care pathways • Goal setting • Self-monitoring, for example use of assistive technology
Choice	• Personalised budgets • Appointment dates and times
Public health	• Information • Health trainers • Peer support

Case study 9.1 Edwin Bates

A safeguarding referral is made by a domiciliary care worker; the referral relates to her finding one of her clients secured to a chair with a belt. Edwin Bates is a 79-year-old man who lives with his wife; he has dementia and a history of recurrent falls. Background information is collated through discussions with health and social care professionals involved in Mr Bates care and a visit is arranged to meet up with Mr and Mrs Bates. The visit includes the client's Admiral Nurse together with the safeguarding nurse from the Primary Care Trust. During the visit it is established that Mrs Bates restrains her husband to enable her to get on with daily chores without having to worry about him falling over and hurting himself. When she is told that she should not restrain him in this way she becomes tearful and says that she is worried about her husband falling and ending up in hospital. She relates a recent experience where her husband sustained a fall; was subsequently admitted to hospital and during his stay became very agitated and distressed.

Following discussion it is agreed that a referral will be made to the Specialist Falls Service to assess Mr Bates and provide advice regarding falls prevention. A discussion takes place regarding opportunities to adapt the couple's daily routine in order to accommodate the needs of both Mr and Mrs Bates, whilst also maintaining Mr Bates' safety. Mrs Bates is also provided with information regarding carer support and voluntary organisations such as the Alzheimer's Association.

Points for reflection

- How can family members acting as carers contribute to the rehabilitation of relatives with dementia?
- How might the needs of carers supporting rehabilitation in the community be addressed?

- The initial investigation revealed that Mrs Bates appeared to be restraining her husband to maintain his safety and prevent him from experiencing harm. Ensuring Mr Bates' welfare must be paramount and it should be ensured that his dignity is maintained by all involved in his care.
- Caring for someone with dementia can be physically and emotionally challenging and can lead to social isolation. Similarly, caring can be positive and rewarding and many carers relate how they get satisfaction from helping the person, and how they continue to have good times together (DH 2007). It is important to recognise the important role and contribution of informal carers in supporting people who have dementia. One of 17 objectives in the national Dementia Strategy (DH 2009c) includes implementing the Carer's Strategy. This includes the right for carers to have an assessment of their needs, together with opportunities for breaks and other support.
- Admiral Nurses are mental health nurses specialising in dementia who work with family carers and people with dementia, both in the community and other settings. Admiral Nurses focus on improving the quality of life for people with dementia and their carers. They employ a variety of therapeutic interventions that help people live positively with the condition and develop skills to improve communication and maintain relationships. (Dementia UK 2010)

Section 3

- People with dementia can suffer accidents and falls which require frequent hospital admissions and may spend longer than is necessary in hospital because they cannot manage in their home without support. A rehabilitation approach that includes occupational therapy, physiotherapy and specialist equipment, plus help with personal care, can maximise independence for people with dementia and reduce their need for hospital admission.
- A risk stratification tool can be used to calculate a risk score for individuals in a given population. This can be applied to people with dementia who are at high risk of being admitted to secondary care (predictive modelling; for further information, see Chapter 8). Use of such tools facilitates a proactive approach to LTC management that allows resources to be targeted at the right people.
- Every year one-third of people aged 65 and above sustain a fall (NHS Choices 2010). Falls can result in serious injury, and loss of independence and confidence. Falls prevention services can provide:
  - assessment and identification of risk factors;
  - support and advice regarding bone health and osteoporosis;
  - recommendations about risk reduction;
  - referral for treatment, physiotherapy, home adaptations, etc.

Further information can be found on the NHS Choices website http://www.nhs.uk/Livewell/Staywellover50/Pages/Fallsprevention.aspx.

Summary

In recent years, the number of people living with LTCs has increased, leading to a corresponding increase in the need for rehabilitation. Health and social care policies increasingly recognise this need and seek to support the provision of rehabilitation in a variety of settings. The need for and value of rehabilitation within community settings is highlighted, as is the requirement for an integrated approach and seamless transition between services. Rehabilitation aims to empower the individual and to enable them to adapt to LTCs and achieve their maximum potential. This presents many challenges, including how best to manage resources in order to maintain and improve services.

Models and theories informing rehabilitation

It is worth considering some of the main theories, models and concepts relating to rehabilitation, and in particular how these apply to LTCs, as they inform the principles discussed later in this chapter. Some, though not all, of the available theoretical frameworks are considered here including the following:

- Disability
- Chronicity
- Illness trajectory
- Disablement-Enablement process
- Adaptation
- Activities of daily living

Section 3

Table 9.4 Models of disability.

Individual	Social	Integrated
Based on the biomedical model, with a focus on the disease process, leading to either cure or death	Where disability is seen as being created by societies attitudes. Society creates barriers to independence.	Intended to integrate the individual and social model. One integrated model developed by WHO is known as *The International Classification of Functioning, Disability and Health* (ICF). This model considers the health or disease of the individual and the effect of this on body structure and functioning, along with personal and environment factors. It is available on WHO website at http://apps.who.int/classifications/icfbrowser.

- Approaches to care delivery including the care pathway approach
- Culture
- Role functions

The World Health Organisation (WHO) (2001) refers to LTCs as 'chronic diseases' and identifies these as a major cause of disability. WHO states that its 'role is to enhance the quality of life, and promote and protect the rights and dignity of people with disabilities', and advocates rehabilitation as one means of fulfilling this role. The two concepts identified here - *disability* and *chronicity* - are used in a number of rehabilitation models, though not necessarily always together.

Disability

Models of disability can be categorised into three types: individual, social and integrated (Lutz and Davis 2008). See Table 9.4.

The WHO (2001) model, The International Classification for Functioning, Disability and Health (also known as ICF), provides one framework to facilitate a shared global understanding of disability and rehabilitation. By taking into account the social, political and cultural aspects of disability the framework encourages a holistic approach to empowering and rehabilitating individuals with disability. The framework is not without its critics and is currently being reviewed by the WHO as part of the 2006-2011 action plan (http://www.who.int/disabilities/publications/dar_action_plan_2006to2011.pdf). However, it is widely used to inform research, to facilitate common understanding between disciplines and to direct care planning.

The ICF framework replaced an earlier model, the International Classification of Impairments, Disabilities and Handicap (ICIDH) (WHO 1980). The revised framework reflects changing attitudes to disability, including a move away from the biomedical model. This more integrated model has developed in parallel with the global increase in the numbers of people living with LTCs who are able to benefit from rehabilitation.

There are detailed codes available within the ICF related to specific problems and conditions. For more detailed information, the reader is directed to the checklists at http://www.who.int/classifications/icf/training/icfchecklist.pdf.

Section 3

Table 9.5   Definitions of ICF terms.

Definition of terms used in ICF checklist version 2.1a (2003)	
Term	Definition
Body functions	The physiological functions of the body systems (including psychological functions)
Body function impairments	Problems in body function as a significant deviation or loss
Body structures	Anatomical parts of the body such as organs, limbs and their components
Body structure impairments	Problems in structure as a significant deviation or loss
Activities	The execution of a task or action by the individual
Participation	Involvement in a life situation
Activity limitation	Difficulties an individual may have in executing activities
Participation restriction	Problems an individual may have in involvement in life situations
Environment factors	The physical, social and attitudinal environment in which people live and conduct their lives

Source: http://www.who.int/classifications/icf/training/icfchecklist.pdf

The ICF codes and checklist can be used to elicit and record information relating to an individual's disability and functioning under the following headings:

- Impairments of *body functions*
- Impairments of *body structures*
- *Activities* limitations and *participation restrictions*
- *Environment factors*

These are explained in more detail in Table 9.5.

Chronicity

The Corbin and Strauss chronic illness trajectory model, (Corbin 1998) is intended as a nursing model for use in a range of chronic (i.e. long-term) conditions. The model identifies the stages an individual passes through from the pre-trajectory stage, where risk factors are recognised (or at least present) to the onset of symptoms and then through various stages leading to the final stage of dying. Though set out as a linear model, in reality the individual with an LTC is likely to move backward and forward between stages as intermittently they experience 'acute on chronic' episodes. At each stage of the model there is opportunity for rehabilitation. The type and purpose of the rehabilitation interventions depend on the stage of the trajectory reached. For example, at the *Pre-trajectory* stage of a condition such as diabetes mellitus, rehabilitation will focus on health promotion and adoption of life style changes. Following *Unstable* phases and *Acute* phases, the aim will be to support return to a *Stable* phase. Disease progression may result in a *Crisis* phase (a critical or life-threatening situation), perhaps as a result of cardiovascular complications, after which rehabilitation will centre on achieving an acceptable quality of life within the limitations of illness/disability (the *Comeback* phase). Further complications leading to increasing disability, for example due to renal or vascular disease, characterise the *Downward* phase. Rehabilitation here will relate to adaptation and psychological adjustment to limitation before the final stage of the trajectory, *Dying*, focuses on the final weeks or days of life, and facilitation to a peaceful death. For more information on the use of the trajectory model and its relationship to rehabilitation in LTCs, the reader is directed to the 'Further reading' at the end of this chapter.

Enabling–disabling process

The Enabling–Disabling process model was developed by the American Institute of Medicine (IOM) and includes the premise that 'Rehabilitation strives to reverse what has been called the disabling process and may therefore be called the enabling process' (Brandt and Pope 1997: 13). The elements of this model are summarised by Remsberg and Carson (2006). The model has five basic concepts:

1. Pathology
2. Impairment
3. Functional limitations
4. Disability
5. Social limitations

As for the ICF, the Enabling–Disabling Process Model can be categorised as an integrated model. The model recognises that the outcome of pathology is not necessarily disability and that for specific impairment the level of disability will vary between individuals. Disability will be influenced by the contextual aspects of disability which include the following:

- Biological factors:
  - Co-morbidities
  - Physical conditions
  - Genetic make-up
- Environmental factors:
  - Societal prejudices
  - Availability of services
  - Reimbursement mechanisms
- Lifestyle factors:
  - Smoking
  - Alcohol use
  - Diet
  - Exercise

Case study 9.2 Bill Jones

Bill Jones is 76-year-old former coal miner. He lives in a bungalow with his 70-year-old wife, Betty. Bill considered himself fortunate to have kept his job at one of the few coal mines to have stayed open following the widespread closures in the 1980s. However, during his last few years before retirement Bill's health deteriorated and he suffered from frequent chest infections. He was diagnosed with Chronic Obstructive Pulmonary Disease (COPD) just as he and Betty were starting to enjoy retirement, spending time with their grown-up children and helping to look after their young grandchildren. Even though his condition is deteriorating and he is increasingly short of breath, Bill will not give up smoking. After several acute chest infections, each leaving him a little more breathless than the last, Bill has become increasingly short-tempered with his family and has been diagnosed with depression. He mostly forgets or refuses to take the antidepressants prescribed, much to Betty's distress. Betty spends much of her time attending to Bill and his needs. She washes and dresses him in the morning, as she claims he is too puffed to do this himself. Then, she settles him into his favourite chair for the day and fetches and carries meals, cigarettes, newspapers, books, and the TV remote control. Their children rely on Betty to help care for their own children, but are reluctant to bring them to the bungalow, asking Betty to go to their homes instead. Recently, Betty has been suffering from frequent headaches, so she goes to see her GP, who finds she is suffering from stress.

Points for reflection

- What can theoretical frameworks offer to staff contributing to the rehabilitation of individuals with COPD such as Bill Jones?
- Consider what cultural issues might influence rehabilitation in LTCs and how professionals might address these?

- It is likely that Betty's concern for Bill and her role in caring for him and her wider family is the cause of Betty's stress. If Bill were to be provided with benefit from appropriate rehabilitation, Betty and the wider family's quality of life may improve. As Bill progresses through the disease trajectory, Betty's role as a carer will be increasingly important if he is to adapt to his limitations and maintain the best possible quality of life. Betty's needs for support must be considered so she can be enabled to continue her role, therefore, a carer assessment should be offered.
- The implications of culture need to be addressed. Culture concerns the values, beliefs and role identity, and is socially constructed (Padilla 2000). Betty may unintentionally hinder rehabilitation, seeing her role as 'taking care of' Bill, providing 'hands on' care. The value of a more 'hands off' approach can be explained to her. Working in a traditional mining culture, Bill is likely to have been frustrated by the onset of COPD and the impact of this on his role and self-image. This may be a contributing factor in depression, and might be anticipated as depression is common in LTCs (Haddad, Taylor and Pilling 2009). Members of the mental health team will contribute specialist assessment and interventions as part of the rehabilitation process.
- Pulmonary rehabilitation should be available to all who need it (National Institute for Clinical Excellence 2004), and therefore should be provided to Bill. It is now recognised that specialist pulmonary rehabilitation should be introduced at an early stage in order to improve functioning and slow disease progression (Gulrajani 2010). However, at the time of Bill's diagnosis it is unlikely this would have been available.
- Pulmonary rehabilitation interventions include smoking cessation support. Bill has so far refused to stop smoking, which creates an ethical dilemma. It may be Bill can be persuaded to reconsider if support is offered. Therefore, the benefits of smoking cessation should be explained. Reasons for continuing to smoke should be explored and strategies for cutting down on or stopping smoking should be explained. However, from an ethical perspective, if Bill chooses to smoke, his autonomy must be respected.

- A care pathway approach will help to structure Bill's care and rehabilitation. A COPD pathway will encourage enablement and self-management as far as possible.

Adaptation

Frequently in LTCs, it is not realistic to expect rehabilitation to return individuals to the same level of health and functioning as they had before the onset of their condition. Rather, the aim of rehabilitation is to help them to adapt to the realities of their situation, and to optimise health and functioning within the constraints they have (for further discussion on adaptation, see Chapter 4). The Roy Adaptation Model (Roy and Andrews 1999) is a nursing model, sometimes used in rehabilitation, which views human beings as 'adaptive systems'. Davis and Madden (2006) relate adaptation to both personal factors and coping styles, and suggest there is, therefore, a commonality between adaptation and the ICF.

Activities of daily living

The concept of 'Activities of Daily Living' (ADLs) is used within both Occupational Therapy and Nursing to inform rehabilitation assessments and interventions. Roper et al. (1990) and Orem (1991) both developed models of nursing based on ADLs and their role in promoting independence.

ADLs are integral to the FIM/FAM model discussed in the 'Outcome measurement' section of this chapter.

Culture

Culture is too complex a concept to explore in detail here. The reader is directed to Padilla (2000) for an in-depth discussion of the impact of culture on rehabilitation. However, everyone has a socially constructed cultural identity which influences the way they view themselves and their role. Cultural identify shapes attitudes and behaviour, and thus approaches to rehabilitation. There are many influences on cultural identity. These include not only the popularly identified issues of ethnicity and religion, but also social class, gender, age, sexuality, health, community, family and profession. Professional culture provides a view of rehabilitation which may be at variance with that of patients and their families (Pryor and O'Connell 2008). Rehabilitation professionals need to show cultural sensitivity, which should be neither predictive nor prescriptive and should recognise that they are under the influence of their own culture (Padilla 2000).

Role functions

The Royal College of Nursing (2007b) identify four role functions carried out by nurses engaged in the rehabilitation of older people, as illustrated in Figure 9.1.

In practice, these role functions and the majority of the components within them have relevance to any professional, regardless of their discipline. These concepts can be related to the rehabilitation of all individuals with LTCs, no matter what age they are. The components of these role functions are summarised in Table 9.6.

Section 3

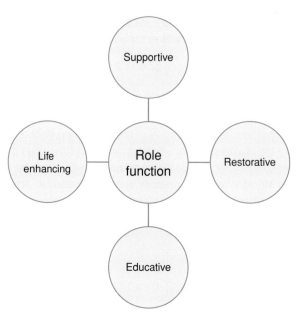

Figure 9.1   RCN role functions.

Table 9.6   Components of RCN role functions.

Role functions	Components
Supportive	• Psychosocial support • Emotional support • Assisting with transition and life review • Enhancing lifestyles and relationships • Facilitating self-expression • Ensuring cultural sensitivity
Restorative	• Aimed at maximising independence and functional ability • Preventing further deterioration and/or disability • Enhancing quality of life • Includes assessment skills • Undertaking essential care elements
Educative	• Teaching self-care (for example health promotion, self-medication) • Facilitating educational activities to increase competence and confidence in activities of daily living
Life enhancing	• All activities aimed at enhancing daily living experience, including, for example: • Relieving pain • Ensuring adequate nutrition

Source: Adapted from: The Royal College of Nursing (2007a) *Maximising Independence: The Role of the Nurse in the Rehabilitation of Older People*. London: Royal College of Nursing

R	Reablement
E	Education
H	Holistic
A	Active engagement
B	Be innovative and creative
I	Interprofessional
L	Life enhancing
I	Individualised
T	Teamwork
A	Advocate
T	Targets
I	Inspiring
O	Outcome based
N	Negotiation

Figure 9.2 Rehabilitation key components model.

Rehabilitation key components model

It is beyond the scope of this chapter to discuss every available rehabilitation theory and model. Some key components of rehabilitation process and approaches are encapsulated in the model shown in Figure 9.2.

Summary

A number of models and theories – some generic, some profession-specific – may be used to underpin rehabilitation. These include biomedical models, social models and integrated models. Theory relating to roles, culture, holism and adaptation also informs rehabilitation practice.

Population changes, along with developments in medicine and technology, lead to increasing numbers of people living with LTCs, may have potential for rehabilitation. Models are developing to accommodate changes in society and its attitudes to disability. This is reflected in the WHO classification system amendments and ongoing discussion around further development of the model.

Teams and teamwork in rehabilitation

Teamwork is essential in rehabilitation. Each member of the team will have their own expertise, but by working together, they are able to see the individual, not as an isolated diagnosis or dysfunctions, such as 'shuffling gait' or 'Parkinson's' but as a whole person (Latella 2000).

Section 3

Table 9.7   Approaches to teamwork.

Multidisciplinary	Interdisciplinary	Transdisciplinary
A team made up of professionals from a number of disciplines (for example, social work, nursing, dietetics, physiotherapy) who work in parallel rather than collaboratively. Each discipline sets thier own goals and works independently within their own discipline-specific boundaries to achieve these. Team members may have limited understanding of each other's asessments, goals and interventions. Team meetings are held to discuss progress. The client has a minimal role.	Team members from different disciplines communicate with each other to collaborate to set and share common goals. They have a good understanding of each other's roles.	Transdisciplinary teams are designed to minimise duplication of service. Team members work flexibly and there is blurring of professional role boundaries, and therefore cross-training is required. Team leaders may be from any of the professions within the team and may be choosen according to the needs of each client.

Source: Based on Reynolds (2005), Latella (2000) and Whitelock (1999)

In rehabilitation, teams may be defined by their purpose or by their approach. The approaches are commonly identified as being either *multidisciplinary, interdisciplinary* or *transdisciplinary* (Smith 1999, Latella 2000) (see Table 9.7). Alternatively, the term '*multiprofessional'* is used, for example by Long et al. (2002). It is argued that the term 'discipline' may be preferable to 'professional' as it allows for a wider membership (Clouder and Smith 2010) and indeed, the latter would exclude some of the potential team member identified below, including the most crucial member, the individual in need of rehabilitation.

An example of a team described by its purpose would be an *accelerated transfer team*, such as one made up of nurses, occupational therapists and physiotherapists. Designed to support a smooth and rapid transfer of joint replacement of patients from home to surgery and home again, the patient is visited by one member of the team at least daily. During the visit, observations are recorded, dressings are checked and replaced if need be, new exercises are taught and supervised, and activites of living are facilitated. One visit may be from an occupational therapist, the next from a nurse. Though named after their purpose, in this case the approach is that of a transdisciplinary team.

In America, some certified nursing assistants have transdisciplinary roles (Latella 2000), working across the boundaries of a number of rehabilitaion professional roles. In the United Kingdom, a similar model is being developed for care assistants undertaking foundation degrees related to an area of care, such as rehabilitation. Arguably, however, if they are working in teams where other professionals stay within their traditional role boundaries, such care assitants, though transdiscplinary workers, will be members of interprofessional rather than transdisciplinary teams.

Depending on the needs of the individuals, there are many potential members in the rehabilitation team (see Figure 9.3), they may be professionals or family members, paid or not, involved for a short time or on a continual basis. Informal carers and voluntary agencies may be as essential to achieving

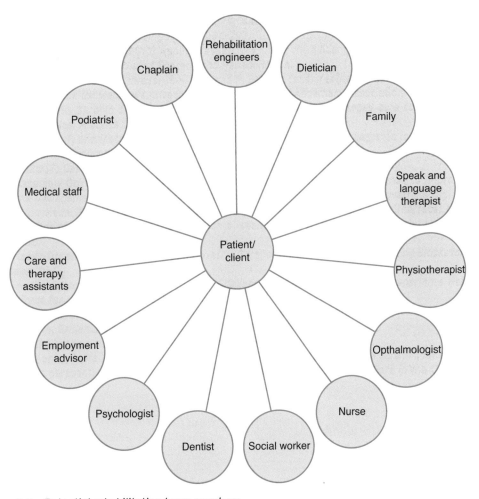

Figure 9.3 Potential rehabilitation team members.

an individual's goals as the professionals; therefore, they must be recognised as team members. Table 9.8 gives examples of team members' roles.

It is widely recognised that in health and social care effective interprofessional teamwork and collaborative practice can improve health outcomes. It has also been recognised that there are barriers to effective teamwork. Interprofessional education is advocated as a means of improving teamwork and overcoming these barriers (WHO 2010). Reynolds (2005) explored the evidence base underpinning interprofessional team working in order to identify strategies for enhancing interprofessional teamwork in rehabilitation. These are summarised as follows:

- Develop clear objectives and goals for the team as a whole.
- Promote ongoing education about professional roles.
- Take part in education about teamwork and group dynamics.
- Work in smaller, more cohesive teams where possible.
- Attend to processes of decision-making in the team.

Section 3

Table 9.8   Role profiles.

Team member	Role profile
Social worker	Have a role in assessment, carer support, setting up care packages to support people living in their own home where possible, provision of adaptations and equipment, and in accessing financial support, such as benefits.
Rehabilitation engineer	Sometimes also called an assistive technologist. Rehabilitation engineers use the clinical application of engineering principles and technology in the provision of services, research, and development to meet the needs of individuals with disabilities. They are involved in the reduction of environmental barriers, and contribute to the restoration or improvement of the physical, mental and social function of a person with a disability. They work in areas including wheelchair services, prosthetics and accessibility. See Chapter 6 for further details.
Psychologist	Psychologists working in rehabilitation provide cognitive and behavioural therapies to both patients and families. They undertake specialist assessment and apply knowledge of psychosocial principles and/or neuropsychology to assist individuals to overcome physical, sociological, cognitive and developmental barriers to functioning related to disability and LTCs. They can contribute to vocational rehabilitation. Psychologists work in both hospital and community settings.
Chaplain	A chaplain provides spiritual and emotional support to individuals who wish to receive it and also for their families. Chaplains are members of the clergy, for example either a priest, pastor, rabbi or imam. They visit individuals who are unable to attend their usual place of worship, for example when they are in hospital. Staff may also be advised by chaplains, particularly when emotionally or ethically challenging situations arise.
Podiatrist	May work in the hospital or community. They treat and prevent foot problems. Those working in the NHS give priority to patients whose mobility is impaired by foot pathologies.
Speech and language therapist	Provide assessment and treatment related to speech, communication and swallowing problems. They have a role in reducing the risk of aspiration during feeding and in interventions to improve speech. They advise patients, families and staff.
Employment advisor	Have a role in vocational rehabilitation. They help to get people back into, and to enable them to stay in, work.
Dietician	Assess nutritional needs and advise on how they might be met. They are involved when enteral feeding is required. Their role includes health promotion.
Ophthalmologist	Contribute to rehabilitation by assessing and, where possible, correcting problems related to vision.

- Have shared assessment strategies, care pathways and systems of record keeping.
- Rotate leadership.
- Attend to 'mundane' barriers to teamwork, such as poor accommodation.
- Give time and attention to team building.
- Regard the patient as a member of the interprofessional team.

In reality, the make-up of the rehabilitation team will be fluid, with membership depending on the needs of individual patients. Latella (2000) suggests that it is the core members of the team, those who work together on a daily basis, who are responsible for developing team processes and operational guidelines. Professionals who, by virtue of their role, work across many teams (for example psychologists or dentists) still need to be able to work effectively within these teams. Interprofessional education at pre- and post-qualifying levels aims to empower all health and social care professionals to overcome barriers to teamwork. Barriers may relate to lack of understanding of role, issues around commitment, conflict and its resolution, philosophical agreement, trust, power, and shared responsibility (Squires and Hastings 2002, Reynolds 2005).

Case study 9.3   Jane

Jane is single, 44-years-old and works in a bank. She developed Type 1 diabetes mellitus as a teenager and while living with her parents, managed her condition well. Fifteen years ago she bought her own house and moved away from her parents. Her job became increasingly demanding, but Jane thought she was coping well, managing the pressure by going out with friends, drinking heavily and occasionally smoking. When she developed a sore on her foot, she ignored it. When it did not heal, she was shocked to be diagnosed with peripheral vascular disease, which led to a recent below knee amputation and Jane being issued with a wheelchair. Jane has also developed retinopathy and renal insufficiency, which she has been warned may progress and result in her needing renal dialysis. Her response was to say that she would never go on dialysis and she just wanted to get on with her life and get back to work. However, she said she would never be able to get around the bank or be able to see over the counter now, because of the wheelchair.

Points for reflection

- How might psychological needs affect rehabilitation of individuals with LTCs such as diabetes and how might these be addressed?
- Consider the focus of rehabilitation for individuals with diabetes at different stages of the chronic illness trajectory. What are the implications of this for vocational rehabilitation?

- Jane's rehabilitation needs are complex (as she has multiple pathologies, Jane will have contact with several medical specialities) and require a holistic approach, taking into account not only physical, but psychological and social aspects as well. Key areas where rehabilitation is required relate to amputation itself, management of diabetes and vocational rehabilitation to enable Jane to return to work.

Section 3

- Preparation for rehabilitation should start pre-operatively, with members of the team including medical and nursing staff, physiotherapists, occupational therapists and dieticians all contributing to care. Smith (1999) highlights the need for professionals working in acute care, including surgery to recognise their role in the rehabilitation process.
- Rehabilitation will continue post-operatively and following discharge back into the community; therefore, different members of the interprofessional rehabilitation team will have their greatest involvement at different stages. Effective teamwork, including communication, is key to providing a seamless service as Jane progresses through her rehabilitation journey.
- Jane had managed her diabetes well in the past, and rehabilitation can enable her do so again. The reasons for her becoming less well controlled should be explored, but may be a result of work-related stress and her chosen coping strategies. As an individual with an LTC, Jane is at increased risk of depression and mental health problems (Haddad, Taylor and Pilling 2009) and there is, possibly as a result of co-morbidity, an increased risk of psychological distress following diabetes-related amputation (Coffey et al. 2009). For further discussion on the management of depression, see Chapter 3.
- Equipment provided through rehabilitation engineering services, including prosthetics and wheelchairs, will be vital in helping Jane return to work. It can be tailored to her specific needs. For example, a wheelchair that can be raised to a high-sitting position so that she can reach counters at work. This would also allow Jane to be at a similar level to friends who are standing, so she can hold conversations more easily in social situations.
- All rehabilitation interventions, including life style management and equipment provision must be agreed in negotiation with Jane and a paternalistic approach avoided, even though she may make decisions about her own care which professionals find hard to accept. Though she will understand the potential consequences of not maintaining good blood sugar control, she may chose not to do so. She has indicated that she would not wish to have dialysis (and thus further rehabilitation adapting to this would require). Should the need arise, Jane should have the information and opportunity for discussion to allow her to make an informed decision. Respecting the principle of autonomy, her decision is accepted.

Summary

Rehabilitation is a team endeavour. This section has discussed approaches to teamwork including multidisciplinary, interdisciplinary and transdisciplinary models of team working. The role of interprofessional education in overcoming barriers to teamwork has been identified. There are many potential members in a rehabilitation team and the actual make-up of it will depend on the needs of the individual requiring rehabilitation. This individual should be recognised as the most important member of the rehabilitation team.

The principles and process of rehabilitation for people with LTCs

It is important to recognise that rehabilitation pathways for people with LTCs will not always follow a linear progression. LTCs are characterised by their chronicity, and therefore rehabilitation programmes need to be dynamic and responsive in order to adapt to periods of regression in the person's physical and psychological health.

Section 3

Principles of rehabilitation

These include:

- Commence rehabilitation as soon as possible after the onset of illness.
- Complete a systematic and holistic patient assessment to use as the foundation for the rehabilitation plan.
- Rehabilitation should be person-centred, and patients and carers should be central to the rehabilitation process at all stages.
- Coordinate the development of an integrated rehabilitation plan with the patient, their carer, and relevant health and social care professionals.
- The integrated rehabilitation plan should include goal setting, interventions by MDT members and clear review dates.
- Provide the patient with appropriate information and literature to inform health, well-being and self-care.
- The rehabilitation approach should be condition specific, evidence based and reflect best practice.

Patient progress should be evaluated regularly – the frequency dependent on their condition.

The rehabilitation process

In practice, the principles and processes of rehabilitation are inextricably linked. However, components of the process are considered separately below.

Holism and the rehabilitation process

Many definitions and models of rehabilitation advocate a holistic approach to the rehabilitation process. The concept of holism is represented by Figure 9.4.

The diagram illustrates the interactions between the various elements, all of which have an influence on rehabilitation outcomes. For example, a person who has an initial hemiplegia following a

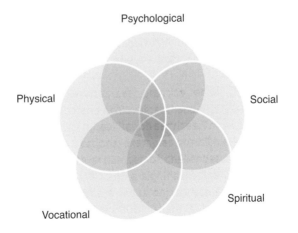

Figure 9.4 Elements of holism.

Section 3

stroke may make a good physical recovery, yet be reluctant to return to independence due to a lack of confidence or motivation. There may be psychological, social or spiritual factors contributing to this, and these need to be identified and addressed as part of a holistic approach.

Case study 9.4 Vera

Vera is a 68-year-old widow and is about to be transferred from a medical ward to IC. Vera has congestive cardiac failure with a poor long-term prognosis. She also has severe pain in her hips and knees due to osteoarthritis, which limits her mobility. She can only move from sitting to standing with assistance and can only walk a few steps at a very slow pace, partly because of her arthritis, but also because she is very short of breath. At 35 stone, Vera is classed as bariatric. It has taken some time to organise suitable transport to take Vera home. There are concerns about the likely ongoing care needs Vera may have, particularly in the longer term and it has been suggested that since at least two carers are needed for each visit and the level of care needed, it would be more cost-effective simply to transfer Vera to a care home.

Points for reflection

- What should be done to facilitate a successful return to the community following hospital admission related to LTCs?
- What processes and tool might be used to set appropriate rehabilitation goals for individuals such as Vera? What elements should be included within these goals?

- As part of effective rehabilitation, discharge planning should be started as soon as possible after admission in order to avoid unnecessarily prolonging hospitalisation. The needs of the increasing population of bariatric patients should be anticipated to prevent delay in providing specialist equipment needed at home. For example, Vera may need a wide walking frame or other equipment.
- An interprofessional home assessment should be undertaken as part of discharge planning so that any issues affecting Vera's ability to carry out activities of living (with support as needed) can be identified and addressed prior to discharge. Liaison between community and hospital services will be essential. Specialist transport, able to transfer Vera in a dignified manner while complying with health and safety requirements must be provided.
- Person-centred goal setting is essential. As her cardiac failure progresses the focus of rehabilitation will be on secondary prevention, adaptation and palliative care. However, with suitable equipment and support Vera may be able to stay at home. Decisions about her future care must involve Vera and from an ethical perspective, her autonomy and rights must be respected.
- Staff caring for Vera must have suitable training to be able to meet her complex needs. This will include pain management, mobility, and use of bariatric moving and handling equipment and cardiorespiratory symptom control. Staff specialising in each of these areas need to work together as part of an interprofessional team to enable rehabilitation.

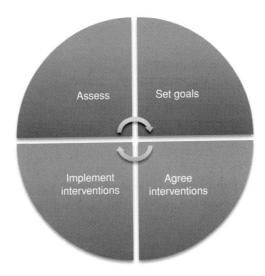

Figure 9.5 Rehabilitation process.

Overview of the rehabilitation process

As shown in Figure 9.5, the rehabilitation process is cyclical. In reality, it is inevitably far more complex than a single diagram shows. An individual with rehabilitation needs will be assessed by many members of the rehabilitation team, not all of whom are necessarily involved from the first step of that individual's rehabilitation journey. Be it in the hospital or community setting, when an LTC gives rise to the need for rehabilitation medical or nursing staff are usually (though not always) the first contact point to carry out an initial assessment. Other disciplines become involved following referral, and each will contribute to assessment, feeding into the process of identifying needs, setting goals, and assessing goal achievement following interventions. Not all goals will be agreed to or interventions instigated at a single point in time. The total rehabilitation programme will contain many goals, interventions and achievement time frames. Inevitably, this creates a potential for confusion, overload, overlap and even conflict (Reynolds 2005). Effective, person-centred goal setting, informed by negotiation which recognises and values the contribution of all team members is key to successful rehabilitation outcomes.

Goal setting

Goal setting will reflect the ethos of each team member and will be influenced by the theories, models and frameworks adopted. Achievement and outcomes will be measured against goals set. Goal setting can be considered in the light of discussions throughout this chapter; therefore, models and outcome measures are not addressed in detail here.

An example of the potential for conflict, with the patient being pulled in all directions, is shown in Figure 9.6. The family may want to show concern by doing everything for their relative and discouraging them from mobilising. The physiotherapist, however, aims to increase mobility to promote independence and allow a person who has lived alone to continue doing so. The family may wish for their relative to move in with them. The social worker may have concerns as to how the family will cope with the realities of this and so consider alternative accommodation. Communication

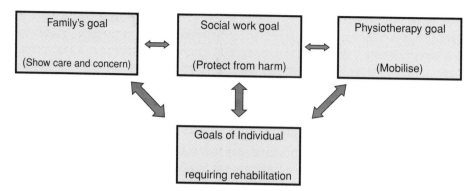

Figure 9.6 Interaction between goals and team members.

between team members is essential to producing compatible goals to which the patient agrees and will, therefore, be motivated to achieve.

Goals must be clearly recorded in a format that is understood by and accessible to all team members. A consistent approach to goal setting is essential. Goals should be individualised and may be long or short term. The SMART approach is recommended, so that goals are:

Specific

Goals should be tailored to the individual, with each goal based on one clear need identified from the assessment. For example, if ADLs are used one goal may relate to mobility and another to economic activity.

Measureable

So that outcome achievement can be gauged and clearly identified goals should be measurable against agreed criteria.

Achievable

Overambitious goals are demotivating. They lead to a sense of failure which may trigger psychological distress and depression. Many long-term goals can be reached via a series of shorter term, achievable goals.

Realistic

Goals must be based on what can be achieved, rather than an unrealistic ideal. For example, an airline pilot who loses their flying licence as a result of limitations caused by a progressive neurological condition cannot realistically expect to fly passenger jets. However, they may be able to retrain for alternative employment which draws on their knowledge and skill.

Time limited

Review dates must be set. These give a target for achievement and a definite point at which goals can be renegotiated. When a goal is not being met, a review date provides an opportunity to introduce an alternative intervention to facilitate achievement. Alternatively, the goal itself may be revised.

Case study 9.5 Katie Lewis

Katie Lewis, a 30-year-old single woman who lived alone and worked as a research scientist, was involved in an accident on her way to work one morning. She sustained multiple fractures and a head injury. Following emergency surgery, she spent several weeks in the intensive care unit where she was ventilated. Whilst she was there, her only sister left her job to be with Katie. Her parents, a retired police officer and a part-time shop assistant who lived 200 miles away, also came to be with their daughter. Once she was no longer ventilated, Katie was transferred to the neuro-rehabilitation unit. At this stage, she could not speak or stand and did not have sufficient coordination to feed herself. After some months of input from physiotherapists, speech and language therapists, occupational therapists and nursing staff Katie was able to wash, dress and feed herself, and could speak. She was discharged to her own home. She still had cognitive impairments, including memory impairment. Following discharge, unfortunately, as a result of her head injury Katie developed epilepsy. In spite of everything Katie returned to work, where she found herself having to relearn processes by using a textbook that she herself had contributed to before her accident. Inevitably, Katie's employers became concerned about her ability to satisfactorily complete research contracts. It became clear that Katie had an ongoing need for rehabilitation support.

Points for reflection

- What members of the interdisciplinary team should be involved in complex long-term situations such as Katie's? What factors need to be addressed to enable the team to work effectively?
- How might the holistic approach inform the rehabilitation process following brain injuries?

- Support for vocational rehabilitation will be essential. Katie may not be able to continue in her current role. Reasonable adjustments may facilitate her doing so; however, redeployment may have to be considered. Katie's rights in relation to this will depend on the nature of her employment contract. Katie's rehabilitation team should include an employment advisor.
- Psychological support is part of the role of all team members; however, in Katie's situation, ongoing specialist support from a clinical psychologist is desirable.
- In complex cases such as Katie's, continuing rehabilitation may be needed over years rather than months.
- The needs of Katie's family, who may now find themselves involved in the care of an adult daughter, must be considered. The family's willingness/ability to be involved will have influenced the goals that can be achieved; for example, the stage at which Katie returned to her own home.
- Following brain injury the risk of epilepsy increases and is around 13% if injury is severe (Ferguson et al. 2009). Katie's driving license will be revoked until and unless her epilepsy is controlled and she is fit free for at least one year, after which she can apply to reinstate it. (http://www.direct.gov.uk/en/DisabledPeople/MotoringAndTransport/Yourvehicleandlicence/DG_10029770)

Section 3

Meanwhile, the impact not driving has on social and vocational rehabilitation should be considered and Katie can be supported to access funding and alternative transport.

Summary

The principles and process of rehabilitation outlined in this section are underpinned by the concepts and theories discussed throughout the chapter. Whatever approach is taken, a key principle is that the person requiring rehabilitation is kept central to the rehabilitation process at all times. Members of the rehabilitation must communicate and work together to ensure a person-centred approach.

Outcome measures and evaluation

Outcome measures are a fundamental part of the rehabilitation process and provide a mechanism with which to evaluate success. It is through evaluation that the success of interventions in achieving individual goals can be measured. This enables monitoring of progress and the identification of areas where goals are not being achieved and so feeds back into the planning and review process. There are a range of tools used to score functioning and measure progress, some of which are explored further in this section. The Royal College of Nursing (2007a) sounds a note of caution regarding the use and interpretation of scores derived from scales. Some scales assume a lower score equates with a lower quality of life, when in fact an individual may have *chosen* to manage an activity of daily living (such as mobility or hygiene) in a way which lowers their score. It is noted while there is a need:

> to use an appropriate range of tools, which have the sensitivity and specificity to discern and evaluate the inputs and outcomes of rehabilitation interventions [however] at the present time none of the central or devolved governments are able to recommend such tools. Royal College of Nursing 2007a: 8

The use of outcome measures is gaining increasing credence in contemporary healthcare driven by the need for the NHS to demonstrate that it is making the most effective use of public money to deliver quality healthcare.

Outcomes, in the context of rehabilitation, can relate to the impact of:

- therapeutic interventions, for example physiotherapy or cognitive behavioural therapy;
- programmes, for example stroke rehabilitation programme or an IC programme;
- policies, for example Transforming Community Services and the shift from acute hospital care to care closer to home.

Outcomes can be measured through the use of standardised tools which assess individual patient outcomes, or be applied more broadly to establish service efficiency, effectiveness and efficacy. Tools can take the form of questionnaires, scales, ratings, etc.

Table 9.9 Rehabilitation outcome measures.

Quality dimension	Description
Effectiveness	Percentage of improvement in independence of daily living as measured by the Nottingham Extended Activities of Daily Living Scale
Effectiveness	Percentage of patients setting and achieving rehabilitation goal as evaluated by the Patient Evaluation Conference System
Effectiveness	Percentage of patients on rehabilitation pathway who have an integrated care plan (content to be defined)
Effectiveness	Percentage of people discharged from hospital and benefiting from IC/rehabilitation enablement still living at home 3 months after discharge from hospital
Experience	Percentage of improvement in self-perceived occupational performance enabling patients to return to work (Canadian Occupational Performance Measure)

Source: Adapted from Department of Health (2009d) *Transforming Community Services Quality Framework: Guidance for Community Services*

'High Quality Care for All' (DH 2008) identified patient safety, effectiveness and patient experience as the three domains of quality, and introduced the quality framework as the national strategy for quality improvement. The first three steps in the quality framework are:

1. To bring clarity to quality
2. To measure quality
3. To publish quality

In order to support quality measurement, Indicators for Quality Improvement (IQI) are being developed to support clinicians to select indicators and facilitate benchmarking.

The Transforming Community Services Quality Framework, for example, includes five suggested outcome measures for rehabilitation; these are outlined in Table 9.9.

Outcome measures in rehabilitation

There is a strong history in the use of outcome measures in rehabilitation. This section provides an overview of some of the more popular tools used in contemporary practice. When selecting an outcome measure, the healthcare professional needs to consider a number of factors which include the following:

- What they want to measure.
- The clinical specialty, for example stroke.
- The rehabilitation setting, for example community or hospital.
- Validity and reliability.

Validity relates to the extent to which a tool measures, what it claims to measure and it is vital for a tool to be valid in order for the results to be accurately applied and interpreted. Reliability refers to the consistency of a measure and a test is considered reliable if we get the same result each time it is administered. For example, if two healthcare professionals independently administered the tool to the same client at the same time, they would be expected to achieve the same result.

Barthel index

The Barthel Index was first introduced by Mahoney and Barthel in 1965; it is one of the oldest outcome measurement tools and is used extensively in rehabilitation, particularly in stroke rehabilitation. The tool is a rating scale based on ADLs that is completed by an observer. A total of ten activities are scored:

1. Feeding
2. Bathing
3. Grooming
4. Dressing
5. Bowels
6. Bladder
7. Toilet use
8. Transfers
9. Mobility
10. Stairs

Values are assigned to each ADL based on the amount of physical assistance required to perform the activity. The Modified Barthel Index includes a maximum score of 20; therefore, the higher the score the greater the independence in ADLs.

The tool is quick and easy to administer and can be applied in all rehabilitation settings, across all age groups.

Limitations of the tool include the following:

- Lack of sensitivity to small differences in functional ability.
- An exclusive focus on physical activities.
- Many areas of functional independence are excluded, for example cognitive ability, language and emotion.

Functional independence measure (FIM) and functional assessment measure (FAM)

The combined FIM + FAM tool is comparatively more sensitive than Barthel and has been developed through a combination of two tools. FIM was developed in the 1980s as a measure of disability. FAM was designed more specifically for use in acquired brain injury and adds an additional 12 areas to FIM that include cognition and psychological aspects; however, it is not a standalone tool, hence the joint use of both tools.

Section 3

Quality of life

Quality of life in the context of health relates to the holistic well-being of an individual person and should, therefore, address physical, functional, psychological and social aspects. EuroQol or EQ-5D is standardised tool for use as a measure of health outcome. EuroQol can be applied to a wide variety of health conditions and treatments, and provides a simple descriptive profile together with a single index value for health status (http://www.euroqol.org/). The tool is relatively easy to use and is designed for self-completion. It is particularly useful for postal surveys and can, therefore, be applied to large numbers of individuals with relative ease.

Case study 9.6   Mina Patel

Mina Patel is a 53-year-old lady who experienced a left-hemisphere stroke four weeks ago; as a result of the stroke, she has aphasia and a right-sided weakness. She displays a slow and cautious behavioural style, and needs ongoing supervision and feedback to complete everyday tasks. Mina has a supportive family who are keen to have her home as soon as she is well enough. Mina and her family live in a three-bedroom semi-detached house with a downstairs toilet. They have an adjoining garage and are planning to apply for planning permission to develop this into a downstairs wet room and sitting room for Mina. Mina's family provide support with daily activities such as washing, dressing and feeding. Prepared food is brought in by her family at most meal times. Mina's mood can be low at times and she is reasonably accepting of people doing things for her.

Points for reflection

- Consider how quality of life issues relate to the rehabilitation process?
- How might outcome measures be used in stroke rehabilitation? What are the advantages and disadvantages of outcome measurement tools?

- In Mina's culture, the right hand is used for eating whilst the left hand is reserved for other toilet-related functions. Eating may, therefore, be an issue for her as it means that, as a result of her right-sided weakness, she needs to rely on her left hand for both eating and toilet purposes.
- Similarly, within Mina's culture the use of running water is the socially acceptable way of maintaining personal hygiene. The offer of a bowl of water or a bath may not, therefore, meet with her approval.
- A slow and cautious behavioural style can often be associated with a left-hemisphere stroke. Ongoing instruction and feedback will, therefore, be required as an integrated part of the rehabilitation process.
- Depression after a stroke is common and healthcare professionals need to be cognizant of the symptoms of depression. Use of a validated screening tool should be utilised where depression is suspected such as the Geriatric Depression Scale.
- It is important to involve family members in the rehabilitation process and support them to recognise and reinforce the importance of promoting self-care. Doing tasks for an individual can have a

negative impact on rehabilitation outcomes and create dependency rather than promoting independence.

Summary

Outcome measures inform care for the individual undergoing rehabilitation. There are a range of measurement tools, some well-validated and others not used by rehabilitation practitioners in order to assess individual's progress and to inform rehabilitation interventions. Outcome measures are also used at policy and service level for purposes of quality monitoring and improvement. Thus, outcome measurement, in various forms, plays an essential role in the delivery of effective rehabilitation.

Conclusion

This chapter has considered the nature of rehabilitation and the essential role it has to play in the care of persons with long-term conditions. Rehabilitation should no longer be seen as a time-limited endeavour taking place only in designated rehabilitation settings. The value of rehabilitation in enhancing quality of life and enabling maximum independence throughout the trajectory of the whole range of long-term conditions is now recognised both by health and social care professionals, and within health and social care policy. Effective, high quality rehabilitation demands a team approach with the numbers and makeup of the team being determined by the individual needs of the client. The team must work together to integrate, as appropriate, the skills and endeavours of a wide range of disciplines in order to assess requirements, develop a rehabilitation plan and ensure this is enacted. Each individual with a long-term condition must remain central throughout the rehabilitation process. This is crucial to successful rehabilitation outcomes.

References

Baker, M., Fardell, J. and Jones, B. (1997) *Disability and Rehabilitation: Survey of Educational Needs of Health and Social Service Professionals*. London: Disability and Rehabilitation Open Learning Project.

Brandt, E. and Pope, A. (1997) *Enabling America: Assessing the Role of Rehabilitation Science and Engineering*. Committee on Assessing Rehabilitation Science and Engineering, Division of Health Policy, Institute of Medicine, Washington DC: National Academy Press.

British Geriatrics Society (2005) Position Paper: Rehabilitation in the NHS and Social Care. Available at: http://www.bgs.org.uk/publications/position%20Papers//psn_rehabilitation_nhs_ss.htm (accessed 28 September 2010).

Clouder, D. and Smith, S. (2010) Interprofessional and interdisciplinary learning. In: A. Bromage, D.L. Clouder, F. Gordon and J. Thistlethwaite (eds) *Interprofessional e-Learning and Collaborative Work: Practices and Technologies*. New York: IGI Global.

Coffey, L., Gallagher, P., Horgan, O., Desmond, D. and MacLachlan, M. (2009) Psychosocial adjustment to diabetes-related lower limb amputation. *DIABETIC Medicine* **26**, 1063-1067.

Corbin, J. (1998) The Corbin and Strauss chronic illness trajectory model: an update. *Scholarly Inquiry for Nursing Practice* **12** (1), 33-41.

Davis, S. (2006) (ed) *Rehabilitation: The Use of Models and Theories in Practice*. Edinburgh: Elsevier – Churchill Livingstone.

Davis, S. and Madden, S. (2006) The international classification of functioning and health. In: S. Davis (ed) *Rehabilitation: The Use of Models and Theories in Practice*. Edinburgh: Elsevier – Churchill Livingstone.

Dementia UK (2010) Admiral Nurses. Available at: http://www.dementiauk.org/what-we-do/admiral-nurses/ (accessed 28 May 2010).

Department of Health (DH) (2000) The NHS Plan. Available at: http://www.dh.gov.uk/en/publicationsandstatistics/publications/publicationspolicyandguidance/dh_4002960 (accessed 28 May 2010).

Department of Health (DH) (2001) National Service Framework for Older People. Available at: http://www.dh.gov.uk/en/publicationsandstatistics/publications/publicationspolicyandguidance/dh_4003066 (accessed 28 May 2010).

Department of Health (DH) (2007) Who Cares? Information and Support for the Carers of People with Dementia. Available at: http://www.dh.gov.uk/prod_consum_dh/groups/dh_digitalassets/@dh/@en/documents/digitalasset/dh_078091.pdf (accessed 28 May 2010).

Department of Health (DH) (2008) High Quality Care for All – NHS Next Stage Review. Available at: http://www.dh.gov.uk/prod_consum_dh/groups/dh_digitalassets/@dh/@en/documents/digitalasset/dh_085828.pdf (accessed 31 May 2010).

Department of Health (DH) (2009a) Transforming Community Services: Enabling New Patterns of Provision. Available at: http://www.dh.gov.uk/prod_consum_dh/groups/dh_digitalassets/documents/digitalasset/dh_093196.pdf (accessed 31 May 2010).

Department of Health (DH) (2009b) Transforming Community Services: Ambition, Action, Achievement – Transforming Rehabilitation Services. Available at: http://www.lp-publicservices.org.uk/Community-Health-News.aspx?title=Transforming%20Community%20Services%20-%20Six%20Transformational%20Guides%20for%20Community%20Services&ID=49 (accessed 31 May 2010).

Department of Health (DH) (2009c) Living Well with Dementia: A National Dementia Strategy. Available at: http://www.dh.gov.uk/prod_consum_dh/groups/dh_digitalassets/@dh/@en/documents/digitalasset/dh_094051.pdf (accessed 28 May 2010).

Department of Health (DH) (2009d) Transforming Community Services Quality Framework: Guidance for Community Services. Available at: http://www.dh.gov.uk/prod_consum_dh/groups/dh_digitalassets/documents/digitalasset/dh_101426.pdf (accessed 28 May 2010).

Department of Health (DH) (2010) The NHS Quality, Innovation, Productivity and Prevention Challenge: an introduction for clinicians. Available at: http://www.dh.gov.uk/prod_consum_dh/groups/dh_digitalassets/@dh/@en/@ps/documents/digitalasset/dh_113807.pdf (accessed 31 May 2010).

Dittmar, S. (1989) (ed) *Rehabilitation Nursing. Practice and Application*. St Louis: Mosby.

Ferguson, P.L., Smith, G.M., Wannamaker, B., Thurman, D., Pickelsimer, E. and Selassie, A.W. (2009) A population-based study of risk of epilepsy after hospitalization for traumatic brain injury. *Epilepsia* **51** (5), 891–898. Available at: http://www3.interscience.wiley.com/journal/122655977/abstract?CRETRY=1&SRETRY=0 (accessed 2 May 2010).

Greenwood, R., Barnes, M.P., McMillan, T.M. and Ward, C.D. (1993) *Neurological Rehabilitation*. Edinburgh: Churchill Livingstone.

Gulrajani, R. (2010) Do people with mild COPD benefit from early pulmonary rehabilitation programs? *Nursing Times* **106** (17), 16–17. Available at: http://www.nursingtimes.net/SearchResults.aspx?qkeyword=Gulrajani (accessed 28 May 2010).

Haddad, M. Taylor, C. and Pilling, S. (2009) Depression in adults with long term conditions.1: how to identify and assess symptoms. *Nursing Times* **105** (48), 14–17. Available at: http://www.nursingtimes.net/nursing-practice-clinical-research/mental-health/depression-in-adults-with-long-term-conditions-1-how-to-identify-and-assess-symptoms-/5009329.article (accessed 28 May 2010).

Hoeman, S. (2008) *Rehabilitation Nursing: Prevention, Intervention and Outcomes*, 4th edn St Louis: Mosby Elsevier.

Jester, R. (2007) (ed) *Advanced Practice in Rehabilitation Nursing*. Oxford: Blackwell Publishing.

Kumar, S. (2000) (ed) *Multidisciplinary Approach to Rehabilitation*. Boston: Butterworth – Heinemann.

Section 3

Latella, D. (2000) Teamwork in rehabilitation. In: S. Kumar (ed) *Multidisciplinary Approach to Rehabilitation*. Boston: Butterworth – Heinemann.

Long, A., Kneafsey, R., Ryan, J. and Berry, J. (2002) The role of the nurse within a multi-professional rehabilitation team. *Journal of Advanced Nursing* **37** (1), 70-78.

Lutz, B. and Davis, S. (2008) Theory and practice models for rehabilitation nursing. In: S. Hoeman (ed) *Rehabilitation Nursing: Prevention, Interventions and Outcomes*, 4th edn. Philadelphia: Mosby Elsevier.

Mahoney, F. and Barthel, D. (1965) Functional evaluation: the Barthel index. *Maryland State Medical Journal* **14**, 61-65.

National Institute for Clinical Excellence (2004) CG12 Clinical Guideline 12. Chronic Obstructive Pulmonary Disease. Available at: http://www.nice.org.uk/nicemedia/live/10938/29302/29302.pdf (accessed 28 May 2010).

NHS Choices (2010) Stay Well Over 50. Available at: http://www.nhs.uk/Livewell/Staywellover50/Pages/Fallsprevention.aspx (accessed 28 May 2010).

Nolan, J. and Nolan, J. (1999) Rehabilitation, chronic illness and disability: the missing elements in nurse education. *Journal of Advanced Nursing* **29** (4), 958-966.

Orem, D. (1991) *Nursing: Concepts of Practice*, 5th edn. Mosby: St. Louis.

Padilla, R. (2000) Cultural diversity and health behavior. In: K. Shrawan (ed) *Multidisciplinary Approach to Rehabilitation*. Boston: Butterworth-Heinemann.

Pryor, J. and O'Connell, B. (2008) Incongruence between nurses' and patients' understandings and expectations of rehabilitation. *Journal of Clinical Nursing* **18**, 1766-1774.

Remsberg, R. and Carson, B. (2006) Rehabilitation. In: I. Lubkin and P. Larsen (eds) *Chronic Illness: Impact and Interventions*. Boston: Jones and Bartlet.

Reynolds, F. (2005) *Communication and Clinical Effectiveness in Rehabilitation*. Edinburgh: Elsevier.

Roper, N., Logan, W. and Tierney, A. (1990) *The Elements of Nursing: A Model for Nursing Based on a Model of Living*. Edinburgh: Churchill Livingstone.

Roy, C. and Andrews, H.A. (1999) *The Roy Adaptation Model: The Definitive Statement*. Norwalk CT: Appleton and Lange.

Royal College of Nursing (2007a) *Maximising Independence: The Role of the Nurse in Supporting the Rehabilitation of Older People*. London: Royal College of Nursing.

Royal College of Nursing (2007b) *Role of the rehabilitation Nurse: RCN guidance*. London: Royal College of Nursing.

Smith, M. (1999) (ed) *Rehabilitation in Adult Nursing Practice*. Edinburgh: Churchill Livingstone.

Squires, A. (2002) The rehabilitation of the older person: past, present and future. In: A. Squires and M. Hastings (eds) *Rehabilitation of the Older Person: A Handbook for the Interdisciplinary Team*, 3rd edn. Cheltenham: Nelson Thornes.

Squires, A., and Hastings, M. (2002) (eds.) *Rehabilitation of the Older Person: A Handbook for the Interdisciplinary Team*, 3rd edn. Cheltenham: Nelson Thornes.

Wade, D. (1996) Designing district disability services – the oxford experience. *Clinical Rehabilitation* **4**, 147-158.

Whitelock, H. (1999) The team. In: S. Davis and S. O'Conner (eds) *Rehabilitation Nursing: Foundations for Practice*. London: Bailliere Tindall.

World Health Organisation (WHO) (1980) *The International Classification of Impairments, Disabilities and Handicaps*. Geneva: World Health Organisation.

World Health Organisation (WHO) (2001) Towards a Common Language of Functioning, Disability and Health. Available at: http://www3.who.int/icf/icftemplate.cfm?myurl=beginner.htm&mytitleBeginner%27%20Guide (accessed 28 May 2010).

World Health Organisation (WHO) (2003) ICF Checklist Version 2.1a. Available at: http://www.who.int/classifications/icf/training/icfchecklist.pdf (accessed 28 May 2010).

World Health Organisation (WHO) (2010) Framework for Action on Interprofessional Education and Collaborative Practice. Available at: http://whqlibdoc.who.int/HQ/2010/WHO_HRH_HPN_10.3_eng.pdf (accessed 28 May 2010).

Resources

In addition to the references provided within this chapter, the following sources provide useful information relating to rehabilitation and long-term conditions. These are by no means exhaustive, and the reader is encouraged to seek out more specific information from other sites as required.

Access to Work Scheme Information Available at: http://www.direct.gov.uk/en/disabledpeople/employmentsupport/workschemesandprogrammes/dg_4000347

Association for Rehabilitation of Communication and Oral Skills Available at: http://www.arcos.org.uk

Alzheimer's Society Available at: www.alzheimers.org.uk

Basket of Scores (Outcomes Measurement Basket) Available at: http://www.bsrm.co.uk/Clinical Guidance/BasketOfScoresWithSCIA%20_2_update2005newref9.pdf

British Lung Foundation Available at: http://www.lunguk.org

British Society for Rehabilitation Medicine Available at: http://www.bsrm.co.uk

COPD International Available at: http://www.copd-international.com

Headway (Brain Injury Support) Available at: http://www.headway.org.uk/home.aspx

International Society of Physical and Rehabilitation Medicine Available at: http://www.isprm.org/

Parkinson's Disease Society Available at: www.parkinsons.org.uk

Thrive (Gardening for Rehabilitation) Available at: http://www.thrive.org.uk

Standards for Rehabilitation Services Mapped to Long-term Conditions Available at: http://www.bsrm.co.uk/ClinicalGuidance/StandardsMapping-Final.pdf

Further reading

In addition to the references provided within this chapter, the following references provide suggestions for further reading relating to rehabilitation and LTCs.

Davis, S. (2006) *Rehabilitation: The Use of Models and Theories in Practice*. Edinburgh: Elsevier.

Disability Discrimination Act (2005) Available at: http://www.opsi.gov.uk/acts/acts2005/ukpga_20050013_en_1

Holm, J. (2007) *Vocational Rehabilitation*. Oxford: Blackwell.

Long-term Conditions Delivery Support Team: Quality Requirements for Rehabilitation Available at: http://www.ltc-community.org.uk/thensf.asp?action=view&id=4613

Mackey, H. and Nancarrow, S. (2006) *Enabling Independence: A Guide for Rehabilitation Workers*. Oxford: Blackwell.

NICE Falls Guidelines Available at: http://www.nice.org.uk/CG21

NICE MS Guidelines Available at: http://www.nice.org.uk/nicemedia/live/10930/46699/46699.pdf

The Scottish Government (2010) Long-term Conditions Collaborative: Improving Care Pathways: Rehabilitation. Available at: http://www.scotland.gov.uk/Publications/2010/04/13103945/8

WHO Action Plan Disability & Rehab 2006–2011 Available at: http://www.who.int/disabilities/publications/dar_action_plan_2006to2011.pdf

Section 3

Chapter 10

Palliative Care in Long-term Conditions: Pathways to Care

Claire Whittle and Jill Main

Learning objectives

By the end of this chapter, the reader will be able to:

- Demonstrate a clear understanding of what is meant by palliative care
- Describe the three illness trajectories
- Discuss end of life care related to people with heart failure, dementia, Chronic Obstructive Pulmonary Disease (COPD) and renal failure
- Outline different models of end of life care which can be utilised when caring for patients with long-term conditions (LTCs)
- Explain what is meant by integrated care pathways
- Describe the main polices informing end of life care

Introduction

This chapter outlines the need for high quality palliative and end of life care for patients who have long-term-conditions (LTCs), and their families. Included in this chapter is the evidence for good practice when caring for patients at the end of life, policy drivers and tools for use to support staff in delivering care. Case studies are used to illustrate different aspects of care and management when supporting patients with LTCs.

What is palliative care?

There is no single agreed definition of palliative care, and the following definition is based on those produced by the World Health Organisation (WHO 1990):

Long-term Conditions: A Guide for Nurses and Healthcare Professionals, First Edition. Edited by S. Randall and H. Ford.
© 2011 Blackwell Publishing Ltd. Published 2011 by Blackwell Publishing Ltd.

Palliative care is an approach that improves the quality of life of patients and their families facing the problems associated with life-threatening illness. This is achieved through the anticipation, management and relief of suffering by means of early identification, impeccable assessment and treatment of pain and other problems. These may include physical, psychological and spiritual needs.

Palliative care:

- provides relief from pain and other distressing symptoms
- affirms life and regards dying as a normal process
- intends neither to hasten or postpone death
- integrates the psychological and spiritual aspects of patient care
- offers a support system to help patients live as actively as possible until death
- offers a support system to help the family cope during the patients illness and in their own bereavement
- uses a team approach to address the needs of patients and their families, including bereavement counselling, if indicated
- will enhance quality of life, and may also positively influence the course of illness
- is applicable early in the course of illness, in conjunction with other therapies that are intended to prolong life, such as chemotherapy or radiation therapy, and includes those investigations needed to better understand and manage distressing clinical complications.
WHO 2009

Comfort care is another term sometimes given to palliative care, and the National Institute for Health and Clinical Excellence (NICE) (2004) in providing guidance for people approaching the end of life described both 'palliative' and 'supportive' care for adults with cancer. However, palliative and supportive care is not just for cancer, but extends to all chronic diseases, and affects carers and professionals, and not only patients.

As described, supportive care is another term that, like palliative care, has a number of different definitions and if palliative care is defined in a narrow way, as being only about pain and other symptom control, then supportive care may include palliative care as well as a range of other care that could be provided to 'support' a person with a life-threatening disease and their family.

However, if palliative care is defined in a wide ranging way, then it may be described as being in two parts: one part being about pain and symptom control, and the other part being about supportive care.

Difficulties caused by different definitions

Having a number of different definitions of both supportive care and palliative care has resulted in a considerable degree of confusion, not only for health professionals but also for patients. Not only are many people unsure about what palliative care is, and when it should be provided, but also that palliative care is in some circumstances part of supportive care, and in other circumstances, it is the opposite way round with supportive care being part of palliative care.

Most people have only heard about palliative care as something that is provided in hospices for people who are dying. So another difficulty that can arise concerns people being offered palliative

Section 3

care early on in the course of a disease. Some people turn down the offer of palliative care believing that to accept will mean that they are terminally ill and going to die. They may also believe that they will no longer be offered any disease modifying or curative treatment. Traditionally, high quality care at the end of life has been mainly provided for cancer patients but this kind of care now needs to be provided for those with a wide range of diseases (World Health Organisation 2004).

High quality end of life care is essential for all people requiring palliative care irrespective of diagnosis. Although attention tends, then, to have been given to cancer care, all patients with chronic, progressive and eventually fatal illness need high quality organised end of life care. This group of patients includes patients with organ system failure such as heart failure or Chronic Obstructive Pulmonary Disease (COPD), stroke, general frailty, dementia and other neurological conditions as well as people with cancer. Research has demonstrated that, while much less likely to access the support afforded to some cancer patients, people with organ system failure suffer significant physical and emotional symptoms very similar to those affected by cancer and would benefit from a palliative approach to their care (Gore et al. 2000, Jones et al. 2003).

This raises many issues for the professionals caring for patients with advanced life limiting disease, and requires the expertise of generalist and specialist palliative care staff in finding support for patients and their families. Most deaths in Europe and other developed countries occur in people over 65, but relatively little health policy concerns their needs in the last years of their lives (World Health Organisation 2004).

Sir Nigel Crisp, the former Chief Executive of the National Health Service (NHS), stated in a parliamentary speech in 2003:

> Better care of the dying should become a touchstone for success in modernising the NHS. This one of the really big issues – we must make it happen.

The issue is that care at the very end of life is only a part of palliative care and people can live with a life-threatening illness for years. Palliative care services need to be designed so they are integrated with other services and are able to meet the wide range of needs of service users, their families and their carers throughout the palliative care phase and into end of life care (The NHS Confederation 2005).

It is now acknowledged that not only people are living longer, with the proportion aged over 65 projected to increase from 16% in 2004 to 21% by 2024 (The NHS Confederation 2005), it is expected that some can expect longer periods of ill-health towards the end of their lives. As a result of recent medical advances, people who previously may have died during an acute life-threatening episode are now living longer with chronic life-limiting conditions.

It has been recognised that while the government is committed to ensure all patients nearing the end of their lives, regardless of their diagnosis, have access to high quality palliative care, the reality is that 95% of referrals to specialist palliative care teams are for patients with a diagnosis of cancer (DH 2003). Cancer, however, accounts for only 25% of deaths (Griffiths et al. 2005).

Although some conditions such as cancer have a relatively predictable journey of illness and decline, others may involve a slower decline over a period of years followed by a number of admissions to hospital and then death. End of life care and palliative care, therefore, overlap with the management of people with LTCs. Increasing numbers of people will be living with organ failure, frailty and dementia and fewer with cancer for which much of the hospice and specialist palliative care has previously been provided. It has been suggested that there needs to be a shift towards the end of life care to incorporate those conditions (The NHS Confederation 2005).

What is end of life care?

End of life care is an important part of palliative care, and usually refers to the care of a person during the last part of their life, from the point at which it has become clear that the person is in a progressive state of decline (Watson et al. 2009).

End of life care is usually a longer period than the time during which someone is considered to be 'dying'. In the United Kingdom, it is mainly healthcare professionals who use the term 'end of life care', whereas patients and their families are more likely to refer to 'terminal illness' and 'terminal care'. The time at the end of life is different for each person, and each person has unique needs for information, for support and for care.

Terminal illness and terminal care

Terminal care is described as the care provided for a patient in the very end phase or terminal phase of their life. But how can it be recognised when this time has come? (Kanabus 2009).

As well as there being many different definitions of palliative care, there are also many different definitions of terminal care. Terminal care can be described as end of life care. In the United Kingdom, many patients and their families will refer to someone being terminally ill when they may have many months or even years to live (Kanabus 2009).

Alternatively, terminal care is sometimes defined as care being provided for someone who is in the 'dying' phase. The difficulty is identifying when someone is in the dying phase. Some people take the view that everyone starts to die from the day they are born. The reality is that it is never known exactly when someone is going to die from a life-threatening disease (Kanabus 2009). Taking this approach of equating terminal care with 'dying', some medical organisations define someone as being terminally ill when it is expected that there is only a short period of time, perhaps a few days or weeks, or at most a month or two, before the person is expected to die (Kanabus 2009).

Illness trajectories

Murray et al. (2005) suggest that the use of the illness trajectories described by Lynne (2004) provide a broad time frame in which to help clinicians plan and deliver care that integrates active and palliative management. They also suggest that an understanding of these trajectories ensure that end of life care is considered at an earlier stage.

Trajectory 1 (Figure 10.1) typically describes the cancer journey with a steady progression and usually a clear terminal phase.

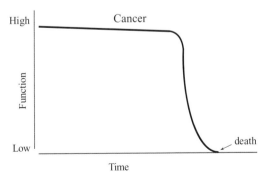

Figure 10.1 Trajectory 1. (Reproduced with kind permission from Lynn, J. and Adamson, D.M. (2003).)

Section 3

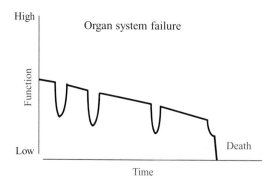

Figure 10.2   Trajectory 2. (Reproduced with kind permission from Lynn, J. and Adamson, D.M. (2003).)

Trajectory 2 (Figure 10.2) describes how those with organ system failure progress towards the end of life with gradual decline, punctuated by episodes of acute deterioration and some recovery, with a more sudden and seemingly unexpected death.

The third trajectory (Figure 10.3) is described by Murray et al. (2005) as 'prolonged dwindling'. Figure 10.3 plots those with a low baseline of cognitive or physical functioning who may die following what may appear to be a minor event. However, these patients typically have very few reserves left, and this relatively minor event can prove fatal.

Patients with LTCs are more likely to fit into the second and third trajectories, typically with a pattern of short-term admission to a hospital for care during an acute exacerbation of their illness. Clark and Seymour (1999) comment that following discharge after these admissions, care at home can often be poorly coordinated and unregulated as a result of over-stretched services.

Murray et al. (2005) point out that episodes of acute deterioration in those with organ failure or minor events for those on the trajectory of extreme frailty or dementia may well result in a hospital admission. Bern-Klug (2004) describes 'the ambiguous dying syndrome'. This refers to the period prior to death during which dying is not acknowledged until the very end when it is too late for the patient and his family to benefit from a palliative approach to their care, even though it is acknowledged they are at high risk of death but the timing is uncertain. This can occur in any care setting, but includes those with chronic illness or co-morbidities in hospital. Clark and Seymour (1999) suggest that while the preferred place of death for most people is home, the majority of those with chronic, degenerative, non-cancer disease, most of whom are elderly, will die in an acute hospital.

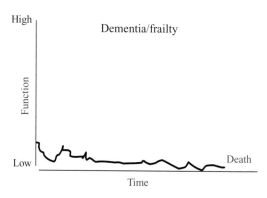

Figure 10.3   Trajectory 3. (Reproduced with kind permission from Lynn, J. and Adamson, D.M. (2003).)

They describe these patients as 'the disadvantaged majority'. Figures from Higginson (2003) confirm that this is still the case, with 56% of people dying in hospital, while 56% would choose to die at home.

Coventry et al. (2005) suggest that most life-threatening diseases have an 'entry-re-entry' death trajectory, which results in frequent acute exacerbations managed in hospital, and while stabilised, there is a steady decline which makes the identification of the palliative phase very problematic. They believe it is difficult to predict the 6 month or less survival rate for those patients with an LTC at the end of life.

Abel et al. (2009) reviewed several studies which explored why the majority of deaths occur in hospital. These include:

- inability to control symptoms;
- inadequate assessment of needs and planning for healthcare response;
- lack of informal carers;
- lack of support for informal carers.

It is interesting to note that these findings are echoed by Munday et al. (2009), who described how issues around admission to hospital at the end of life continue. They reported that preferences for place of death frequently changed over time and were often ill defined or poorly formed in patients' minds. Preferences were often inferred by the health professional without direct questioning or receiving a definitive answer from the patient.

'This uncertainty then challenged the practicality, usefulness, and value of recording a definitive preference resulting in a limited effectiveness of palliative care delivery' (Munday et al. 2009: 1).

Family and carers

The experience of those caring for someone is often one of extreme disadvantage in terms of health and social care provision, particularly specialist palliative care, in spite of the fact that their needs are often similar to those with advanced cancer.

The Neurological Alliance (n.d.) has identified that approximately 850,000 people in the United Kingdom care for someone with a neurological LTC. They point out that carer's health is often compromised, with about half suffering physical injuries such as back strain and half experience stress-related illness. Carers may be elderly as well, with healthcare problems of their own, which can affect their ability to care for others. Families and carers must be supported to look after their own health and well-being. Having to come to terms with the fact that someone they love is dying is stressful enough, but the effort of caring that this requires can lead to carer's breakdown. This can result in a potentially unnecessary acute hospital admission. Initiatives such as regular planned respite can help alleviate this.

The Carers Equal Opportunity Act (Great Britain Parliament 2004), which came into force in 2005, places a duty on local councils and social services departments to offer an assessment of carers' needs, with the intention that there should be greater collaboration between councils and the health services to provide support for carers to enable them to carry on this invaluable role.

There are:

- between five and six million unpaid carers looking after a relative or friend at home (Carers UK 2009);
- another six thousand people who take on a caring responsibility every day;

Section 3

- carers who provide considerable unpaid care by looking after an ill, frail or disabled family member, friend or partner;
- approximately 24% of carers over the age of 75 years providing 50 hours or more (per week) of informal care (Department of Work and Pensions 2008);
- 2.8 million people aged 50 and over providing unpaid care;
- 5% of people aged 85 years providing unpaid care (Office for National Statistics 2004).

This represents a huge saving in the UK economy of an estimated £87 billion a year, a value of unpaid care which is often not recognised (Carers UK 2007). These carers undoubtedly support their loved ones throughout the whole of their illness right through to death. This means there is a huge requirement for bereavement and after death care for this group of people.

Dying from LTCs

Dying from dementia

Dementia is a progressive illness which results in a decline in many areas of function including memory, reasoning and communication skills, and the skills needed to carry out the activities of daily living (DH 2009b). Current projections suggest while there are currently around 700,000 people in the United Kingdom with dementia, this figure is likely to rise to 1 million by 2025 and to 1.7 million by 2051 (DH 2009b).

The prevalence of dementia rises with age, with 'one person in five' over 80 years of age affected rising to 'one person in three' over the age of 90 affected. 'One in three' people over 65 will die with dementia (Knapp et al. 2007).

While these numbers and the associated costs are certainly daunting, it must be remembered that the impact of the disease is profound for those who care for a person with dementia. Dementia results in the progressive decline in a number of areas of that person's life from a decline in memory, reasoning and communication skills to an inability to carry out simple activities of daily living. Care can be further complicated if the person develops behavioural or psychological problems such as depression, aggression or wandering. As the prevalence of dementia rises with age, often those caring for them are elderly themselves and may have health problems of their own. This can result in a very poor quality of life as they struggle to cope. While dementia is a terminal condition, people can live with it for up to 12 years (DH 2009b).

Case study 10.1 illustrates the impact of dementia and the difficulties experienced by carers and the difference that appropriate help and support can make.

Case study 10.1 Frank and Betty's story

Frank and Betty had been married for 40 years and enjoyed a very happy life together. Betty was a retired school teacher and Frank had worked in the NHS as a radiologist. Over a period of time, Frank began to notice that Betty was doing some odd things. They seemed silly at first, like trying to find the ham to put on their sandwiches when they were already made. Then Frank came into the kitchen a couple of times to find the kitchen floor flooded as the taps had been left full on and the sink overflowing. The knob on the dimmer switch in the living room was frequently missing and Frank came to realise that Betty had taken it off but no longer remembered how to put it back so would deny touching it.

As Betty's behaviour became increasingly strange and she became more and more forgetful, Frank spoke with his General Practitioner (GP) about what might be the matter. A brain scan showed nothing unexpected but was referred to a psychiatrist who suggested that Betty was in the early stages of dementia, which was most likely to be Alzheimer's disease. The diagnosis came as shock. Frank had worked in the NHS for many years and had come into contact with people with dementia but never thought it could affect him. Frank was determined to care for Betty himself at home and for a time did indeed manage to do this, resenting anyone who suggested that he might have 'outsiders' coming into the house to help.

However, Frank eventually realised that he could not cope on his own. A visit to a local carer support office put him in touch with the Alzheimer's Society, which is a UK charity that offers support for people with dementia, their carers and families. A visit from a member of the Alzheimer's Society, Alison, gave him both practical and emotional support to get the help he was entitled to. Indeed, Alison became a friend and frequent visitor over the years that Frank was caring for Betty.

Frank learned that he could access funds called direct payments. Direct payments are local council payments for anyone who has been assessed as needing help from social services. They can be used to buy services from an organisation or to employ somebody to provide assistance. This proved difficult initially and he felt he was battling with the 'red tape and bureaucracy' but through perseverance and the continued support of Alison eventually managed to get some funding.

Betty's condition continued to deteriorate relentlessly as the years progressed. She no longer recognised Frank although she was happy for him to care for her. In fact, if she was left on her own she would shout for him. She was mobile and used to go out for a walk or to the park with him and seemed to enjoy these outings. While not physically aggressive, she happily told people exactly what she thought about them or what she didn't like about them, something the old Betty would never have done.

The money from the direct payments allowed Frank to employ a personal assistant, Susan, who came in every weekday morning to help Frank get Betty up in the morning. Frank was also put in touch with an organisation called Crossroads who provide support for carers and those they care for. For 12 hours a week, a Crossroads visitor would sit with Betty allowing Frank to go out for a break. Betty did not seem to mind Frank not being there as long as she was not left on her own. Frank came to see all those supporting him as his family, as old friends stopped visiting and gradually vanished.

A unique respite package was put in place using the direct payments, which involved Susan living in the family home for a week to give Frank a holiday, something he had not had for over 10 years. However, during the second of the planned respites, Betty's condition suddenly got much worse. She became physically more frail and in a short period of time she was unable to move independently. Her speech became more and more incoherent. She also became incontinent and no longer able to feed herself. While he had been determined not to let Betty go into a nursing home, he finally accepted that he could no longer look after Betty himself and reluctantly arranged for her to go onto a local nursing home. She was only there a couple of

Section 3

weeks when she was admitted to hospital with a chest infection. Following a 3 hour wait in the emergency department, she was admitted to a general medical ward. Although Frank himself felt that she was dying, active treatments and intravenous antibiotics were commenced. Betty died one week after she was admitted.

Frank had cared for Betty for 13 years before she died, but felt he had lost her twice. He first lost her many years before when the old Betty left him and she longer knew who or where she was. Frank keeps himself busy to help him deal with the death of Betty. He continues to work for the Alzheimer's Society and also works for other local support groups. He finds the weekends particularly difficult, so he bought a season ticket for his local football team and now spends Saturday afternoons on the terraces.

This case study is based on a true story, although the names have been changed.
It has been reproduced with the kind permission of 'Frank'

Points for reflection

- What charitable organisations are available to support people with Alzheimer's disease and their families?
- How might Frank have been better supported as a carer?
- How would the use of the Liverpool Care Pathway have supported Betty's end of life care?

Heart failure

Heart failure has been described as not just a disabling condition, but also as the end stage of most chronic diseases that affect the heart (While and Kiek 2009) and is a major cause of morbidity and mortality. It has a poor prognosis, worse than several major cancers, including colon cancer in men and breast cancer in women (DH 2000) (as illustrated in Figure 10.4 below). It also carries with it a high risk of sudden death. The incidence of heart failure is approximately one new case per 1000 population per year and is rising at about 10% per year. This increases with age to more than 10 cases per 1000 population in those 85 years and over, with the average age of clinical presentation being 76 years (DH 2000). Heart failure accounts for about 5% of medical admissions to hospital and people with heart failure are frequently readmitted to hospital.

Dying from neurological conditions

It is estimated that there are 10 million people in the United Kingdom living with a neurological disorder, of which 1 million are disabled by their condition and a further 350,000 require help for most of their daily activities (The Neurological Alliance n.d.).

Stroke is the third biggest cause of death (DH 2009a). It is also the largest single cause of disability. It is estimated that each year, more than 110,000 people in England will suffer from a stroke. Of those, about a third are likely to die in the first 10 days, about a third are likely to make a recovery within a month, but a third are likely to be left with a significant disability. Therefore, the incidence of stroke is high and a significant number of people who have a stroke will die.

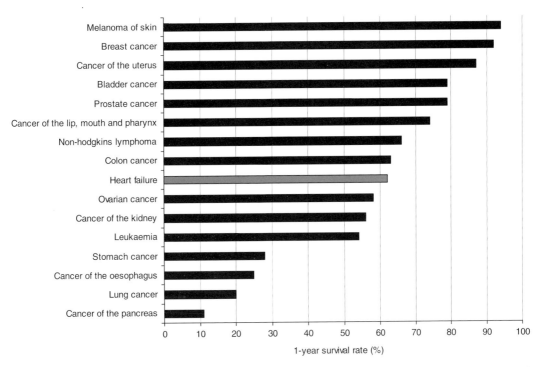

Figure 10.4 1-year survival rates, heart failure and major cancers compared, mid-1990s, England and Wales. (Cowie et al. 2000.)

Of the neurodegenerative diseases, including multiple sclerosis, motor neurone disease, Parkinson's disease and Huntingdon's disease, there is a variation in presentation and life expectancy but there are similarities in the need for symptom management and services.

Indeed, the National Service Framework (NSF) for long-term (neurological) conditions explicitly calls for the need for a palliative care approach for neurological conditions at the end of life (DH 2005). A subsequent document in 2008 (DH 2008b) reviewing implementation of the original NSF, points out the difficulty in making an accurate prognosis of end of life in those with neurological LTCs, refers to the use of prognostic indicators to try to help health professionals initiate discussions around end of life (National Gold Standards Framework Centre 2008).

Dying from COPD

COPD tends to develop over a number of years with many people developing symptoms in mid-life or later. The most important causative factor is smoking – but others include occupational exposures to fumes, chemicals and dusts, as well as genetic susceptibility and environmental pollution (Health and Safety Executive 2005).

COPD is responsible for a large number of deaths in Great Britain: it has given rise to between 25,000 and 30,000 deaths each year over the last 25 years. It is the fifth biggest killer in the United Kingdom (National Statistics 2006a). It is difficult to establish the number of people suffering from the disease at any given time because of different definitions of the disease and under-diagnosis. Results from a survey in 2001 estimated the prevalence of COPD, as defined by lung function test,

Section 3

to be much higher than this: an estimated 13.3% of those aged over 35 years in England had COPD (Shahab et al. 2006), equivalent to 3.4-3.8 million cases. In 2005, COPD killed more women than breast cancer: 11,302 died of COPD, 10,969 died of breast cancer (National Statistics 2006b), and therefore the care and management of this large group of people at the end of life needs careful consideration.

End of life symptoms and management of symptoms

The primary aim of symptom management in palliative care, regardless of diagnosis, is to control any symptoms which are distressing to the patient and focused entirely to the patient's needs. All treatment must be individualised and based on the most recent evidence for the management of any specific symptom (Abu-Saad 2001). There are a number of clinical guidelines developed by expert working parties and the World Health Organisation, one example being the guideline for pain relief: the 'pain relief ladder' (WHO 2005) (see Figure 10.5 below). While originally developed for those suffering from cancer, as has been already noted, many of the symptoms suffered by those with LTCs are similar to those of cancer patients, as end of life symptoms are similar regardless of the predisposing disease. As long as the patients are able to swallow and aspiration is not considered to be a risk, the oral route for medication is the preferred option. Otherwise the subcutaneous route should be used.

The management of pain, a common symptom at the end of life, should be tailored to each individual and the WHO three-step analgesic ladder can be used to provide the most appropriate pain relief, progressing as the pain becomes more difficult to control (see Figure 10.5) (WHO 2005). The effect of the medication must be continually monitored to ensure it is effective, there are no unacceptable side effects and whether new pains are developing that may need different treatment.

The underlying principle is that there should be good pain assessment, a good knowledge of a small number of analgesics, and a simple approach should bring pain relief in most patients (Faull et al.

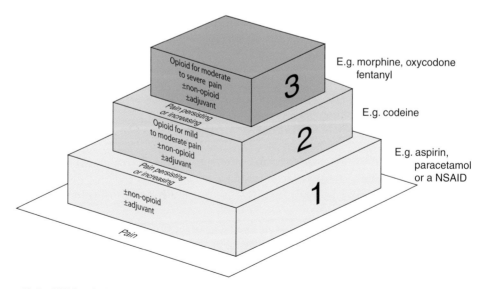

Figure 10.5   WHO pain ladder. (WHO 2005)

1998). However, when pain relief becomes difficult to control, the advice of the specialist palliative care teams can be invaluable.

Policies

There is now an increasing awareness amongst care professionals that healthcare policy needs to recognise and plan for the consequences of the ageing population. Most people will now die of the chronic diseases of old age and conditions other than cancer. The need for the provision of palliative care beyond cancer will inevitably grow due to the rise of long-term chronic and degenerative diseases, and policy must reflect this.

The National Service Framework for LTCs

In March 2005, the DH published the National Service Framework (NSF) for Long-term Conditions. This NSF outlines 11 quality requirements aimed at transforming the way social and healthcare services support people with long-term neurological conditions, aiming to promote independent living for as long as possible. Although the NSF focuses on people with long-term neurological conditions, much of the guidance can be applied to anyone living with an LTC (DH 2005). In the guidance, Quality Requirement 9 relates to palliative care stating that:

> People in the later stages of long-term neurological conditions are to receive a comprehensive range of palliative care services when they need them to control symptoms, offer pain relief, and meet their needs for personal, social, psychological and spiritual support, in line with the principles of palliative care.
>
> *DH 2005: 5*

This was further supported 3 years later when the DH (2008a) published the 'End of Life Strategy'.

End of life strategy

In 2008, the DH produced the 'End of Life Strategy', which outlined the key areas to be addressed to ensure that all people at the end of life regardless of diagnosis have access to high quality services in all locations (DH 2008a).

The strategy recommends a structured whole systems approach to care and the use of Integrated Care Pathways to deliver on this. The Strategy (DH 2008a: 17) outlines how the end of life care pathway involves the following steps:

- Identification of people approaching the end of life
- Initiating discussions about preferences for end of life care
- *Care planning*: assessing needs and preferences
- Agreeing a care plan to reflect these and reviewing regularly
- Coordination of care
- Delivery of high quality services in all locations
- Management of the last days of life
- Care after death
- Support for carers, both during a person's illness and after their death

Section 3

The National Institute of Health and Clinical Excellence (NICE 2004) recognise, a number of programmes that have made an impact in meeting these objectives including Preferred Priorities of Care (PPC), the Delivering Choices Programme, run by the Marie Curie organisation, Liverpool Care Pathway for the Dying Patient (LCP) and the Gold Standards Framework (GSF). These tools (PPC, LCP and GSF) have been identified by the National Institute of Clinical Excellence (NICE 2004) to ensure best practice in end of life care.

Models of care

Hospice care

Hospice care aims to relieve pain and other symptoms and provides the best possible quality of life at a time when the underlying disease can no longer be treated or cured. Hospice care is a term that first came into widespread use in the 1960s when St. Christopher's hospice in London was opened. St. Christopher's provided care for people who were dying of advanced cancer.

Hospice care is a philosophy of care which has been described by Cecily Saunders (the founder of the modern hospice movement) as follows:

> You matter because you are you. You matter to the last moment of your life and we will do all we can not only to help you die peacefully but to live until you die.
>
> *Saunders n.d.*

In more recent times, hospice care is no longer provided only for inpatients at hospices but now many hospices now provide a 'hospice at home' service (Kanabus 2009).

Liverpool care pathway (LCP) (Ellershaw and Wilkinson 2003)

The LCP recognised the excellence of hospice care at the end of life and uses that model to enable staff across a number of healthcare settings to deliver care to patients when it appears that they are in the final few days of their lives. It prompts good communication with the patients and their families, addressing their care in a holistic manner (Main et al. 2006).

The use of the LCP is triggered at a point when the person is in the terminal phase of their illness, is no longer able to swallow adequately and may be bed-bound and semi-comatose. The care facilitated by the LCP also focuses on what are often considered to be the four main end of life distressing symptoms: pain, agitation, breathlessness and nausea. The LCP provides a framework for assessment and treatment of these symptoms which promote comfort and dignity for the dying person, and also gives a reassurance to family and carers that optimal care has been given at a very difficult time.

The gold standards framework

The Gold Standards Framework (GSF) (National Gold Standards Framework Centre 2008) aims to improve palliative care provided by the whole primary care team. It enables those approaching the end of life to be identified within General Practice in the community. It enables GP to plan care for those patients who are thought to be in approximately the last year of life and to ensure that information about their needs is known to any other who may be involved in their care.

The Gold Standards Framework focuses on improving continuity of care, teamwork, advanced planning (including out of hours), symptom control and patient carer and staff support. The key processes are:

- To identify patients in need of supportive/palliative care
- To assess their needs and preferences
- To plan their care
- To communicate across all relevant agencies throughout

Although developed for use in primary care with cancer patients GSF can be used in other settings and for all disease groups.

National End of Life Care Programme n.d.

The following stories (Case studies 10.2 and 10.3) highlight how the differing models of care can be used to facilitate good end of life care.

Case study 10.2 Mary's story

Mary is a 75-year-old lady who was diagnosed with hypertension 15 years ago. Two years ago, she had a myocardial infarction. She has been suffering from increasing breathlessness and was admitted to hospital on a number of occasions as her symptoms worsened, and during one of these she was given the diagnosis of heart failure.

Over the last year, Mary has become increasingly depressed as she feels her quality of life is becoming poor. She used to regularly take care of her granddaughter for her son, but her breathlessness has meant that she can no longer do this. She is also becoming socially isolated because her mobility is now affected by the increasing levels of breathlessness, and she has lost confidence in her ability to go out on her own. Stewart and McMurray (2002) also document that people with heart failure, most of whom are elderly, often have extremely poor quality of life.

Mary was admitted once again to hospital after falling at home, and taken to an elderly care ward. Here the staff, familiar with the kinds of ailments that older people suffer from and how they interrelate, looked at Mary's needs as a whole, rather than just addressing her presenting symptoms. The consultant geriatrician felt that Mary's heart failure had progressed significantly and he considered that she was now in the final stage of her life, and though not imminently dying, she should now be considered for palliative care. This is often a very difficult decision to make and others have commented on the problems of making such a decision due to the unpredictable nature of the heart failure illness trajectory (Stewart and McMurray 2002, While and Kiek 2009).

The staff talked to Mary and her family about the question of resuscitation. While initially very anxious about this, it was explained that it did not mean that she would not be given any more treatment, but the actual act of cardio pulmonary resuscitation (CPR) would not be initiated, as it was unlikely to be successful given the degree of heart failure. Mary and her family were reassured that she would continue to be given active care but the focus was now about improving the quality of her life and they understood that her life was now time-limited.

Section 3

This decision not to attempt resuscitation in the future was clearly documented in her case notes and passed to all appropriate members of staff. This information was passed to Mary's GP in a comprehensive discharge letter sent by the consultant after Mary went home.

Mary was also referred to the heart failure specialist nurse, who visited her on the ward to offer advice and support, both while she was in hospital and after she was discharged home. The specialist nurse also left Mary her card with a contact phone number should Mary need to see or speak with her in between regular visits.

Before she was discharged Mary had a home visit with the physiotherapist and the occupational therapist to see how she was able to manage at home, and whether any aids or adaptations might be able to be put in place to make life easier for her.

As Mary's condition continued to deteriorate, Mary was referred to her local hospice which worked closely with her heart failure nurse to provide joint care in a model similar to that described by Daley et al. (2006). The knowledge and expertise of the hospice nurses in addressing issues around advance care planning and the often difficult conversations about end of life wishes were complemented by the heart failure nurse's specialist knowledge of heart failure management.

Mary expressed a wish to die at home and this was facilitated by the local district nursing team who visited her at home and provided skilled care when she required a medication to be given subcutaneously in a syringe driver in order to control her symptoms. Mary and her family developed a good relationship with all the healthcare professionals involved in her care as they had confidence in their ability and desire to make sure Mary was kept as comfortable as possible and her wishes to stay at home respected.

However, as her symptoms worsened, Mary felt frightened to be at home and asked if she could be admitted to the hospice where trained staff would be there to help and provide care 24 hours a day. Shortly after her admission there, Mary died a comfortable and peaceful death with her family at her side.

Points for reflection

- How does the survival rate for heart failure compare to some cancer diagnoses?
- Mary died in a hospice. How might this have improved the quality of her end of life care?
- Which illness trajectory best fits Mary's illness journey?

Case study 10.3 Tom's story

Tom is a 60-year-old retired security guard who was brought into hospital complaining of a severe persistent cough for two weeks. He has been experiencing difficulty breathing and is finding it more difficult to mobilise from his bed to the chair. Tom admits to smoking two packets of cigarettes per day which he has done for the last thirty years. Tom was recently diagnosed with severe COPD, a slowly progressive condition of the airways which although preventable is not curable. Nearly 900,000 people have been diagnosed with COPD within the United Kingdom, with half as many again thought to be living with the disease (National Collaborating Centre for Chronic Conditions (NCCCC) 2004). Sullivan et al. (2000) predict that by 2020 COPD will be the third leading cause of death and the fifth leading cause of disability worldwide.

Tom lives with his daughter Sonia who cares for him. She has become increasingly worried about her father, who now sleeps downstairs as he can't climb the stairs to his bedroom.

Tom is a regular visitor to hospital and has had three admissions in the last six months. Tom has been on long-term oxygen therapy for 9 months. Each time Tom comes into hospital it is as a result of his COPD becoming exacerbated by a chest infection. The frequent admissions are causing Tom to become more anxious and depressed. It is recognised that patients with COPD who are moving towards the end stage of the disease often present with a complicated picture of psychological issues as well as physical illness symptoms, social care requirements and spiritual factors (Barnett 2008). During this admission Tom was treated with a combination of pharmacological and non-pharmacological interventions to improve his symptom control. Firstly, Tom was given salbutamol, a bronchodilator therapy, to reduce the sensation of breathlessness by reducing the hyperinflation of the lungs and allowing his lungs to move and work more effectively (McAllister 2002). He was also given ipatropium bromide (an anticholinergic drug) to cause bronchodilation, and mucolytics to increase the expectoration of sputum by reducing the viscosity of the sputum. Unfortunately, the bronchodilator therapy failed and Tom required Oramorph (an opioid which relieves symptoms of breathlessness when bronchodilators don't have an effect).

Tom remained in hospital for 3 weeks during which time he became more depressed. Depression is a common symptom in patients with COPD as patients have a poor quality of life. van Manen et al. (2002) reported that patients with severe COPD are at increased risk of developing depression. The results of their study underscore the importance of reducing symptoms and improving physical functioning in patients with COPD. Therefore, as well as pharmacological interventions, Tom was given non-pharmacological support. With the assistance of the physiotherapist he was encouraged to enhance his breathing control, and was encouraged to adopt a position most comfortable for him, which eased his discomfort and reduced the breathlessness slightly.

During his admission, Tom was cared for by the consultant in charge and the multi-professional team. It is essential that communication is central to the effective care of patients with any LTC (Barnett 2008), none more so than when caring for a patient with COPD. Indeed, Curtis et al. (2002) stress that physicians should target patients with COPD to improve patient education not only about their disease but also about end of life care. During one conversation with the consultant, Tom outlined how he didn't want to be resuscitated should he become so ill that he couldn't make his wishes known, and that he didn't want to be ventilated when he became too weak to breathe without help.

During Tom's admission the multi-professional team spoke to him regarding his wishes for future care. Communication regarding death and dying can produce some awkward barriers for both patients and healthcare professionals, and where possible these conversations should take place when the patient is well and not in an acute life-threatening situation (Barnett 2008). Tom's daughter Sonia had discussed Tom's future care several times with the nursing team

Section 3

throughout his admission, as she felt that caring for Tom at home was becoming increasingly difficult as he was becoming more ill. Prior to discharge Tom was referred to the social care team and the district nursing team for assessment at home with a view to more support being provided. The district nursing team were made aware of this on discharge and Tom was registered by his GP on the Gold Standards register.

Tom's condition continued to deteriorate and with support from the district nursing team and a COPD outreach specialist nurse Tom died peacefully at home. His final few days care was managed using the Liverpool Care Pathway. Tom's death was managed well and his end of life symptoms were well controlled. Evidence suggests that this may not always be the case as the end of life phase is difficult to recognise in patients with COPD. In a study undertaken by Gore et al. in 2000, COPD patients were highlighted as receiving poorer end of life care than patients with lung cancer despite suffering similar symptoms which often lasted longer. By using established and validated tools to support care at the end of life, it is hoped that palliative care becomes increasingly recognised as a vital component in caring for patients with end stage COPD.

Points for reflection

- How did being on the Gold Standards Framework (GSF) register improve Tom's end of life care?
- How can the ultidisciplinary team enhance quality care at the end of life?
- Previously, why might people like Tom have had difficulty accessing good palliative care at the end of life?

The preferred priorities for care (PPC)

Previously known as Preferred Place of Care, this is a document that individuals hold themselves and take with them if they receive care in different places. It allows them to record their thoughts and feelings about their care and choices including, if possible, where they would want to end their life. This information, therefore, can be made available so that anyone involved in their care is aware of what matters to them and assists with seamless care. As care needs change, the PPC can be updated to reflect this. It is never too early to start a PPC plan, particularly for people with LTCs who can live with their deteriorating condition for many years. Identifying each person's Preferred Place of Care was also highlighted as important by Lord Darzi who reported that the 'sick and elderly should have the right to choose to die at home' (DH 2007).

Preferred Priorities for Care (PPC) documentation can include Advanced Care Plans (ACPs), which are plans that are developed following discussions with anyone who has a life-limiting illness. The ACP is a voluntary process of discussion between a person with a life-limiting illness and their carers (irrespective of discipline). The ACP outlines in detail what the person would like or not like to happen at the end of life when they are no longer able to communicate their wishes. If the person wishes, their friends and family can be involved in the discussion too.

Section 3

An ACP discussion might include:

- the individual's concerns;
- their important values or personal goals for care;
- their understanding about their illness and prognosis;
- preferences for types of care or treatment that may be beneficial in the future and the availability of these.

National end of life care programme (n.d.)

One other aspect of care which can be included in an ACP is the person's wishes regarding resuscitation and advanced directives.

The following story (Case study 10.4) highlights how important ACP is in end of life care.

Case study 10.4   David's story

David was diagnosed with adult nephrotic syndrome secondary to chronic renal failure when he was 20 years old. By the age of 26, he had received two unsuccessful kidney transplants. After each failed transplant, David became more reluctant to receive further treatment. Following a hospital admission 12 months ago, David had declined specialist input and was receiving care from the conservative management team and community outreach nurses. His mental health was good and he was settled at home.

He had stated that when his time to die came, he wanted to be at home. He was offered the PPC model of support. Following much discussion with his family, friends and carers, he outlined in writing his end of life care plan in the PPC documentation. This advanced care plan was reviewed regularly over the next few months as part of his ongoing assessment to ensure that David's plans for his end of life care were as he wished them to be.

One Friday evening, his condition deteriorated. His parents called the Out of Hours nursing staff who were reluctant to administer the anticipated end of life drugs. The Out of Hours GP was contacted who visited and said David would have to be admitted to hospital so the GP contacted the paramedics. However, when they arrived, David's mum, Anne, met them at the door, and forced them to read what David had written on the PPC.

The paramedics requested that the doctor revisit and a different doctor then called who set up a syringe driver. David settled after this. He was lucid and calm, with no complaints other than some dyspnoea. David died at home, as he wished, with all his family and friends in the room, his cat on the bed, and his beloved mobile phone still in his hand.

Points for reflection

- David died at home, as was his wish. Why might other people who wish to die at home die in hospital?
- How did the advanced plan of care guide the multiprofessional team in their care of David?
- What are the key policy drivers for end of life care?

Section 3

Table 10.1   Required elements of an ICP.

It is a plan of expected clinical care along some form of timeline, whether that is days, hours or stages.
It is a multi-disciplinary document.
It forms the actual clinical record.
It incorporates evidence-based guidelines.
It is a system to review performance.
It should be able to cross-organisational boundaries.
It is never 'cast in stone' and is a evolutionary and dynamic tool.

Integrated care pathways

Life-limiting, non-malignant LTCs increase the demands on palliative care professionals. Patients with diseases other than cancer, who tend to be over 65 years, can experience disadvantage in the provision of specialist palliative care. However, it is recognised by Coventry et al. (2005) that generalist palliative care has a vital role to play in the delivery of high quality clinical care supporting both physical and psychological health to all at the end of life, regardless of diagnosis or prognosis.

Nurses have a key role in managing and coordinating palliative care for those with LTCs and there is a need for tools to support their practice and promote multidisciplinary working. One solution is the use of an integrated care pathway (ICP). This approach is supported by the British Geriatric Society (BGS) (2009) as a helpful way to deliver planned palliative care for this specific group of patients. ICP methodology highlights practice which is evidence based, from which variations occur as healthcare professionals continue to use their professional judgement.

Croucher (2005) also describes the required elements of an ICP. These are outlined in Table 10.1.

The fundamental principle of the ICP is to ensure that the most appropriate and evidence-based care is delivered to the patient by the right person, doing the right thing, at the right time, in the right pace to ensure the right outcome. It also addresses policy drivers such as clinical governance as a way of improving the quality of care for those groups of patients for whom it has been designed (McAloon et al. 2005).

In addition to developing a pathway within the broad principles of ICP methodology, it has been recognised that an ICP also needs to be able to demonstrate core standards which stand up to scrutiny, in order to gain credibility (Croucher 2005). To this end, the Supportive Care Pathway has been developed and is being audited against the Integrated Care Pathway Appraisal Tool (ICPAT) (De Luc and Whittle 2002). The ICPAT is a nationally validated tool designed not only to evaluate the content of ICPs but also the quality of the development, implementation and maintenance of ICPs (McDonald et al. 2006a, McDonald et al. 2006b).

The British Geriatric Society (2009) suggest that 'Advanced planning and Integrated Care Pathways enhance the quality of end of life care'. A further example of such an integrated care pathway is the Supportive Care Pathway.

Supportive care pathway
The Supportive Care Pathway (SCP) is a holistic document addressing the physical, psychological and spiritual needs of patients and their families, and draws upon elements of the three existing tools described earlier (PPC, LCP and GSF). Those patients who are considered suitable for commencement on the pathway are those with advanced organ system failure, advanced dementia, those who are

generally extremely frail and debilitated as well as those with metastatic or advanced cancer. The SCP is an integrated care pathway for all people with advanced life-limiting illness who are thought to be in the last of life.

The SCP was built on the following principles: patient involvement, empowerment and continued assessment. It has two variable end points and is easy to use, plus it encourages interprofessional communication (Main et al. 2006). The 'End-of-Life Strategy' (DH 2008a) recognises that many health and social care staff have difficulty in recognising those people who are reaching the end of life, communicating with them and delivering optimal care. The SCP was designed to help staff recognise the high percentage of patients who would benefit from a palliative care approach to their care and who, previously, might not have been identified by encouraging staff to commence people on the pathway before what appears to be the terminal event.

Spirituality

The concept of spirituality has traditionally been the subject of debate and numerous attempts at definition (Kellehear 2000). In addition, the spiritual needs of patients are often unrecognised by healthcare professionals who may feel uncomfortable about talking about spiritual needs. However, the following definition (Cancer Research n.d.) is offered:

> Spirituality can be defined as whomever or whatever gives a person meaning in life. It is often expressed as religion but can also refer to other things – nature, energy, belief in the good of all or belief in the importance of family and community.

Religion is a more structured belief system that provides a framework for making sense of the meaning of our existence. Religious rituals provide a way of expressing spirituality.

Spirituality can be seen as the way in which a person understands the meaning and purpose of life. Their beliefs and values can affect how a person might cope with illness, particularly when facing life-limiting illness. They need to find a way to make sense of their situation as they come to terms with living with an LTC which will end their life. Spiritual 'pain' can result if they lose that meaning or lose hope. It can also happen as they lose their identity due to lost roles or lost independence.

Healing can occur if hope can be renewed and the person can find meaning in their present situation, perhaps drawing on what had previously sustained them. Renewing hope means being realistic about the disease and prognosis. Hope now moves from hope for a cure to that of a good and dignified death. However, maintaining hope can be very challenging, so how can the nurse help?

Points for reflection

Be real and honest with the person. Listen to them and be with them but acknowledge that you don't have all the answers or will always be able to fix things. If physical symptoms are addressed and the person is pain free and comfortable, spiritual pain is lessened. The healthcare professional must always respect that person's belief systems, regardless of their own feelings with regard to religion or spirituality.

If appropriate, the services of a religious advisor should be offered.

Section 3

Giving spiritual care for patients with LTCs, who are considered to be in the palliative phase, may be to help give them hope as described above, provide companionship or advocacy, or just to let them know someone is there with them on what can be a difficult and sometimes frightening journey.

Conclusion

It is increasingly accepted that palliative care services have a role in the care of those with progressive non-malignant LTCs. Traditionally, it was thought that palliative care and hospice services were only for the dying or those with a cancer diagnosis, but it is increasingly being understood that they must expand to incorporate care much earlier in the illness trajectory.

However, problems do exist where clinicians have difficulty or reluctance to identify at what point the person is perceived to be in the palliative phase of their illness and where that illness comes into the category of a chronic LTC. Often the last few days of that person's life is more likely to be in an acute hospital and more likely to have life prolonging treatments than cancer patients.

Our increasing ageing population means that palliative care services must expand to meet that need. Very few people die unexpectedly, and open and honest communication between all involved should result in early discussions about choices – about treatment decisions and options and where that person may want to be cared for. However, these choices must be revisited regularly with the patient, his family and carers as choices may change as the illness progresses.

People living with a long-term chronic illness or disability should be able to expect good quality care in comfortable surroundings, being treated with dignity and respect. The tools and models of care described in this chapter can enable this to happen, although the unpredictability of the illness trajectories for those with LTCs will always be a challenge in terms of delivering that care.

References

Abel, J., Rich, A., Griffin, T. and Purdy, S. (2009) End of life care in hospital: a descriptive study of all inpatient's deaths in 1 year. *Palliative Medicine* **23**, 616-622.

Abu-Saad, A. (2001) *Evidenced based Palliative Care: Across the Lifespan*. Oxford: Blackwell.

Barnett, M. (2008) Management of end stage chronic obstructive pulmonary disease. *British Journal of Nursing* **17** (22), 1390-1394.

Bern-Klug, M. (2004) The ambiguous dying syndrome. *Health & Social Work* **29** (1), 55-66.

British Geriatric Society (2009) Palliative and End of Life Care of Older People. Guide 4.8. Available at: http://www.bgs.org.uk (accessed October 2009).

Cancer Research (n.d.) Spirituality and Palliative Care. Available at: http://www.cancer-research.umaryland.edu/spirituality (accessed 30 September 2009).

Carers UK (2007) Valuing Carers – Calculating the Value of Unpaid Care, 2007. Carers UK, ACE National and the University of Leeds. Available at: http://www.carersuk.org/Professionals/ResearchLibrary/Profileofcaring/1201108437 (accessed September 2009).

Carers UK (2009) The Voice of Carers. Available at: http://www.carersuk.org/Information (accessed September 2009).

Clark, D. and Seymour, J. (1999) *Reflections on Palliative Care*. Buckingham: Open University Press.

Coventry, P., Gunn, G., Richards, D. and Todd, C. (2005) Prediction of appropriate timing of palliative care for older adults with non-malignant life-threatening disease: a systematic review. *Age and Ageing* **34**, 218-227.

Cowie, M.R., Mosterd, A. and Wood, D.A. (2000) The epidemiology of heart failure and major cancers compared. *Heart* **83**, 505-510.

Crisp, N. (2003) Parliamentary speech March 2003.

Crossroads Organisation (n.d.) Crossroads Care. Available at: http://www.crossroads.org.uk (accessed 30 September 2009).

Croucher, M. (2005) An evaluation of the quality of integrated care pathway development in the UK national health service. *Journal of Integrated Care Pathways* **9**, 13-16.

Curtis, R., Wenrich, M.D., Carline, J.D., Shannon, S.E., Ambrozy, D.M. and Ramsey, P.G. (2002) Patients' perspectives on physician skill in end-of-life care· differences between patients with COPD, cancer, and AIDS. *Chest* **122** (1), 356-362.

Daley, A., Matthews, C. and Williams, A. (2006) Heart failure and palliative care services working in partnership: report of a new model of care. *Palliative Medicine* **20** (6), 593-601.

De Luc, K. and Whittle, C. (2002) An integrated care pathway appraisal tool: a "badge of quality". *Journal of Integrated Care Pathways* **6**, 13-17.

Department of Health (DH) (2000) *National Service Framework for Coronary Heart Disease: Modern Standards and Service Models.* London: HMSO.

Department of Health (DH) (2003) *Building on the Best.* London: HMSO.

Department of Health (DH) (2005) *The National Service Framework for Long-term Conditions.* London: HMSO.

Department of Health (DH) (2007) *Our NHS Our Future: NHS Next Stage Review - Interim Report.* London: HMSO.

Department of Health (DH) (2008a) *End of Life Care Strategy - Promoting High Quality Care for Adults at the End of Life.* London: HMSO.

Department of Health (DH) (2008b) *The National Service Framework for Long-term Neurological Conditions: National Support for Local Implementation.* London: HMSO.

Department of Health (DH) (2009a) Stroke. Available at: http://www.dh.gov.uk/stroke (accessed October 2009).

Department of Health (DH) (2009b) *Living Well with Dementia: A National Dementia Strategy.* London: HMSO.

Department of Work and Pensions (2008) Family Resource Survey 2006/7. Available at: http://research.dwp.gov.uk/asd/frs (accessed October 2009).

Ellershaw, J. and Wilkinson, S. (2003) *Care of the Dying: A Pathway to Excellence.* Oxford: Oxford University Press.

Faull, C., Daniel, L., Carter, Y. and Woof, W. (1998) *Handbook of Palliative Care.* Oxford: Wiley Blackwell.

Gore, J.M., Brophy, C.J. and Greenstone, M.A. (2000) How do we care for patients with end-stage Chronic Obstructive Pulmonary Disease (COPD)? a comparison of palliative care and quality of life in COPD and lung cancer. *Thorax* **55** (12), 1000-1006.

Great Britain Parliament (2004) *Carers* (Equal Opportunities) Act 2004 Chapter 15 (Act of Parliament) London: HMSO.

Griffiths, C., Rooney, C. and Brock, A. (2005) Leading causes of death in England and Wales- how should we group causes? *Health Statistics Quarterly* **28**, 6-17.

Health and Safety Executive (2005) Chronic Obstructive Pulmonary Disease (COPD). Available at: http://hse.gov.uk/statistics/causdis/index.htm (accessed October 2009).

Higginson, I. (2003) *Priorities for End of Life Care in England, Wales and Scotland (Conducted by the Cecily Saunders Foundation)* London: National Council for Palliative Care.

Jones, A., O'Connell, J. and Gray, C. (2003) Living and dying with congestive heart failure: addressing the needs of older people with heart failure. *Age and Ageing* **32** (6), 566-568.

Kanabus, A. (2009) Definitions of Palliative Care. Available at: http://www.avert.org/palliative-care.htm (accessed 4 September 2009).

Kellehear, A. (2000) Spirituality and palliative care: a model of needs. *Palliative Medicine* **14**, 149-155.

Knapp, M., Comas- Herrera, A., Somani, A. and Banerjee, S. (2007) *Dementia UK: Report to the Alzheimers Society.* London: Kings College, London and London School of Economics and Political Science.

Section 3

Lynne, J. (2004) *In Palliative Care: The Solid Facts Europe.* Geneva: World Health Organisation.

Lynn, J. and Adamson, D.M. (2003) *Living Well at the End of Life: Adapting Health Care to Serious Chronic Illness in Old Age.* Santa Monica, California: RAND Corporation. Available at: http://www.rand.org/pubs/white_papers/WP137/

McAllister, J. (2002) Special focus on chronic obstructive pulmonary disease. *Nursing Times* **98** (35), 41-44.

McAloon, M., Tolson, D. and Reid, W. (2005) Overview of the development of a generic integrated care pathway in a department of medicine for the elderly. *Journal of Integrated Care Pathways* **9** (3), 130-136.

McDonald, P., Whittle, C., Dunn, L. and De Luc, K. (2006a) Shortfalls in integrated care pathways part 1: what don't they contain? *Journal of Integrated Care Pathways* **10** (1), 17-22.

McDonald, P., Whittle, C., Dunn, L. and De Luc, K. (2006b) Shortfalls in integrated care pathways part 2: how well are we doing? *Journal of Integrated Care Pathways* **10** (1), 17-27.

Main, J., Whittle, C., Treml, J., Woolley, J. and Main, A. (2006) The development of an integrated care pathway for all patients with advanced life limiting illness - the supportive care pathway. *Journal of Nursing Management* **14** (7), 521-528.

Munday, D., Petrova, M. and Dale, J. (2009) Exploring preferences for place of death with terminally ill patients: qualitative study of experiences of general practitioners and community nurses in England. *British Medical Journal* **339**, b2391.

Murray, S., Kendall, M., Boyd, K. and Sheikh, A. (2005) Illness trajectories and palliative care. *British Medical Journal* **330**, 1007-1011.

National Collaborating Centre for Chronic Conditions (NCCCC) (2004) Chronic obstructive pulmonary disease. National clinical guideline on management of chronic obstructive pulmonary disease in adults in primary and secondary care. *Thorax* **59** (1 suppl.), 1-232.

National End of Life Care Programme (n.d.) Gold Standards Framework. Available at: http://www.endoflifecareforadults.nhs.uk/eolc/gsf.htm (accessed 4 August 2009).

National Gold Standards Framework Centre (2008) The Gold Standards Framework Prognostic Indicator Guidance. Available at: http://www.goldstandardsframework.nhs.uk/Resources/Gold%20Standards%20Framework/PIG_Paper_Final_revised_v5_Sept08.pdf (accessed 30 September 2009).

National Institute for Health and Clinical Excellence (2004) *Improving Supportive and Palliative Care for Adults with Cancer National Institute for Clinical Excellence.* London: NICE.

National Statistics (2006a) Trends in Mortality from Alzheimer's Disease, Parkinson's Disease and Dementia. Health Statistics Quarterly 30. Available at: http://www.statistics.gov.uk/downloads/theme_health/HSQ30.pdf (accessed 30 September 2009).

National Statistics (2006b) Death registrations in England and Wales: 2005, Causes. Health Statistics Quarterly 30. Available at: http://www.statistics.gov.uk/downloads/theme_health/HSQ30.pdf (accessed 30 September 2009).

Office for National Statistics (2004) Focus on Older People. Available at: http://www.statistics.gov.uk/downloads/theme_compendia/foop05/Olderpeople2005.pdf (accessed 30 September 2009).

Saunders, C. (n.d.) A Tribute to Dame Cecily Saunders. Available at: http://www.stchristophers.org.uk/page.cfm?link=900/GoSection=4 (accessed 23 January 2010).

Shahab, L., Jarvis, M., Britton, J. and West, R. (2006) Prevalence, diagnosis and relation to tobacco dependence of chronic obstructive pulmonary disease in a nationally representative population sample. *Thorax* **61**, 1043-1047.

Stewart, S. and McMurray, J. (2002) Palliative care for heart failure. *British Medical Journal* **325** (7370), 915-916.

Sullivan, S.D., Ramsey, S.D. and Lee, T.A. (2000) The economic burden of COPD. *Chest* **117** (2 suppl.), 58-95.

The Neurological Alliance (n.d.) Living with a Neurological Condition. Available at: http://www.neural.org.uk/ (accessed 30 September 2009).

The NHS Confederation (2005) *Leading Edge - Improving End-of-Life Care.* London: NHS Confederation Publications.

van Manen, J.G., Bindels, P.J.E., Dekker, F.W., Ijzermans, C.J., van der Zee, J.S. and Schadé E. (2002) Risk of depression in patients with chronic obstructive pulmonary disease and it's determinants. *Thorax* **57**, 412-416.

Watson, M., Lucas, C., Hoy, A. and Back, I. (2009) *Oxford Handbook of Palliative Care.* Oxford: Oxford University Press.

While, A. and Kiek, F. (2009) Chronic Heart Failure: Promoting Quality of Life. *British Journal of Community Nursing* **14** (2), 54–59.

World Health Organisation (WHO) (1990) *Cancer Pain Relief and Palliative Care 11 (World Health Organisation technical report series 804).* Geneva: World Health Organisation.

World Health Organisation (WHO) (2004) *Palliative Care: The Solid Facts Europe.* Geneva: World Health Organisation.

World Health Organisation (WHO) (2005) WHO's Pain Relief Ladder. Available at: http://www.who.int/cancer/palliative/painladder/en/ (accessed 10 February 2010).

World Health Organisation (WHO) (2009) Palliative Care. Available at: http://www.who.int/cancer/palliative/en/ (accessed 30 September 2009).

Resources

Alzheimer's Organisation Available at: www.alzheimers.org.uk
Crossroads Organisation Available at: www.crossroads.org.uk

Further reading

Carrier, J. (2009) *Managing Long-term Conditions and Chronic Illness in Primary Care.* Routledge: Abingdon.

Main, J., Whittle, C., Treml, J., Woolley, J. and Main, A. (2006) The development of an integrated care pathway for all patients with advanced life limiting illness – the supportive care pathway. *Journal of Nursing Management* **14** (7), 521–528.

Watson, M., Lucas, C., Hoy, A. and Back, I. (2009) *Oxford Handbook of Palliative Care.* Oxford: Oxford University Press.

Section 3

Index

Long-term Conditions: A Guide for Nurses and Healthcare Professionals, First Edition. Edited by S. Randall and H. Ford.
© 2011 Blackwell Publishing Ltd. Published 2011 by Blackwell Publishing Ltd.